NATIVE INTOXICANTS OF NORTH AMERICA

NATIVE INTOXICANTS OF NORTH AMERICA

SEAN RAFFERTY

The University of Tennessee Press
Knoxville

First Edition.

LIBRARY OF CONGRESS CATALOGING-IN-PUBLICATION DATA

Names: Rafferty, Sean M. (Sean Michael), author.

Title: Native intoxicants of North America / Sean Rafferty.

Description: First edition. | Knoxville : The University of Tennessee Press, [2021] | Includes bibliographical references and index. | Summary: "This book discusses the cultural significance that narcotics, stimulants, and hallucinogens had on prehistoric societies, whether used for ritual, medicinal, or even recreational purposes. Rafferty notes that prehistoric intoxicants can be found in sites ranging throughout North America, and their use, though varied, presents a near-universal human disposition toward the use of drugs to achieve certain social and spiritual goals and states of consciousness"— Provided by publisher.

Identifiers: LCCN 2020056676 (print) | LCCN 2020056677 (ebook) | ISBN 9781621906308 (hardcover) | ISBN 9781621906315 (adobe pdf)

Subjects: LCSH: Indians of North America—Drug use—History. | Indians of North America—Tobacco use—History. | Indians of North America—Alcohol use—History. | Calumets—North America—History. | Indians of North America—Rites and ceremonies. | Indians of North America—Antiquities.

Classification: LCC E98.N5 R34 2021 (print) | LCC E98.N5 (ebook) | DDC 970.01—dc23

LC record available at https://lccn.loc.gov/2020056676

LC ebook record available at https://lccn.loc.gov/2020056677

CONTENTS

ILLUSTRATIONS

NATIVE INTOXICANTS
OF NORTH AMERICA

INTRODUCTION

Every culture has found chemical means of transcendence, and at some point the use of such intoxicants becomes institutionalized at a magical or sacramental level; the sacramental use of psychoactive plant substances has a long history and continues to the present day in various shamanic and religious rites around the world (Sacks 2012).

Humans are endlessly surprising in their cultural variability. Once you move beyond the basic requirements for life, very few human behaviors are universal. One universal human trait is experiencing altered states of consciousness (ASCs), usually through ingestion of intoxicants (Withington 2014:10).

A recent article (Wadley 2016:138) states:

> It is a remarkable thing, easily overlooked because it is so commonplace, that a very small dose of a chemical can change the way someone thinks and feels. Furthermore, this subjective change can be so compelling that a desire to repeatedly experience it motivates individuals and groups to carry out complex plans that play out over timescales ranging from hours to decades.

Another writer (Saniotis 2010:482) elaborates on the adaptive value of intoxicants:

> Such substances have served several purposes, such as inducing ASC for religious and recreational purposes, cognitive enhancement, strengthening group identity, reproductive success, and food. Given their current prevalence, psychotropic and mood-altering substances will continue to have a considerable impact on future human societies.

Experiencing ASCs is not merely a recreational practice. It is a default state of human cognition, an evolved trait selected for, and continually reinforced, in the human population.

This volume is an investigation of the role intoxicants have played, and still play, in Native cultures of North America. This is hardly the first volume to address this topic (see Fitzpatrick 2018, Rafferty 2018), and the author is indebted to the work of several key figures. The work of Peter Furst (e.g., 1972a) among peyote-using cultures of Mexico, as well as his edited volume on the topic of intoxication in numerous cultures, springs immediately to mind. Richard Schultes (e.g., Schultes and Hofmann 1987) also has published extensively on the role of intoxicants in both Old World and New World settings. Michael Winkelman has written extensively on the archaeological correlates of shamanism and of hallucinogenic intoxicants in a range of cultural contexts. Mycologist R. Gordon Wasson has written extensively about the cultural role hallucinogenic mushrooms have played across the globe. Åke Hultkrantz conducted foundational research on the religious frameworks that structured Native American cultures, and Robert Hall has been prolific in applying such structures toward the understanding of the archaeology of North America. The work of these seminal researchers, as well as many others, has been fundamental to the creation of this volume.

This volume does stand apart from earlier work in two key respects. First, it is focused on the Native cultures of North America, a region that has historically been underrepresented in studies of intoxication. North America in this sense is meant culturally rather than geographically, excluding Mesoamerica. Much existing research on intoxicants has been directed to the traditional cultures of Asia, Africa, Mesoamerica, and South America. While this is understandable given the far greater range of intoxicant plants found in those regions in comparison with North America, it has left a sizeable gap in the documentary record. Table 1 lists the major intoxicants used in North America and covered in this volume. Second, the coverage in this volume is holistic, in that it investigates all classes of intoxicants, whereas past research has largely been focused on hallucinogenic intoxicants, or, in the Old World, opium or cannabis. These are compounds that have some of the most dramatic physiological and psychological effects on their users, so this focus is not surprising. However, it again leaves a gap in the research, particularly with respect to milder stimulants or substances such as tobacco whose effects are difficult to characterize in a single term. These types of compounds are particularly prevalent in North America, and so feature prominently in this volume.

It should also be made clear at the outset that the content of this volume is in no way meant to comprise an endorsement or encouragement of the use of intoxicants today, by the reader or anyone else. Two points can be stressed here. First, intoxicants intoxicate because they are *toxic*. While human physiology has adapted to many intoxicant compounds, they are still poisons, and while toxic doses vary widely, none of the compounds discussed are likely to be beneficial given long-term use. Some can be harmful or fatal even in small doses. Second, traditional cultures have developed a range of cultural practices, prescriptions, and proscriptions for intoxicants that have formed checks on abusive use in most settings. These checks are largely absent when intoxicant substances are removed from their traditional cultural context, as is the case for most modern intoxicant use in the developed and developing world. Absent the vital cultural setting an intoxicant is far more likely to be harmful and abused.

TABLE 1. NATIVE AMERICAN INTOXICANTS

SOURCE(S)	COMPOUND(S)	EFFECTS	DISTRIBUTION
Red "Mescal" Bean	Cytisine	Severe toxicity, hallucination	Southwestern US, Northern Mexico
Peyote	Mescaline	Hallucination	Southwestern US, Northern Mexico
Datura "Jimson weed" species	Scopolamine, Atropine	Severe delirium, amnesia	Throughout Temperate North America
Psilocybin species	Psilocybin	Hallucination	Mesoamerica, West Coast
Amanita species	Muscimol, Ibotenic acid	Hallucination	West Coast, Great Lakes
Ilex species, Theobroma species	Caffeine, Theobromine	Stimulation, emetic	Southeastern and Southwestern North America
Fermented starchy plants	Ethyl Alcohol	Euphoria, loss of coordination	Southwestern US, Northern Mexico
Nicotiana Tobacco species	Nicotine	Stimulation/ relaxation; hallucination in high doses	Wild: Southwestern US, Great Plains Domesticated: Throughout North America

The reader might also question why the term "intoxicant" has been chosen over other, more common terms. Intoxicant is a term for any mind-altering substance, referring to the fact that mind-altering substances are generally plant-derived toxins. Withington (2014:12) notes:

> Unlike that of drugs, the vocabulary of intoxication is etymologically and semantically precise, having always depicted artificial alterations of consciousness. It is relatively neutral, certainly without the ideological connotations of drugs. It is encompassing, accounting for all substances with demonstrable physiological and neurological impact. And it depicts a cognitive and social condition (intoxication) as well as the substances that induce it (intoxicants).

The word "drug" is vague and pejorative and can refer to medicinal substances. "Mind-altering substance" is unwieldy. Some use the overly abstruse term "entheogen." Popular sources and legal statutes often use the term "narcotic" which is confusing, as narcotics are a particular class of intoxicant, those that cause euphoria and drowsiness, such as various opiates. This class of drugs is absent in the Americas and using the term as a general term for intoxicants is simply erroneous.

Prior to discussing the details of Native North American intoxicant use, we must first address the key question: why do humans use intoxicants in the first place?

EVERYBODY MUST GET STONED: EVOLUTION, SOCIETY, AND INTOXICATION

Hypotheses abound as to the origin of intoxication. Perhaps early humans observed animals that had consumed intoxicants and emulated the behavior. Perhaps early foragers were experimenting with food sources and got more than they bargained for but liked what they found. Perhaps altering consciousness is a widespread behavior of many mammals, and humans are just better at it. Intoxicants have been described as "psychotechnology" with which we hack our consciousness (Calabrese 1994). This author uses the term "neurotechnology" in discussing intoxicants and other human developments designed to manipulate neurologic processes.

Whatever the origin of intoxication, the use of mind-altering substances is a fundamental aspect of human behavior. Froese (2015:90) connects this modern ubiquity and past behavior: "Intentional alterations of normal waking consciousness are so widely prevalent in today's world that it is difficult to think why they should not have previously played a role." Intoxicants play a huge role in modern society. In 2012, the United Nations Office on Drugs and Crime (UNODC) estimated that in the prior year some 5% of the adult population, 230 million people, had used some form of illegal drug (UNODC 2013:iii), which is a fraction of those using legal intoxicants. Over a *trillion* dollars was spent on alcohol alone across the globe in 2017 (Jernigan and Ross 2020). Global tobacco production has decreased in recent years, but production in 2010 was estimated at over seven billion tons (United Nations Food and Agriculture Organization 2004).

Annual spending on illegal drugs is similarly huge, if difficult to measure. According to the United Nations (UNODC 2008), drug seizures in 2006 included 104 metric tons of heroin and 705 metric tons of cocaine, representing a fraction of the total amount actually used. The same document estimated 165.6 million cannabis users and 24.7 million amphetamine users. Intoxicants are hugely popular and represent a significant portion of the international legal and illegal economy.

Most efforts at limiting or banning intoxicants have been failures. Prohibition breeds smuggling and black markets, not to mention an often less pure, more dangerous product. Illegal drugs become sources of wealth for a criminal elite. The wealth of these cartels is such that they are able to buy their way out of most criminal prosecution. Criminalizing drug use and possession is similarly ineffective and serves only to fill prisons with nonviolent offenders. Decriminalization and treatment programs have more potential to yield positive results.

One could argue based on these figures that intoxicant use is a recent phenomenon. However, several facts argue against an interpretation of a recent origin of intoxicants. Archaeology shows intoxicants were among resources utilized by prehistoric societies. The archaeological record of intoxication is limited due to (1) small amounts of drugs used in comparison with food plants and (2) limitations of organic preservation. Despite these limitations, when we have good preservation, we find intoxicants alongside food. Intoxicants may even have been a better initial choice for domestication than food plants, as there is relatively little risk in the failure of nonfood plant crops (Asch 1994:26). There has been speculation that the domestication of intoxicant plants predates that of food plants (Braidwood et al. 1953; Smalley and Blake 2003).

Intoxicant use is ubiquitous among human cultures regardless of economic development. West Africans chew kola nuts for their caffeine (Lovejoy 1980); Amazonian farmers take hallucinogenic *yopo* snuff (Torres and Repke 2006).

Qat (*Catha edulis*), a stimulant, is endemic in the Horn of Africa and Arabian Peninsula (Giannini et al. 1986; Manghi et al. 2009). Betel nut, another mild stimulant, is consumed by nearly 200 million people in the Western Pacific and East Asia (Norton 1998). Kratom (*Mitragyna speciosa*), an evergreen from Southeast Asia, has a substantial history of use due to opium-like qualities (Hassan et al. 2013). And your average American drinks beer and coffee, possibly smokes tobacco, or indulges in cannabis. People everywhere have long since scoured their environment for substances that can alter their consciousness.

Every culture has its drugs of choice. The truly interesting question is why. Some researchers have hypothesized that animal models show the phenomenon is not a coincidence:

> Are we dealing with another unfortunate mismatch between animal brains and their botanical environments that evolution by natural selection has been unable to remove from populations? Or could there even be selective advantages conferred by this seemingly unusual behaviour? The idea of pure coincidence can be ruled out by taking a closer look at the chemical substances and neurotransmitter receptors that are involved in the effects of psychoactive plants. On the contrary, the highly specific ways in which these plant substances interfere with animal neurotransmitters is suggestive of a co-evolutionary relationship that is millions of years old [Froese 2015:90].

Several suggestions for the selective advantage conveyed by intoxicants have been proposed. One possibility is that at least one intoxicant (alcohol) is used by animals besides humans and must be an adaptive trait (McGovern 2009). Alcohol depends on concentrations of fermentable sugars and would have indicated a nutritious food. Intoxication, in this interpretation, is a side effect. This idea is bolstered by genetic evidence that a single mutation in our primate ancestors increased the ability to metabolize alcohol, allowing access to a new food source (Dudley 2014).

There are other examples of animal intoxicant use (Samorini 2002). Gorillas and chimpanzees have been observed ingesting plants that have a range of properties (Cousins and Huffman 2002; Huffman et al. 1996). Gorillas consume kola nuts and have been observed ingesting *Tabernanthe iboga*, which contains the hallucinogenic compound ibogaine. *T. iboga* is used by the indigenous Gabonese Metsogho-Massango and Bapinzi in religious initiation ceremonies. Chimpanzees drink fermented palm sap, and even utilize crude leaf sponges while doing so (Hockings et al. 2020:52). Lab mice can possess genes that encourage alcohol consumption (Fuller 1985). Cows will pursue "locoweed" preferentially to the point of starvation. Dolphins have been observed consuming puffer fish, becoming intoxicated on toxins in their tissue. Lab primates have been trained to smoke tobacco. Bighorn sheep will risk death on nearly vertical outcrops, gnawing on narcotic lichens, grinding their teeth to the gum (Siegel 2005:50). It should be noted that these are largely observational studies, not controlled experiments, and are often anecdotal as well.

It is plausible that animals with complex nervous systems might derive adaptive benefit from intoxicants. Researchers have looked at ASCs as playing a significant psychological role. Bateson (1972) took a view of consciousness where psychological elements (e.g., conscious brain versus unconscious) interacted with each other in a complex interplay. Altered states, particularly trance-like states, could allow the conscious mind access to concepts mediated by the unconscious. Other hypotheses have been suggested that drugs can provide a sense of attaining a goal when real goals cannot be achieved, may offer protection against parasites, or reduce stress levels (Wadley 2016).

Others have suggested a neurological explanation. Mammals have complex brains, especially in regions that enable complex behavior and decision making. This is most elaborated in humans. Examples of intoxicant use in animals have tended to be among those with complex brains and behaviors. Perhaps brain stimulation by intoxicants is valuable to animals with complex nervous systems. Research on artificial neural networks lends this some support (Woodward et al. 2015). Disrupting neural networks, simulating intoxication, increased their complexity. This agrees with Winkelman's (2010) suggestion that ASCs could increase our early ability to conceive of and manipulate symbols.

However, while these hypotheses are all plausible, it is equally possible that the correlation between intoxicant use and neurologic complexity indicates correlation in the other direction. Perhaps intoxicant use did not contribute to the development of brain complexity, but instead animals with complex brains are more likely to indulge in intoxication. Regardless of whether intoxication is an adaptive strategy, a maladaptive trait retained with adaptive uses of the same pathways, or a side effect of neurologic complexity, drug use likely goes back to mammalian origins. It should come as no surprise that intoxicants are ubiquitous among humans and widespread among closely related animals. Intoxicants are a technology through which we manipulate our own cognition and emotions and should be seen as technological adaptations no different than domesticated crops.

Another way intoxicants might confer adaptive advantage is by aiding dissociation. Dissociation is a suppression of awareness and sense of self. While dissociation is a coping mechanism in cases of mental trauma, Lynn (2005; Lynn et al. 2010) has shown it can have a positive effect, correlating with a decrease in stress hormones. Since dissociation is an effect of many intoxicants, controlled use of such substances could have a stress-reducing effect.

Other adaptationist hypotheses have focused on how intoxicant use might be a side effect of existing neurology. Evolutionarily adaptive behavior is reinforced through reward pathways in the brain that cause pleasure. Since many intoxicants appropriate these pathways, their use may be a side effect of our neurology and can lead to maladaptive outcomes such as addiction (Nesse and Berridge 1997). Perhaps these compounds may have had adaptive effects earlier in human history, enhancing emotional states that encourage adaptive behaviors. But these behaviors may now be rendered maladaptive by modern social, economic, and technological circumstances (Saniotis 2010:480). An alternative view is that many intoxicants are plant toxins. In that view, humans have evolved a counter-exploitation of plant neurotoxins (Saniotis 2010:480; Sullivan et al. 2008). While not implausible, these hypotheses suffer from a common problem in evolutionary psychology: they may be untestable and thus ultimately speculative.

However, while it is plausible that intoxicant use has adaptive value for an individual animal, human or otherwise, humans are unlike other animals in one primary effect. Humans are the ultimate social animal, to a degree of complexity that hugely exceeds any of our closest nonhuman primate relatives. All humans are members of social groups, and individuals are defined in relation to the group to which they belong. Group membership is vital for survival as is the solidarity of that group. One probable factor in the evolution of human brain complexity is a corresponding social complexity. Accordingly, in understanding the universal human drive to intoxication, we must also examine the social implications of intoxication.

Any trait contributing to group solidarity will have adaptive value for that group. Intoxication is likely to become widespread when it encourages social solidarity and likely to be pathologized when it leads to antisocial behavior. So, when a scholar of Native American tobacco posed the question: "How and why did a solanaceous weed [tobacco], apparently of no advantage to human subsistence or survival, come to have a conspicuous presence in the vast majority of Amerindian cultures on both continents" (Von Gernet 1992:171)? The most likely answer is that there is a group survival advantage to the use of such substances.

Research supports this. In a review of intoxicants in society, Wadley (2016) noted: "It is likely that the association between socializing and drugs is built upon their pharmacological properties. Many drugs influence an individual's perceptions of and interactions with other people. Prosocial behavior is facilitated through mechanisms such as reduction of anxiety, enhancement of self-confidence, suppression of fatigue, and disinhibition of communication." Wadley identifies seven areas where intoxicants lead to adaptive, prosocial behaviors: (1) they stimulate economic production of the substance and associated material culture; (2) they are used to facilitate certain actions; (3) they can serve as tools to motivate groups of people to act toward a common goal; (4) they can encourage general prosocial behavior and mediate social status; (5) they stimulate effort and allow a user to delay the gratification of physical needs such as hunger; (6) they can create new, meaningful cultural experiences; and (7) they stimulate trade (in the intoxicants) within and beyond their native region. But this list omits, or has buried within its categories, the most significant aspect of intoxicant use in traditional societies for the purposes of enhancing social solidarity: their common role in religious, magical, and spiritual ritual practices, as is discussed in the following section.

If the social aspect of intoxication is as highly significant as suggested, we would expect to see some predictable outcomes. For example, those intoxicants that are the most amenable to social use should be the most widespread within any particular culture. Specifically, intoxicants that create a manageable degree of social disinhibition and/or mental stimulation would be socially beneficial and more likely to become widespread in their use. This would include substances like caffeine, nicotine, or moderate doses of alcohol, all of which are not mentally or physically debilitating and are typically consumed in social settings. Intoxicants that are less amenable to commensal settings, with effects that prevent socializing or are potentially dangerous, should be more likely to be culturally regulated and restricted, if not forbidden. We would expect more potent hallucinogenic substances, powerful stimulants, or narcotics to belong to this category. We will return to these predictions in the concluding chapter to this volume, where we see whether the data regarding specifically North American intoxicants support these predictions.

There are less benign aspects to intoxicants, such as when used to aid in violence. Viking warriors would ingest hallucinogenic mushrooms and alcohol and enter berserker frenzy in battle (Fabing 1956). The medieval Nizari *hashshashin* are purported to have used hashish to spur themselves to violence. While these are extreme examples, there are uncontested examples of militarized intoxication. Stories of soldiers drinking alcohol to suppress fear are as old as writing about war. Modern armies run on tobacco and caffeine. Access to coffee was vital to military operations during the American Civil War (Billings 1993). Intoxicants were the first performance-enhancing drugs when it came to the enabling of organized human violence. It should be noted that these situations are still uses of intoxicants to form social connections, or to enable users to take uninhibited actions in social interactions, albeit social interactions of a decidedly aggressive form. A military force that enhances unit cohesion through the controlled use of intoxicants is likely to have an advantage over opponents that do not.

Intoxicants have a long history; they enhance cognition, provide stimulation, enable sociability, and aid in physical activities. However, the most significant role intoxicants have played is not evolutionary, or practical, but spiritual.

INTOXICANTS AND SHAMANISM

A recurrent theme for intoxicants is their role in rituals. The connection between intoxicants and ritual is fundamental yet often overlooked. A recent volume on the archaeology of ritual (Insoll 2011) makes little mention of intoxicants. Winter (2000d:265), in his study of Native American religious use of tobacco, identified a three-part classification of Native American practices that could be generally applied. He discusses the "religious importance" at "three basic levels": "individual use . . . by shamans, medicine men, other religious practitioners, and the ordinary members of their tribes; group use by voluntary, sometimes secret societies; and formal, institutionalized use by priests and other elites." The first category is important: the connection between intoxicants and shamanism.

Shamans, defined in Siberian ethnographies (e.g., Shirokogoroff 1935), refers to individuals who communicate with spirits while in a trance: "Shamanism is precisely one of the archaic techniques of ecstasy—at once mysticism, magic, and 'religion' in the broadest sense of the term" (Eliade 2004:xx). Eliade's conception of shamanism was based on traits he identified in shamanic traditions. Chief among these is the shaman as psychopomp, mediating between spirits and the living (Aldenderfer 1993). Other traits include trances (possibly induced by hallucinogens), bird/flight symbolism, animal-human/human-animal transformations, physical/physiological abnormalities and gender ambiguities, and the shaman's role as spiritual warrior (Winkelman 2002). Shamans are involved in healing, divination, magic, and jurisprudence, and protect their group against spiritual threats. Clottes wrote: "This word [shaman] has entered Western languages and is now applied to similar ritual specialists around the world who, like the Tungus shamans, go into a trance—frenzied or passive—to heal the sick, change the weather, foretell the future, control the movements of animals, and converse with spirits and spirit-animals" (Clottes and Lewis-Williams 1996:11). Clottes and other researchers have underlined the role intoxicants play in shamanic trances. Intoxicant use is found in many shamanic societies (Harner 1973; Mentzner 1998; Saniotis 2010:481; Winkelman 1996). Wiercinski (1989:22) argues that the discovery of hallucinogens was related to the development of shamanism.

Researchers differ in their definitions of shamanism, from narrow, relevant only to Central Asia, to broad, applying to any individual engaging in any spiritual activity (Bourguignon 1973, 1989; Jones 2006:11). Use of the term has varied, with some modern researchers using outmoded definitions. The use of the term lacks "coherence and consistency" (Dobkin de Rios and Winkelman

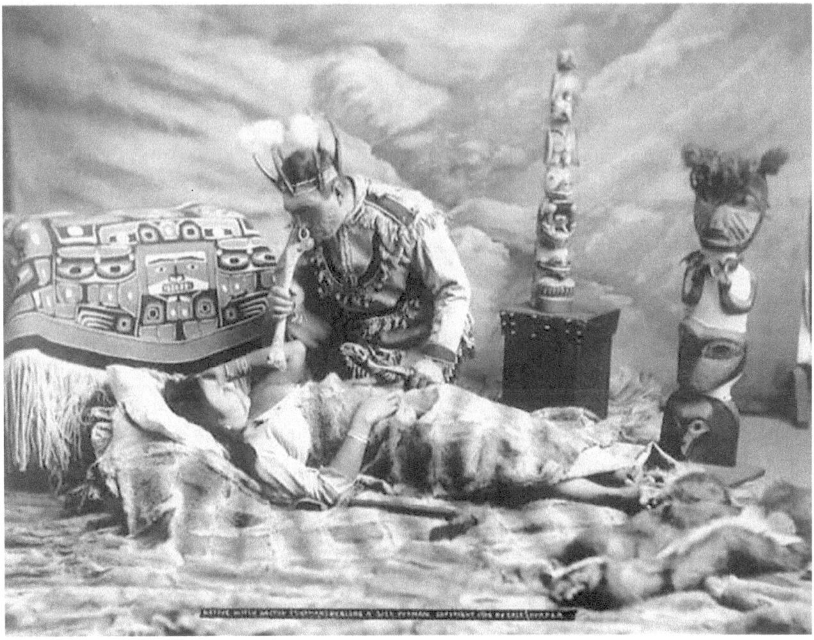

FIGURE 1 Tlingit Healer, 1906. (National Anthropological Archives.)

1989:1). Some have critiqued expansion of the term, which should be applied only to individuals achieving specific neuropsychological states. Some (e.g., Kehoe 2000) have dismissed the term outside of its initial area as "intellectual racism." While "shaman" has been applied uncritically, it is useful provided one keeps in mind there is significant variability in the term's use. Despite this, common trends occur in shamanic traditions, the most salient being ASCs.

"Shamanism" can be defined as the relatively unstructured, undogmatic, and unspecialized religious practices of traditional societies. While typically modeled as specific to foraging societies, it need not be, as many concerns of foraging groups are relevant to agricultural or pastoral groups (Malotki 1999:108): "The adaptive character of shamanism is confirmed by its ubiquitous appearance around the world, not only in hunter-gatherer and fishing societies, but in centralized societies as well" (Krippner 2000:93). In societies where spiritual authority is monopolized by elites, shamanism is typically replaced by formal religion; even then, religious leaders often retain shamanistic tendencies.

Shamans' occupation involves interceding with spirits using ASCs:

> The neuropsychological basis of shamanism is manifested in cross-cultural similarities in shamans' characteristics. These include visionary experience, soul journey, guardian spirit quest, healing practices, and self-transformation experiences such as death and rebirth. Cross-cultural research reveals that shamans are charismatic social and religious leaders in hunter-gatherer (or simple agricultural and pastoral) societies where political integration and leadership is limited to the level of the local community [Winkelman 2002:72].

Shamans' social role is to interact with spirits while in an ASC (Hultkranz 1968), which is what distinguishes a shaman from a priest.

Emerson (2003:136) comprehensively frames the definition:

> Shamans are essentially society's servants who communicate with the spirit world on behalf of individuals and their communities to heal, to propitiate or battle injurious spirits, to increase game and other resources, to find objects, or to ascertain future events. This is possible because this ritual practitioner envisions a universe in which the body and soul are separate and in which the soul can travel to spatially, culturally, or spiritually distant places . . . those who through the aid of ASCs travel to other worlds literally to battle with spirits or evil shamans to reclaim lost souls and banish evil.

Some scholars suggest a diaspora of hallucinogen-using shamans out of Central Asia (e.g., Furst 1976a, LaBarre 1972). However, similarities among shamanic traditions is more likely due to similar practices proving adaptive for similar groups (Hultkranz 1966; Winkelman 1992), as well as human neurologic tendencies (Shermer 2008). These include dualistic thinking (where "mind" is seen as distinct from body), pattern recognition (seeing cause and effect between human action and natural events), and agency attribution (ascribing human thought to natural or nonexistent phenomena).

Shamans tend to have an animistic worldview, defined as: "attributing an essence with mental qualities like those of humans to imaginary or natural phenomena, is exemplified in anthropomorphism, attributing human-like 'mind' characteristics to gods, spirits, and nonhuman entities, particularly animals" (Winkelman 2002:75). Animists apply agency to natural elements, including animals, landscape, weather, and manufactured objects. Wallis (2013:22) states shamanism is: "a relational ontology according to which the world is filled with people, only some of whom are human." Intoxicating plants particularly are often viewed as possessing agency, as are paraphernalia associated with their consumption.

Shamanistic, as opposed to shamanic, practices are when someone achieves an ASC to interact with spirits, but this is not the person's primary social role (i.e., the individual is not a shaman):

> It is suggested that the term "shaman" and the derivation "shamanic" be reserved for those trance practitioners found in hunting and gathering societies, as well as the empirically similar practitioners found in slightly more complex horticultural and pastoral societies. The term "shamanistic"... can be used to refer to other practitioners who utilize deliberately induced trances as part of their functions [Dobkin de Rios and Winkelman 1989:2].

ASCs are a tool by which a shaman contacts spirits. An ASC implies a substantial departure from normal cognition. Winkelman (1989:18) offers a precise definition:

> A variety of trance-induction procedures share common physiological characteristics by replacing the normal physiological condition of sympathetic dominance and desynchronized fast-wave activity of the frontal cortex with a parasympathetic dominant state characterized by cortical synchronization and high-voltage slow-wave electroencephalographic activity originating in the hippocampal-septal area.

This refers to mental states where the parasympathetic nervous system (which regulates resting processes) dominates the sympathetic system (which regulates fight or flight responses) and where the prefrontal cortex (impulse control and rational thought) is suppressed. There are many ways to enter an ASC: physical trauma, sensory deprivation, rhythmic sounds, fasting, exhaustion, and of course, intoxicants (VanPool 2009:180).

Intoxicant use is found in many shamanic societies (Harner 1973; Mentzner 1998; Saniotis 2010:481; Winkelman 1996). Wiercinski (1989:22) argues that the discovery of hallucinogens was directly related to the development of shamanism. The ability to invoke spirits could have an anxiety-reducing effect, offering a cause for the widespread distribution of shamanism and intoxicant use (La Barre 1972:262). Von Gernet (1992:173) writes: "It has become axiomatic that the original immigrants who peopled the New World carried with them the ideological baggage now known as shamanism. Moreover, it is widely accepted that this baggage included a cultural predisposition for the use of psychoactive plants to attain the ASCs and visions so important in the religion of hunter-gatherers."

Shamanism is part of the broader phenomenon of rituals. Bell (1997) identifies six categories of ritual: rites of passage; calendric rites; rites of exchange and communion; rites of affliction; feasting, fasting, and festivals; and political rites (Bell 1997). Early approaches to ritual emphasize preservation of cultural equilibrium, by maintaining equilibrium between society and environment (Rappaport 1968; Rappaport 1992), reaffirming values and mediating conflict (Evans-Pritchard 1969:152; Turner 1968:5), or providing social order (Lévi-Strauss 1963). Such approaches are largely limited to material concerns (Bloch and Bloch 1986:8) or focus on symbols out of social context (Lewis 1980:18). More nuanced perspectives treat ritual as communication: ritual communicates ideology, maintaining a social status quo (Godelier 1986).

Two aspects of intoxicant use contribute to their role in rituals. A drug must be consumed, and consumption is often collective and amenable to ritualization. Many feast practices include group consumption of intoxicants. This is more likely to be the case for intoxicants like alcohol or tobacco than for hallucinogens. Also, rituals often take the participants out of their normal social context; rules are suspended, altered, even reversed (Turner 1969). Many intoxicants alter their user's perceptions so that liminality is not simply agreed upon but directly experienced (Saniotis 2010:481). Most importantly, rituals provide a controlled context in which the social-solidarity-enhancing properties of intoxicants discussed previously can be effectively channeled.

Intoxicants often feature in rites of passage (Bell 1997:94). For example, some West African religions use hallucinogenic iboga in male coming-of-age rituals (Fernandez and Fernandez 2001; Pope 1969). Chapter 1 presents several instances of the use of hallucinogenic jimsonweed (*Datura* sp.) in Native North American coming-of-age rituals. A common effect of hallucinogens is suppression of self and a sense of "oneness" with the social and natural world, putting the user in an ideal mindset for the ritual. Funeral rituals include intoxicants as well. Herodotus records use of cannabis during Scythian funerals (Touw 1981; Zuardi 2006:154). Alcohol consumption during funerals can be found in numerous ethnographies (e.g., Huntington 1973; Lomnitz 1969:270; Van den Berghe 1978:132; Zolnikov 2013:1–2). Fijians use narcotic kava (*Piper methysticum*) in funerals (Turner 2012). Kava, alcohol, and cannabis are used in some aboriginal Australian funerals (Clough 2001). Chapter 5 includes numerous examples of the use of tobacco, or of smoking pipes, in Native North American funeral rituals and burials.

While the ethnographic evidence is compelling, archaeological evidence shows such practices have a lengthy history. A range of intoxicants have been found in Old World prehistoric contexts. Cannabis has a long history. Cannabis makes a useful comparative case for Native North American tobacco (Chapter 5) since their method of consumption is similar and both are relaxants with mild hallucinogenic properties. The geographic origin of *Cannabis sativa* is in Central Asia (ElSohly 2007:8; Rudgley 1998:44; Warf 2014:418). There is evidence of religious use of cannabis in India, Central Asia, Persia, and China (Clarke and Merlin 2013). It has been suggested that cannabis goes back to 12,000 BCE (Abel 1980), though evidence in Central Asian burials dates as early as 3000 BCE (Godwin 1967; Merlin 2003:313). In northwest China, a shaman buried with cannabis was dated to 2475 ± 30 BP (Jiang et al. 2006). Examples of the ritual use of cannabis become common after 2000 BP in the Near East, Europe, and Asia.

Another Old World example is opium. The opium poppy (*Papaver somniferum*) is native to Central and Eastern Europe. The poppy contains morphine, codeine, and thebaine. These compounds cause sedation, suppress pain and appetite, induce euphoria, and depress respiration. Addiction and overdose are possible. The earliest opium seeds are from 5700 BCE in southern Europe (Merlin 2003). The oldest site with evidence of opium is from the Italian Neolithic (Guerra-Doce 2015:99). It is thought that the poppy was domesticated during the sixth millennium BCE. Analysis of a Spanish skeleton from the fourth century BCE indicates opium used by at least that date (Guerra-Doce 2015:99; Juan-Tresserras and Villalba 1999). Poppies are shown in Egyptian art and have been found in pottery dating from 1540 to 1307 BCE (Emboden 1979a:25). A recent study used gas chromatography–mass spectrometry (GC–MS) to identify morphine and codeine in Bronze Age vessels from the Eastern Mediterranean (Bisset et al. 1996; Koschel 1996). These vessels are commonly recovered in temples (Chovanec 2013).

Based on these brief descriptions, we can conclude intoxication is an ancient and widespread practice. In the following chapters, I will investigate how it has featured in the Native cultures of North America. Before I present evidence for intoxicant use in North America, I must briefly discuss what types of evidence there are to study.

TYPES AND STANDARDS OF EVIDENCE

Archaeological evidence for intoxicants comes in several forms. The strongest evidence is botanical remains or organic residues from a dateable context. This standard is rarely met due to poor preservation and a past lack of interest in collecting such data. More durable evidence are artifacts associated with intoxicant use such as pipes, enema tubes, or snuff trays. However, it is often not clear what substances an artifact was used to ingest. Many substances can be smoked in a pipe, for example. The situation is more confusing for ceramic vessels used in intoxicants storage, processing, or consumption, which may be identical to food-related ceramics.

Ethnographic observation of intoxication can inform on past practices, especially if there is a historic connection. Likewise, historic documents can illuminate past behavior. However, the meanings of any practice, intoxication included, can change dramatically over time, so a researcher must maintain skepticism.

The hardest type of evidence to interpret is iconographic. Images or depictions of the intoxicant plants can be straightforward to interpret, such as representations of datura in Southwestern rock art (discussed in Chapter 2). However, artistic abstraction often makes interpretation speculative. Most subjective are supposed representations of hallucinations induced by intoxicants (Lewis-Williams and Dowson 1988).

In the following chapters, I will describe the most prevalent examples of intoxicants that have been used by Native Americans, beginning with a general discussion of one of the most remarkable classes of intoxicants: the hallucinogens.

1 HALLUCINOGENS

HALLUCINOGENS ARE "AGENTS [THAT ALTER] PERCEPTIONS WITHOUT major autonomic or metabolic changes" (Abraham et al. 1996:287) or that produce "hallucinations, false perceptions, which have a compelling sense of reality in the absence of relevant stimuli" (Winkelman 1996:17). There are three classes of hallucinogen based on molecular structure (Abraham et al. 1996:287; Schultes 1976; Winkelman 2010). While there are differences in effect among these classes, all three induce an ASC analogous to shamanic trances. A hallucinogen alters perception, but does not induce confusion, amnesia, or disorientation. Compounds that do, such as datura, while herein discussed as hallucinogens, are technically referred to as deliriants, and typically include potentially lethal side effects.

HALLUCINOGENS, HALLUCINATIONS, AND CULTURE

Hallucinogens have an ancient pedigree. Researchers have even argued hallucinogens played a role in the origin of art and religion (La Barre 1972; Schultes and Hofmann 1987:62). Others have argued for the reverse:

> This is a generalization that can hardly be acceptable if we cling to the hypothesis that man's sense of another reality is the foundation of religious awareness. On the other hand, this awareness may be concretized in visionary experiences. . . . It seems obvious . . . that the idea of the supernatural preceded the use of drugs in religion and granted them their supernatural quality [Hultkrantz 1997:152].

It is plausible that hallucinogens were used to accommodate an innate sense of the supernatural.

As defined above, hallucinogens substantially alter perception and cognition (Glennon 1994). It is worth discussing what a hallucination is. At one end of a continuum are subtle alterations or enhancements of perceptions. Colors are more vivid, sounds more impactful, odors and tastes more evocative, touch more sensitive. An intermediate level includes perception of images such as dots, lines, or other geometric combinations. There can also be blurring or trailing effect of moving objects. At both this intermediate and the level of simple sensory enhancement, a subject is generally aware that what they are perceiving is not real.

At the most intense end of the spectrum are full hallucinations completely divorced from reality. Hallucinations this extreme are rare but can be the goal of those who consume hallucinogens in rituals. The nature of the hallucinations varies based on psychology, cultural context, or the hallucinogen's specific properties. Research indicates that hallucinatory imagery is based on prior experience (Teufel et al. 2015). However, even if hallucinations are based on personal concepts, they are not congruent with external reality.

Extreme hallucinations are more isolating than the effects of other intoxicants, which are often consumed in groups. But hallucination is a subjective phenomenon. Even when taken in groups, hallucinations are not shared. Sacks (2013) notes that hallucination lacks "consensual validation." This makes hallucinogens more amenable for some types of ritual contexts than others. Rites of passage might more readily incorporate hallucinogens than rituals of social inclusion, where all participants should be "on the same page" cognitively.

Hallucinogens differ from other intoxicants in that they do not amplify or degrade cognitive states but instill qualitatively different states of consciousness and perception. They induce more severe changes in personality and behavior than other intoxicants. Since their effects tend to be the most extreme, their use tends to be the most restricted socially. Explanations for such proscriptions based on safety are insufficient, as hallucinogens are not easy to overdose on. However, social rules and laws exist to maintain social cohesion, and by entering a hallucinatory state, one temporarily leaves that cohesion.

North America is notable in its lack of hallucinogenic species (Driver 2011:105). South American hallucinogenic plants and fungi have been extensively used by traditional societies and have a substantial history. The two best known are ayahuasca (*Banisteriopsis caapi*), an Amazonian vine used in shamanistic rituals in Peru and Brazil (Dean 2009), and San Pedro cactus (*Echinopsis pachanoi*), native to the Andes with a prehistoric use dating back to the Moche (Carod-Artal and Vázquez-Cabrera 2006).

North American hallucinogens are less common. A list of 28 hallucinogens from around the world includes only eight from North America, five of which were limited to Mesoamerica. Since Mesoamerica has a distinct cultural history from the rest of North America, Mesoamerican intoxicants will be referenced only tangentially in this volume. Toxicity has also limited the use of native North American hallucinogenic plants. Of the North American hallucinogens, red (mescal) bean and datura are highly toxic, and their use has a potential for fatal overdose. Their use was likely limited to those with expertise.

Three hallucinogenic plants from North America exhibit sufficient evidence to warrant discussion. Those include red bean (*Dermatophyllum secundiflorum*), jimsonweed (*Datura* sp.), and peyote (*Lophophora williamsii*). Also considered are hallucinogenic fungi and limited use of hallucinogenic fauna. While tobacco does have hallucinogenic properties, since its use was so pervasive in Native culture, it is discussed in its own chapter. The discussion begins with one of the oldest known intoxicants in North America.

RED BEAN (*DERMATOPHYLLUM SECUNDIFLORUM*)

The red or mescal bean is the seed of Texas mountain laurel. Once classified as *Sophora secundiflora*, red bean has been reclassified as *Dermatophyllum secundiflorum* (Gandhi et al. 2011). Mountain laurel grows along riverbanks throughout southern Texas and the northern Mexican highlands. Red bean comprises some of the oldest known evidence for New World hallucinogens (Furst 1972a) due to favorable preservation.

The name "mescal bean" has sown confusion. The plant has no relation to the Mesoamerican alcoholic beverage mescal which is derived from fermented and distilled Agave (*Agave americana*). Adding to confusion, the red bean also does not contain the hallucinogen mescaline, the active agent in peyote (discussed below). Complicating matters further is the fact that some Southwestern cultures, such as the Apache, are reputed to have added red bean to mescal. Peyote

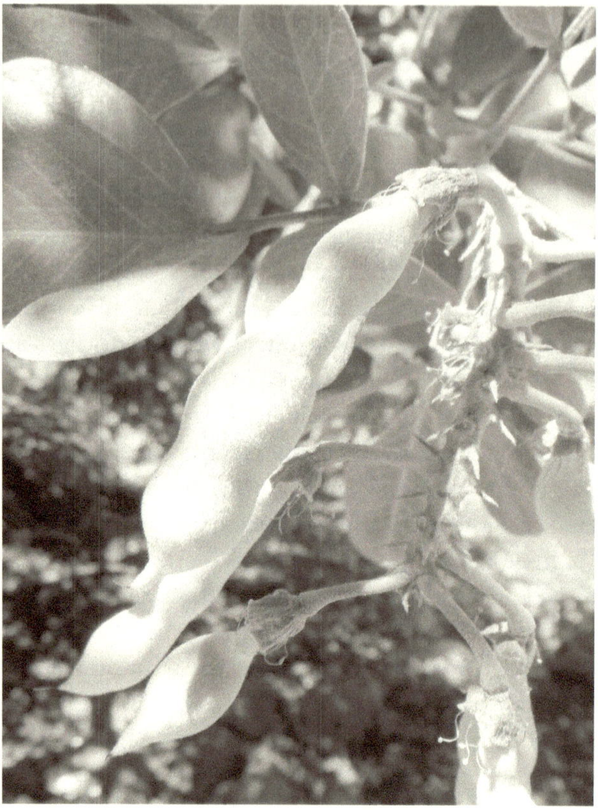

FIGURE 2 Red "Mescal" Bean (*Dermatophyllum secundiflorum*).

has itself been erroneously referred to as "mescal" (La Barre 1938:225; 1960:45; Stewart 1987:4). It is possible that the habit of decorating ritual clothing for peyote rituals with red beans may have contributed to this confusion (Emboden 1979a:87). Red bean is used here to avoid further confusion.

Red beans contain cytisine, which is similar to nicotine (Emboden 1979a:86). Like nicotine, cytosine is not technically a hallucinogen, but its properties can mimic "true" hallucinogens (Devereux 1997:107; Schultes et al. 1998:75). Cytisine is used in smoking cessation therapy (West et al. 2011), despite relatively high toxicity (Merck 1983). Effects of cytisine include mild intoxication and hyperawareness of color. Side effects include nausea, headache, chest pains, and even respiratory failure.

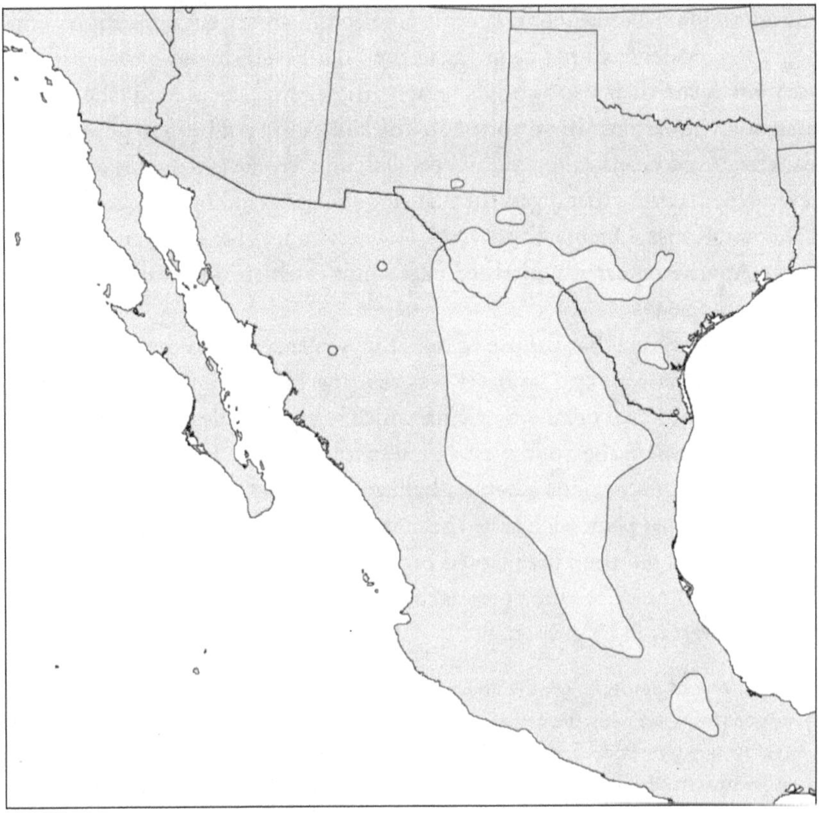

FIGURE 3 Mescal Bean Range.

Some researchers (e.g., Gonzalez Davila 2012) have argued that red bean can have hallucinogenic effects. Others have argued that red beans do not induce hallucinations, but that cytosine leaves the user susceptible to secondary ASCs (Merrill 1977) or that cytosine in sufficient doses induces delirium (Devereux 1997:107). The effect of red bean on color perception would qualify it as a hallucinogen, even if that is a minor effect. There have been incidents of individuals ingesting red beans expecting the effects of peyote, with dire medical consequences due to the plant's toxicity (Wiegand and Smollin 2007:344).

The earliest European to observe red beans was Cabeza de Vaca in 1539 (Schultes 1963), who noted their use as trade items in Texas. Early-to-mid-eighteenth-century Spanish reports from Texas also mention their trade

(Swanton 1946; Troike 1962). There is nineteenth- and twentieth-century ethnographic evidence of red bean use in the Southwest, though many of these accounts relate their use as beads (among the Kiowa), or as medicine, rather than as an intoxicant (Boyd 2003:89). The Kiowa use red bean in peyote rituals. Use of red beans as intoxicants persists, and Troike (1962:946) identified several Plains tribes that ingest them during rituals, including Apache, Comanche, Iowa, Kansa, Omaha, Oto, Osage, Pawnee, Ponca, Tonkawa, and Wichita. Some Apache reportedly used red beans into the historic period (Gonzalez Davila 2012:264).

La Barre argued that the use of red bean was ancestral to the historic peyote cult (La Barre 1957). La Barre was refuting Howard's (1957) hypothesis that "mescalism" had northern origins, which is implausible given the range of *D. secundiflorum* in the Southwest and northern Mexico. The connection with peyote is speculative, but a benign hallucinogen such as peyote replacing a potentially lethal plant such as red bean is plausible. Troike (1962:958) argued that the use of red bean preadapted populations for later peyote. Hultkrantz (1997:95, 164) describes the potential circumstances by which red bean might have been replaced by peyote:

> What caused peyote to get the upper hand over mescalism? There were probably two reasons for this. Firstly, the mescal bean belonged to a closed society, its consumption was not open to everybody. Secondly, it has been described as five times stronger than peyote. A person who drinks the mescal tea sees the world intensely red, loses his sensibility and falls in a coma that may last for hours. This was obviously not a means for bringing man in touch with the supernatural world in an easy way.

And also:

> Some anthropologists consider it probable that the taking of peyote has supplanted the earlier use of intoxicating or cleansing drugs, such as the black tea of the Southeast, or the mescal bean of the Southern Plains. This is quite possible, but difficult to prove. It seems certain however that the ritual pattern of Peyotism qua a Southern Plains ritual pattern has been similar to the Mescal Bean ritual pattern. It is probable that the ritual consumption itself owes some of its outlines to the mescalism consumption pattern. The peyote took over from the Mescal Bean because of its milder physiological consequences.

Stewart (1980) argued that the association of red beans and peyote was spurious, that there is little evidence of red bean use south of the Rio Grande, and that peyote's significance was independent of red bean. He (1980:297) writes:

> The absence of references to mescal beans in either Spanish or Mexican literature . . . makes me wonder if there really was any important relationship between mescal beans and Peyote

> except to use mescal beans to decorate clothing or wear as jewelry. The fact that the use of the term mescal bean to designate the red seed of *Sophora secundiflora* began only in 1914 further casts doubt on the importance of the relationship between mescal beans and Peyote.

Stewart attributes the association to the aforementioned linguistic confusion, and to the two being conflated into a fictional single substance "mescalito" by Castaneda.

Ethnographic documentation of red bean use indicates that a simple replacement of one plant by another is not a sufficient explanation. Use of both plants over time, for differing cultural purposes, is a more likely scenario. Ethnographic accounts show that when red beans are used as an intoxicant, it is in conjunction with peyote. While peyote was the more pervasive intoxicant historically, there is substantial evidence that points to the use of red bean as well.

Havard (1896:39–40) cites a nineteenth-century observer of red bean use:

> According to Bellanger, the Indians near San Antonio formerly used it as an intoxicant, half a bean producing "delirious exhilaration followed by a sleep which lasts 2 or 3 days," and it is asserted that a whole bean would kill a man. I am not aware however that it was used in infusion or decoction, or added to other drinks, although this is likely enough, the bean being very hard and difficult to chew.

Castetter and Opler (1936:54) report such a practice, adding red beans to corn-based fermented beverages by the Chiricahua and Mescalero Apache, though the practice was discontinued.

Howard (1957:76) describes a "mescal bean cult" present among many of the Plains cultures noted by Troike. He cites early twentieth-century ethnographies and concludes that red bean ceremonialism came in two forms. One is similar to peyote rituals (discussed below) and often included peyote. These ceremonies took the form of ingesting red beans and then engaging in physical feats. Descriptions point to this being a male-only practice for establishing social hierarchies through demonstration of physical prowess. Skinner (1915:44–45) describes such an event among the Iowa:

> This ceremony was held in the spring when the sunflowers were in blossom on the prairie, for then nearly all the vegetable foods given by wakanda [the Great Spirit] were ripe. The leader, who was the owner of a medicine and war bundle called mankncutzi waruhawe connected with this society, had his men prepare by "killing" the beans by placing them before the fire until they turned yellow. Then they are taken and pounded up fine and made into a medicine brew. The members then danced all night, and just past midnight they commenced to drink the red bean decoction. They kept this up until about dawn when it began to work upon them so that they vomited and prayed repeatedly, and were thus cleansed ceremonially, the evil being having been driven from their bodies. Then a feast of

> the new vegetable foods was given them and a prayer of thanks was made to wakanda for vegetable foods and tobacco.

Skinner goes on to describe the symbolic power of the beans: "Members of the society tied red beans around their belts when they went to war, deeming them a protection against injury."

The second form of red bean ritual is a ceremony symbolically related to deer hunting where beans were "shot" into participants who then "withdrew" them, prior to ingesting them. Troike (1962:947) argues this had eastern, Algonquian roots. This is a classically shamanistic ritual relating to interaction with animal spirits. The symbolic shooting of foreign objects and their symbolic removal is common in shamanic rituals (Eliade 2004; Harner 1972:158). This involved sleight-of-hand by performers to "remove" objects from a victim (Stein and Stein 2011). Howard suggests that red bean rituals predate peyote, though it is unclear if this is based on evidence other than his own impressions. Troike (1962:947) identifies red bean societies in the Iowa, Kansa, Omaha, Oto, Osage, Pawnee, and Wichita. In these groups, use of the substance is separate from peyote. These societies also focused on deer symbolism, which is similar to symbolic associations for peyote.

Archaeological evidence indicates a significant prehistory for the practice. Winkelman (1996) places the earliest use in the late Pleistocene, though this is not supported by evidence. *D. secundiflorum* has been identified at sites in Texas and northern Mexico. Campbell (1958) notes 12 Archaic (ca. 7000 BCE–1000 CE) cave and rockshelter sites in Texas that contained red bean. Adovasio and Fry (1976) describe nine similar sites from the same region. The contexts and associations of these specimens indicate *D. secundiflorum* was used in shamanic rituals involving the ingestion of intoxicants and the creation of artwork.

Frightful Cave in northern Mexico yielded red beans as well as Texas buckeye seeds (*Ungnadia speciosa*), which may have euphoric effects but are toxic in large doses (Adovasio and Fry 1976:95; Selmar et al. 1990; Taylor 1972:175). Texas buckeye could have been used as a poison, but Adovasio and Fry (1976:94) note that it is "invariably" found with red bean and argue the two were related. Both were recovered in sealed fiber containers. Similar discoveries in Texas and Mexican caves indicate that the two were likely used early as 7000 BCE.

Campbell (1958) notes numerous rockshelters along the Pecos River show similar patterns. Horseshoe Ranch Cave yielded numerous red beans in a fiber bundle, including stone tools, pigments, animal bones, and Texas buckeye (Boyd and Dering 1996; Campbell 1958:157). The bag was placed on a rabbit fur robe. In addition to the red beans and buckeye seeds, the bag included materials commonly associated with shamanistic practices, including bones of small animals (in this case jackrabbit), a turtle shell rattle, and raw materials for the creation of wall art (hematite and a grinding stone). Horseshoe Ranch Cave shows many traits associated with shamanistic practices: subterranean context, percussion instruments, artwork, animal bones, animalistic costumes, and intoxicants.

Red bean predates the Archaic period in Texas. Bonfire Shelter, among the earliest sites in the region, yielded red bean in association with Paleoindian projectile points and radiocarbon dates as early as 8440 BCE (uncalibrated), as well as the bones of extinct bison (Adovasio and Fry 1976:95). Considered with evidence that Paleoindians were using wild tobacco (discussed in Chapter 5), this shows intoxication was found among North America's earliest inhabitants. This supports Furst's (1972b) hypothesis that early migrants to North America readily exploited new intoxicants as they encountered them.

As discussed, it is likely red bean was used with other intoxicants including peyote, and it is to that substance that we now turn.

PEYOTE (*LOPHOPHORA WILLIAMSII*)

> [T]he Peyote religion seeks in its ethics to achieve a good life for the Indian both in this world and in the world after death. Its main goal is to establish man's harmony with his fellow-men and God, and it will promote man's general wellbeing, deliverance from diseases, and protection in times of stress and need [Hultkrantz 1997:31].

Peyote is a spineless cactus native to the northern Mexico/southern Texas desert. The name is derived from the Nahuatl word *peyotl*. Peyote flesh contains substantial concentrations of alkaloids, notably mescaline. Alkaloids as a class of compounds account for most intoxicants globally. They are produced as toxins in a range of plants and fungi, and in a few animals (McBride 2000). Alkaloids are organic molecules containing nitrogen (Roberts and Wink 1998:2; Waterman 1998:87–88). Many have biological effects when ingested due to structural similarity to various neurotransmitters.

Mescaline is similar to LSD or psilocybin. There are 55 different alkaloids in peyote (Schultes 1972) of which only mescaline has been substantially studied. The effect of peyote is likely due to the influence of many compounds, though mescaline is the primary component. Other alkaloids in peyote are similar to strychnine or to morphine. The addition of these alkaloids explains peyote's

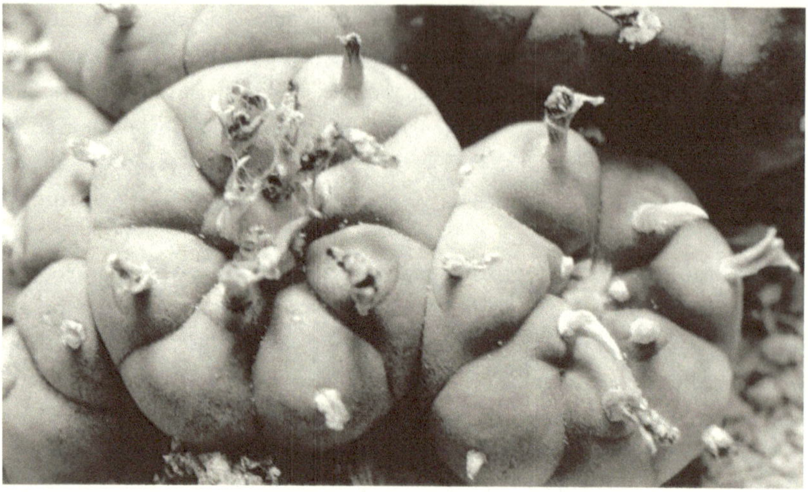

FIGURE 4 Peyote (*Lophophoria williamsii*).

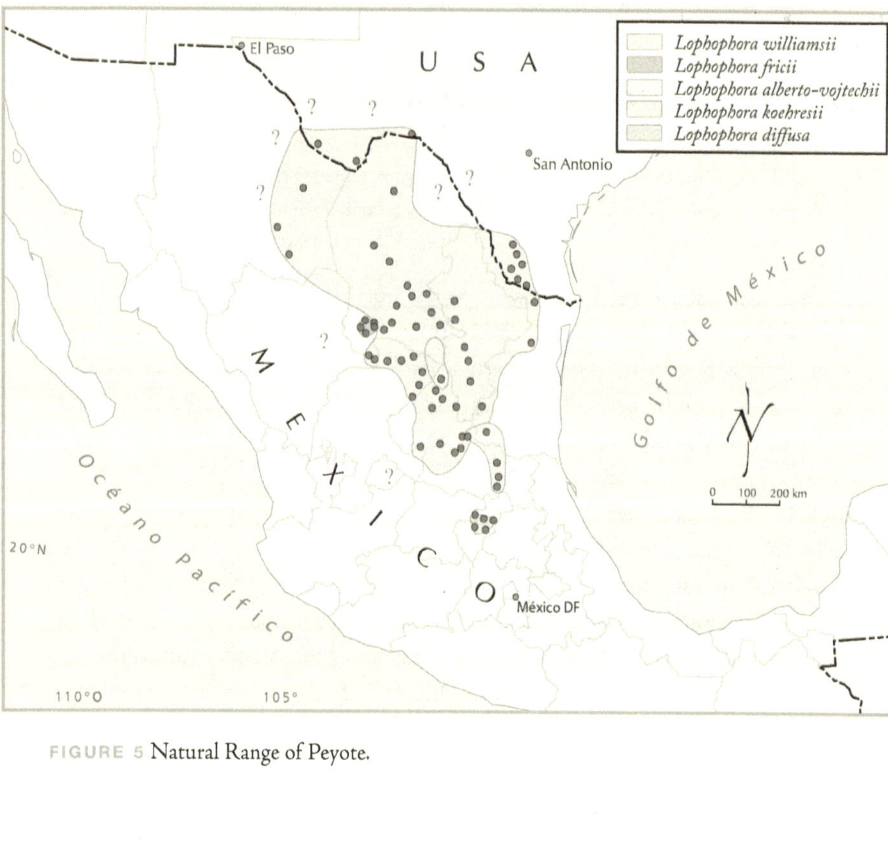

FIGURE 5 Natural Range of Peyote.

complex effects. Peyote users, when taking pure mescaline, report the two experiences are very different, preferring the cactus.

Peyote is typically chewed, can be drunk as a tea or fermented beverage, smoked, added to incense (Rätsch 2005:329), and taken as an enema (Emboden 1979a:85). Eating was generally preferred in North America. The taste is unpleasant, once described as "eating mud" (Hultkrantz 1995:59). There are two phases of intoxication. An initial phase may last up to three to four hours and includes sweating, nausea, and heart palpitations. Once this passes, a subject experiences hours of euphoria, exhilaration, visions, synesthesia, and sensory distortion (Anderson 1995:372). Mescaline hallucinations tend to be relatively mild, featuring geometric imagery, exaggeration of light or colors, or audiovisual synesthesia (Diaz 1996; Giannini and Slaby 1989).

Some have reported that colors perceived with peyote are indescribable (Ellis 1898; Klüver 1966). VanPool (2009:183) suggests color in Native art relates to the hallucinogens that inspired it. MacLean (2001:307) states: "Color visions seem to be part of the experience associated with shamanic states of consciousness, particularly using hallucinogens. These color visions have been described verbally and through paintings and drawings." MacLean ties Huichol art to peyote. The Huichol make brightly colored embroidery, and MacLean cites informants who stated patterns and colors chosen were inspired by peyote visions.

Driver and Massey (1957:270) describe two stages of peyote intoxication thusly:

> In [the] first stage, the drug allays hunger and thirst on the march or out hunting, gives courage in war, and endurance in dancing and racing. This is followed by a second stage of depression and hallucinations, in which the individual may feel fear or hostility to the point of becoming dangerous or, on the contrary, experience euphoria and partial anaesthesia. Among the hallucinations which appear, color visions are the most frequent, with auditory sensations next, and taste and smell somewhat less common.

Others have reported the effect of peyote to be more intense:

> At first there may be only simple images in both pattern and coloring, which constantly change in shape; they are always brightly colored. This early phase of the vision experience is usually followed by one in which there are vividly colored fantasies or hallucinations. These visions may not be able to be distinguished from reality and all of the senses are involved. No longer are there simply geometrical forms, but in this phase brilliantly illuminated scenes and figures appear, constantly changing and filling the mind with a confusion of colors. [Anderson 1995:373]

There is also this relation of an Omaha peyote ritual:

> After I have taken 12 peyote I saw a mountain with roads leading to the top and people dressed in white going up these roads. I got very dizzy, and I began to see all kinds of colors, and arrows began to fly, all around me. I began to perspire very freely. I asked to be taken out of doors. At that time it was 20 degrees below zero. I felt better when I got out of doors. When I went in again I began to hear voices just like they came from all over the ceiling, and I looked around in the other room and thought I heard women singing in there; but the women were not allowed to sing in the meetings usually, and so this was kind of strange. After eating 36 of these peyote I got just like drunk, only more so, and I felt kind of good, but more good than when I drink whisky; and then after that I began to see a big bunch of snakes crawling all around in front of me, and it was a feeling like as if I was cold came over me. The treasurer of the Sacred Peyote Society was sitting near me, and I asked him if he heard young kittens. It sounded as if they were right close to me; and then I sat still for a long time and I saw a big black cat coming toward me, and I felt him just like a tiger walking up on my legs toward me [Safford 1917:404].

Not all who use peyote frame it as a positive experience. Radin (1923) cites a Winnebago informant who experienced anxiety, fear of imminent death, visions of snakes, and monstrous, horned and clawed humanoid monsters under the influence of peyote. John Rave experienced traumatic hallucinations his first time ingesting the drug (Radin 1923:389–391):

> Suddenly I saw a big snake. I was very much frightened. Then another one came crawling over me. . . . There at my back there seemed to be something. So I looked around and I saw a snake about to swallow me entirely. It had legs and arms and a long tail. The end of its tail was a spear. Then I looked again in another direction and I saw a man with horns and long claws with a spear in his hand. He jumped for me and I threw myself on the ground. He missed me.

This went on all night. Undaunted, he ate seven buttons the next night and went on to become a peyote priest. While most describe peyote as a mild intoxicant, what the user brings to the experience psychologically could alter its effect. Rave reported that the experience was positive, perhaps in the same way one might find a horror film cathartic.

Complicating analysis is "false peyote," *Ariocarpus fissuratus*. This superficially similar cactus overlaps peyote's range. While rarely ingested, there are references to its use as a peyote substitute. *A. fissuratus* does not contain mescaline, and its pharmacological effect is unclear. Rätsch (2005:68) relates a Huichol shaman's words regarding false peyote: "When you eat it, you become crazy; you fall into the canyons, you see scorpions, snakes, dangerous animals, you are unable to walk, you fall, you often fall to your death by falling from the cliffs." The Huichol believed people hunting for peyote who were not properly purified might be beguiled by false peyote. Ingesting false peyote was seen as spiritual penance. "If one comes not having been cleansed of everything, then this false [peyote] will discover it. This . . . is like a sorcerer, it acts upon one in this manner. It is going to bring out that which is evil in one, that which frightens one, all those bad thoughts" (Furst 1971:184). False peyote hallucinations are less pleasant and more intense, reportedly full of fear and images of danger, as opposed to the peaceful and placid euphoria. Another species, *Pelecyphora aselliformis*, is also referred to as false peyote or *peyotillo* and has also been used by Natives as a peyote substitute. While it does contain mescaline (Neal et al. 1972), the effects are weaker and not as unpleasant as for *A. fissuratus*.

Researchers tend to focus on the visual aspects of ASCs at the expense of other senses. Some report an auditory component of peyote hallucinations. Micheaux (1963:57–59) reported mescaline intoxication stimulated music perception: "It was music, more insatiable than any monster, the possessed music of the mescalinian demon, given over to its devastations, to its twists and turns, and giving over to them." Music plays a prominent role in many shamanistic rituals, and the fact that peyote interacts with musical perceptions is another reason why it is relevant to the study of shamanism.

In addition to visual and auditory hallucinations, many consumers report alterations in self-perception. Subjects report a sense of oneness with the world and a suppression of identity. There can be "out-of-body" experiences. Some might say that they "died," that their body was occupied by another, and that they were later revived. It is common to report unseen presences, what neuroscientists call "sensed presence anomalies." Such presences can be induced through exertion, such as is experienced by long-distance runners or cyclists, by mountain climbers, or by the rigors of a vision quest. Physiologically this can be attributed to conflict in body schema or mind schema, where the mind, under stress, is tricked into sensing itself as a separate agent (Shermer 2011:104). Peyote, and other hallucinogens, likely excite and/or suppress function in brain regions in the same way as extreme exertion, leading to a subjectively real but objectively false perception of lack of self and presence of unseen others.

Some have argued that hallucinogenic compounds are only partly contributing to the ASCs "peyotists" experience:

> My own experiences in eating peyote have tended to confirm my belief that the auditory and visual hallucinations supposedly so important in the diffusion and perpetuation of the religion . . . are actually rather rare phenomena. In fact, I suspect that many of the "visions" attributed to the consumption of peyote by American Indian peyotists are as much a result

> of the lack of sleep, the hypnotic eighth-note drumbeat, and the habit of staring into the sacred fire, as to the hallucinogenic properties of the plant [Howard 1967:2].

This is anecdotal, based on personal experience, by someone working to rehabilitate public views of peyote. It is not an uncommon perspective, however: "It is my impression that the more intelligent members of the religion tend to consider [peyote visions], at best, as means of learning from peyote; at worst, as distractions resulting from not concentrating on proper subjects, as well as from physical and spiritual impurity" (Slotkin and McAllester 1952:569).

The intensity of significance of hallucinations likely varies among individuals and depends on how much an individual ingests. Most eat a few peyote buttons (less than 10), but some eat more, with higher doses of peyote alkaloids and more intense hallucinations.

Much literature about Native peyote has focused on its role in the Native American Church. Peyote rituals were first observed anthropologically by the ethnologist James Mooney (1897), who was one of the first to record details of the Ghost Dance. La Barre (1960:45) contends that the peyote-centered religious practices arose as an alternative to the Ghost Dance, as a less contentious form of "crisis religion." Peyotism provided many of the same ideals as the Ghost Dance without the bellicosity and anti-white sentiment. Some attribute the greater success of peyotism as due in part to it being a symptom of "passive acceptance" of the new status quo (e.g., Barber 1941:669). I would point out that simply because peyotism did not encourage violence does not make it any less a form of resistance: "[Peyotism] is not an attempt to flee from reality, but rather an attempt to deal with it in another form" (Wagner 1975:201).

Peyote rituals were also more amenable to Christianity, and some groups who adopted them incorporated Christian symbols. Hultkranz (1997:4–5) writes: "It is obvious that Peyote Indians . . . have dismissed Christian missionary programs but at the same time incorporated salient features of Christian thought and ritual in their own religion. . . . We are here facing a basically Mexican Indian religious complex that has become integrated with North American ritual elements, absorbed some important European ideas and been transformed into a sectarian movement." And in a comparison with the Ghost Dance movement Hultkrantz (1997:169) wrote:

> Peyotism was on the whole a better answer to the needs of the Plains Indians at the time. It referred to traditional patterns of religious expression, and it mediated an immediate relation to the supernatural. At the same time it was able to integrate important aspects of the new value systems and organizational forms promoted by Christianity and white civilization in general. It represented a middle way between traditional tribal religion and

> Christianity. And it had a flexibility and simplicity that made it easy to adopt and to adapt to different cultural systems—it became the herald of pan-Indianism.

Not only was peyotism less contentious, it also decreased intertribal conflict by creating a shared ideology that superseded tribal affiliations. Brant (1950:212) stated: "Informants stated that inter-tribal participation is the rule rather than the exception. In this connection the view is frequently expressed that peyote's power has brought all the tribes into friendly association and has mitigated old hostilities and hatreds." Hayes (1940:35) related the opinions of a peyote chief in Utah during the 1930s:

> He wonders why some white people frown on the use of peyote and why some Indian Service officials try to stamp it out. He knows that the constitution grants religious freedom and is perplexed that anybody should resent the peyote church which he feels will establish the Indians as a progressive people—unite them as well as heal them in mind and body.

Ironically this support of intertribal engagement may have contributed to the decline of Native languages in favor of English among peyotists (Hultkrantz 1997:175).

Despite its contribution to intertribal solidarity, peyotism was largely limited to the Great Plains. While peyotism did make inroads in the Northeast, Southeast, and West, this was in groups that had traditions of vision quests and were preadapted to peyotism. In some cultures, existing traditions of other intoxicants, primarily datura, limited peyote's appeal. In those settings, within California and parts of the Great Basin, peyote was superfluous and foreign.

Another reason for the adoption of the peyote ritual is that users typically report feelings of personal significance and harmony with the natural world (Aberle 1991:6; Driver 2011:112): "All the participants radiate an inner harmony and friendliness . . . we all seem to be cocooned in the same unit" (Hultkrantz 1995:60). It is easy to see how this would be comforting in a time of cultural upheaval. Peyote use is:

> An adaptation to conditions created by the contact situation and the degraded status which resulted. Peyotism provided internal peace and harmony instead of competition and conflict, and a reference group with close relations which met needs for approval and esteem. Peyotism offers status, and assertion of self-worth, and a means of countering the effects of prejudice by providing validation of the separate identity [Schultes and Winkelman 1995:225].

Peyote does all this while reproducing a distinctly Native ideology, eschewing acculturation.

The Native American Church originated in the late 1800s largely through

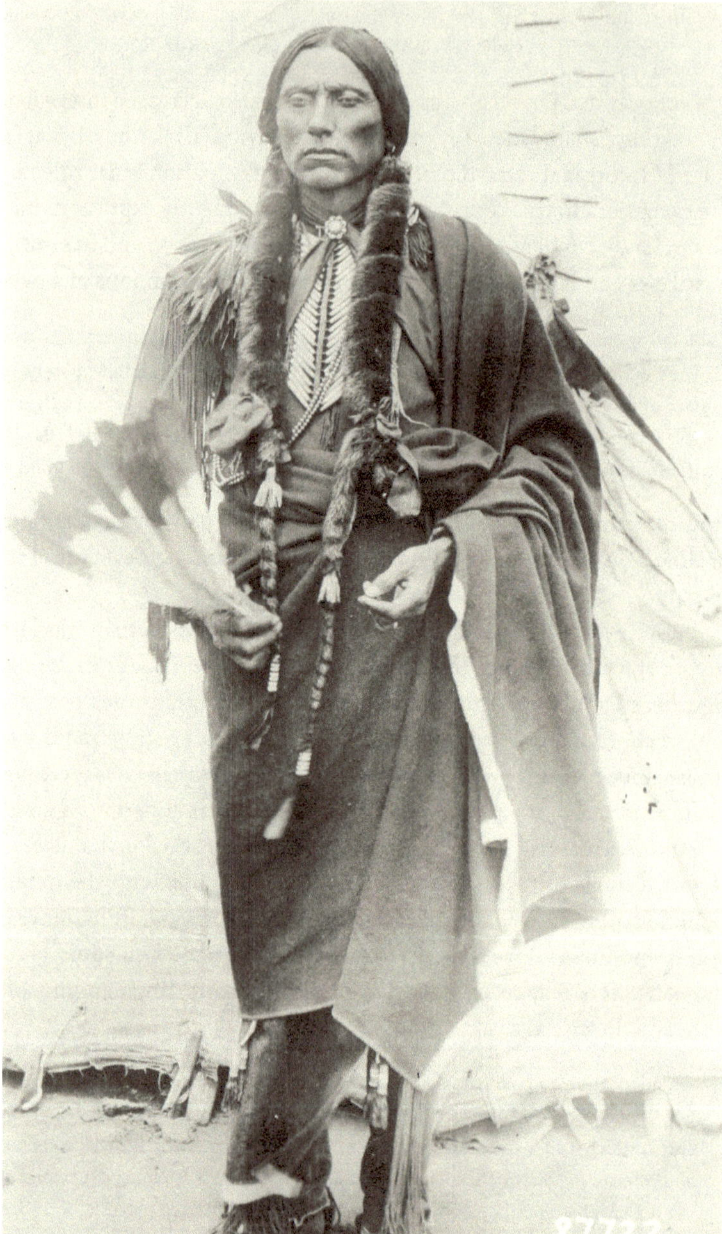

FIGURE 6 Quanah Parker, ca. 1880.

the efforts of a Comanche named Quanah Parker (ca. 1845–1911). Parker was a hero of the Indian Wars. His mother was a captured white settler who was married to a Comanche. After spending years resisting white encroachment, Parker moved to a reservation in 1875 (Stewart 1987:70). There he made a fortune in cattle trading and supported Presbyterian missionaries. He opposed the Ghost Dance in the 1880s and was seen as a model acculturated Native by the Bureau of Indian Affairs (BIA) agents. Parker first tried peyote in 1884 to treat an intestinal ailment and may have seen it administered to treat a fever. Some compounds in peyote show antibacterial properties (McCleary et al. 1960), so peyote may have had some benefit for Parker's illness.

Peyote has been used medically in many cultures; the substance was used for fever among the Aztec and Huichol of Mexico. The Kickapoo used peyote for headache and sunstroke, and it has been used in the Native American Church to treat alcoholism (Rätsch 2005:333). An early Kiowa proponent of the Native American Church embraced the practice when peyote allegedly "cured" his tuberculosis (Hultkrantz 1997:82). Peyote consumption and healing rituals were taking the place of what would have been done by shamans prior to the contact period, with healing power embodied in peyote rather than a human agent (Stewart 1982:202). In some tribes, shamanic practices have remained within peyotism, with the ritual leader, or "road man" for example, sucking out sickness. Shamanistic practices are apparent in several peyotist traditions, among the Mescalero Apache, the Caddo, the Kiowa, and the Southern Ute.

In some tribes, such as the Washoe or Northern Arapaho, relations between peyotists and traditional medicine men were antagonistic (Aberle and Stewart 1957), each seen as a usurper of the other's role. In some cultures, practitioners of either sort coexisted with little friction, with some participating in both practices. Stewart (1956) mentions a Northern Paiute who was active in peyotism, traditional healing, and the Episcopal Church. He argued this was not an unusual case, and that the idea of being raised in a single religion would not have made sense to many Natives, who might belong to many religious traditions over their life. Hultkrantz (1997:162) notes: "it has been characteristic for the Indians not to throw away old religious traditions when accepting new ones." In any event, it was the hallucinogenic effects of peyote that lead Parker and others to embrace its potential as a ritual drug. Parker became a regularly practicing member of the "Half Moon" or "Little Moon" variety of the peyote ceremony and used his prominence among Native and white society to popularize the religion and lobby against its prohibition.

Several churches in the Oklahoma region were using peyote as early as the late 1800s (La Barre 1960). The use of Christian symbols in peyote rituals increased over time from the 1880s into the early twentieth century (Stewart 1987:66). Peyotism was able to incorporate elements from other religions, both Native and Christian. Many Christian concepts were adopted, such as representations of Jesus, or baptism. Peyotists recognize a triple pantheon, with a Great Spirit, then peyote, and then a less clearly defined entity that communicates between the other two, which easily connects with the Catholic trinity. Peyotism recognizes subsidiary spirits which have been equated to angels (Hultkrantz 1997:33). Eating peyote and drinking water during the ritual itself has been likened to the bread and wine of the Sacrament, and repetitions of the number twelve (posts in the tipi, feathers in a ritual fan) evoke the apostles. The post-ceremonial breakfast has been likened to the last supper (Howard 1967:17). And, Christian churches served as a model for how the peyote religion was structured and implemented.

The peyote ritual often involves confessions, but according to La Barre (1947:302) confession was precolumbian, an example of convergence rather than adoption. Radin attributed confession among the Winnebago peyotists as a continuation of an older practice (Stewart 1942:81). While the practice is similar, the intent is different. In Christian traditions, confession is a means to repair one's relationship with God. In Native traditions, confession is a means of reestablishing harmony within the community. La Barre connects the catharsis of confession to the physical expurgation of vomiting, a common effect of peyote. He notes that you see confessions co-occurring with vomiting among Southeastern Natives consuming ilex "black drink" (see Chapter 3). In some settings, such as in California/Nevada, the vomiting associated with peyote consumption was seen to have physical as well as spiritual benefits, with individuals vomiting out disease-causing substances (Merriam and D'Azevedo 1957:618).

Opinions differ whether these Christian aspects are later additions or were central to the early peyote churches. La Barre views Christianity as "thin and superficial" over a purely Native practice, while Stewart saw Christianity as a fundamental element to peyotism (Hultkrantz 1997:28). Some believe the Bible mentions peyote in the Book of Romans 14:2 (Brant 1950:219), though this passage ambiguously refers to unspecified herbs. Parker's mother, a white woman, may have inculcated some Christian dogma into her children, and these ideas may have influenced the later development of the peyote ritual.

There was a second tradition of peyotism in the Southwest, known as the "Big Moon" tradition, promulgated by John Wilson, who was of Caddo, Delaware, and French extraction. Wilson was also active in the Ghost Dance movement. Wilson adapted practices of the Little Moon tradition, incorporating additional Christian concepts. The Big Moon tradition's most obvious characteristic was permanent altars in wooden buildings, as opposed to the ephemeral structures associated with the Little Moon practice. The Big Moon ritual became dominant among Natives in Oklahoma Territory, including the Delaware, Quapaw, and Osage. Several churches of both traditions joined to form the Native American Church, in part to avoid persecution from the white majority (Anderson 1996:47). Estimates of the number of Natives active in the church ranged as high as 250,000 in the late twentieth century (Anderson 1996:48); current estimates are difficult to come by as members may be less willing to self-identify in the current political climate.

Much research has been conducted on the rapid spread of peyotism in the late nineteenth and early twentieth centuries. Mooney (1897) argued it was the properties of the drug which led to its widespread adoption. What specific properties were emphasized varied, including hypothetical (and erroneous) addictive properties. Addiction-centered ideas are now largely rejected in favor of more experiential interpretations: "In Peyotism it is the religious experience, not Peyote as such, that is important, although due to its miracle-promoting efficacy the Peyote herb itself may become divinized" (Hultkrantz 1997:156).

Others have emphasized the confinement of Natives to reservations and the resulting social disruption. Some of the impacts peyotists were reacting to, such as telegraphs, postal services, and railways, also contributed to the spread of peyotism (Hultkrantz 1997:66), while use of English minimized language differences (La Barre 1975). Hultkrantz (1997:184) notes several stages: (1) "A pre-Columbian tribal and shamanic peyotism, integrated with the harvesting year among seed gatherers and horticulturists"; (2) "Basic peyotism in North America" where shamanism was largely superseded by the "democratic pursuit of visions"; (3) "The Peyote religion of the first reservation time" where the ritual spread through the Plains; and finally (4) "The modern Peyote development" embodied in the Native American Church.

Historical uses of red bean or datura have also been cited as providing fertile ground for peyotism to take root, as Aberle (1991) has argued for the Navajo. However, the distributions of datura, peyote, and ilex are largely distinct from one another (see Driver and Massey 1957), indicating cultural preferences for specific intoxicants was more the rule. Only tobacco seems to have widely coexisted with other intoxicants.

More nuanced proposals have included historical events, peyotist proselytization, social disruption, conflict with white society, the need for defined social units, and the practice's contribution to identity (Gerber 1982:302). Anderson (1996:48) summarizes: "The Peyote Ceremony has considerable influence on the Indian's life, it offers him prayer for his soul, food for his stomach, health for his body, prestige and self-expression. It allows for the venting of certain aggressive feelings and, to a degree, soothes the ever-present sense of cultural loss." Peyotism spread rapidly in cultures that emphasized individual's visions and vison quests (Shonle 1925:58). Some traditionalists have cast aspersions on such peyote-induced visions, essentially considering it cheating (e.g., Lame Deer and Erdoes 1972:217), though this ignores the history of intoxicant-induced vision seeking.

Religious power in peyotism is individual and accessible to anyone, and the rituals associated with peyotism did not require substantial training. Even prayers in peyote ceremonies are less formalized than in traditional practices (Howard 1967:19). It is worth quoting Hultkrantz at length:

> The simpler structure of Peyote ritualism is expressed in its short duration (one night), its lack of standardized song contents, its few ritual gestures and opportunities for individual digressions. . . . To those who were not fixed in their old traditional beliefs it offered a simpler way of experiencing an encounter with the supernatural—simpler than the vision quest which required abstinence and suffering and often involved spirit powers of a tricky or even dangerous disposition [Hultkrantz 1997:115–117]. . . . Through the use of psychotropic drugs like Peyote psychically ungifted persons were able to partake in supernatural experiences. Peyote contributed in this way to the democratization of shamanism (154). Long fasting periods were no longer needed, nor of course self-torture. The sometimes painful loneliness in the wilderness was replaced by the joyful togetherness in the Peyote tipi. Everybody could receive visions, not just the few favoured by the spirits, or strong enough to withstand the attacks of wild animals or bad spirits. Faith was restored to those whose religious stability was shaky after the loss of guardian spirits in the vision quest. Indeed, some Peyote visions seem to have been stronger and more compelling than their vision-quest counterparts (173).

Finally, there is peyote's safety in comparison with other ways of inducing ASCs, primarily physical stress, red bean, and datura. Datura did dominate in the Great Basin and California. Peyote by comparison required little specialist training, nor much durable material culture. The closest parallel is tobacco, which also allowed a democratization of spirituality after the development of clay pipes. Had peyote enjoyed the same tolerance as tobacco, it may have spread even farther. Peyotism is a very democratic practice in comparison with shamanic systems and organized religions, be they traditional or Christian. An informant from the Menomini explained (Slotkin and McAllester 1952:579) that, since it was impossible to know what parts of the Bible were the true words of God, it was better to take peyote, which provided the word of God directly. This personalized access explains peyotism's appeal and its occasional suppression.

A brief presentation of peyote ritual is necessary. Meetings may be held for many reasons, such as for healing the sick, for honoring the dead, to recognize major holidays, or for significant birthdays. The Native American Church ceremony is formulaic (Anderson 1996:55–59; Brant 1950; La Barre 1975:43–56, 1979:35–36), though there is regional variation. Stewart (1942:77–78) notes the ritual had changed relatively little despite the area over which it had spread.

The ritual established during the late nineteenth century begins when officials enter a purpose-built tipi or dedicated frame building and sit in a circle around a fire. The tipi represents the cosmos, and the fire is in the shape of a crescent or full moon (or an altar of that shape is created in front of the fire). The crescent versus full moon shapes are reflected in the names of the "Half Moon" as opposed to the "Whole Moon" (or "Big Moon") forms of the ritual. A peyote button (referred to as "father" or "grandfather") is centrally placed, and may represent a traditional deity, or Jesus Christ, depending on the degree of Christian acculturation.

The road man or "peyote chief" prepares the site in advance. He directs the ritual, leading songs and dictating actions, and manages ritual paraphernalia. Other officials manage the fire, burn incense, tend to participants, and dole out the peyote. These officials include a "drum chief" (a chief drummer), a "fire chief" (who manages the fire), and a "cedar chief" (who burns cedar incense). Participants then enter and sit around the fire. Peyote rituals in general, even outside of the Native American Church, are group endeavors (Emboden 1979a:85).

As the ritual commences, tobacco is smoked by all participants, who rub incense onto their bodies. Peyote is then passed around and eaten. Additional incense burning follows, along with drumming and singing. Smoking and drumming duties move around the circle clockwise, and there are repeated gestures to cardinal directions and associated winds. Bird symbolism is common, in the form of eagle feathers or as bird effigies formed from the ashes of the fire. These symbols represent spirits who transmit prayers.

Individuals offer prayers throughout the ceremony. Occasionally peyote juice is rubbed onto the body. Peyote consumption, drumming, and blowing of eagle bone whistles continues into the morning and culminates in a ritual breakfast. Most groups allow any adult to participate, but some limit participation to men; or if women are involved, they must be postmenopausal (Goggin 1938; La Barre 1960:56).

Lakota medicine man Leonard Crow Dog describes the ritual's purpose (Rätsch 2005:331):

> Grandfather Peyote unites us all in love, but first he must separate us, cut us off from the outer world in order to bring us to look into ourselves. . . . A new understanding dawns within you—joyful and hot like the fire, or bitter like the peyote. . . . You will see people that bend themselves into a ball, as if they were still in the belly of their mother, remember things that happened before you were born. Time and space grow and shrink in an inexplicable manner—an entire lifetime of being, learning, understanding, compressed into a few seconds of insight, or time stands still, does not move at all, a minute becomes an entire lifetime.

There have been variations upon this theme (Stewart 1987:xiii). Some variations forgo the use of tobacco (e.g., Hayes 1940:34), while for most, tobacco is integral. There is significant variation within individual traditions in terms of internal interpretation. Menomini peyotists conformed to a set of practices, but individual interpretations of what they meant varied (Slotkin and McAllester 1952:567). Stewart (1942:65) states of the Northern Paiute:

> Hallucinations obtained from eating peyote are extremely varied and individually interpreted. In such visions, the teachings of peyote, all manner of warnings and recommendations, as well as punishments or rewards for past actions, are received. Peyote is said to reveal to the faithful all knowledge essential for life, the price being continued devotion.

Peyote rituals include essential material culture in addition to peyote. La Barre's (1975:66) summary of peyote ritual notes the following items: a satchel (containing peyote), a gourd rattle, a deer hide drum, a staff (used by the leader), feathers, a bone whistle, tobacco, leather bags, and sage incense. This paraphernalia is often standardized (Wiedman 1985). All of these items are perishable and unlikely to be recovered archaeologically. Also, structures in which peyote rituals were conducted can be ephemeral, such as a tipi erected for a single use and then removed. This would leave a negligible archaeological footprint.

The exception is smoking pipes; the passing of a pipe is central to the ritual.

We tend to consider tobacco separately, but in groups using peyote, tobacco might be a lesser aspect of ritual intoxication. Among the Shoshone and Kiowa, tobacco smoke carries prayers during peyote rituals, but the prayers are imbued with power by peyote (Howard 1967:8; Hultkranz 1997:46). Similar practices have been observed for Puebloan groups (Adams and Toll 2000:151). The use of cigarettes complicates archaeological investigation as tobacco use would be invisible.

Tobacco is commonly associated with peyote use. Among the Huichol tobacco is smoked prior to collecting or ingesting peyote:

> Shamanism is at the heart of Huichol culture and religion, and the shaman is able to communicate with the deities through peyote-induced hallucinations. Shamans also use tobacco to induce visions by violently inhaling and swallowing large quantities of smoke, which results in stupor and intoxication. During ceremonial periods the smoking is carried out almost continuously for up to four days by the shamans and other men [Winter 2000d:277].

It would be more accurate to say Huichol rituals are centered on both peyote and tobacco, though peyote gets the greater share of attention. Ironically the Huichol suffer a significant health burden due to labor on industrial tobacco farms (Díaz-Romo and Alvarez 2000).

Schaefer (1996) observes tobacco is "integral" to Huichol peyote use, citing the belief that both were created by the "Deer Person." Huichol taking part in the peyote hunt carry a tobacco bag deemed vital to a successful hunt. The leader of a hunt must distribute tobacco at the outset of the hunt, and that bundle is seen as so powerful that non-Huichol, or Huichol women, cannot come into contact with it. They believe tobacco facilitates peyote's effect. While recreational smoking occurs, the need for using tobacco in peyote rituals is paramount. In addition, the Huichol drink fermented beverages in conjunction with peyote and tobacco.

In addition to using peyote, tobacco, and alcohol, the Huichol use datura. However, as mentioned previously, peyote and datura generally have mutually exclusive distributions (Driver 2011:113), and peyote never became popular in California or the Great Basin (Driver and Massey 1957:273). These areas do see heavy use of tobacco, complementing datura in the same way as for peyote to the west and south. Tobacco, as we will discuss in Chapter 5, is either the primary intoxicant in North America, or it is a complement to more powerful hallucinogens.

For much of the Native American Church's history, peyote has existed in legal limbo, and its use was often suppressed. Peyote was viewed by whites with suspicion, and there were repeated "grass roots" attempts to associate it with early twentieth-century temperance movements. White opposition goes back to contact; it was forbidden by the Spanish Inquisition in 1620, who were as concerned about Spanish colonists using the substance. There are Inquisition documents from the early 1600s where Spanish colonists are held to account for using peyote for healing illness or alleviating the effects of witchcraft (Leonard 1942; Slotkin 1955:214; Stewart 1987:20–21). Some of the venues in which peyote was used by Natives impinged upon Spanish authority:

> The purposes of prophecy and of establishing guilt which peyote was apparently serving brought the matter clearly within the sphere of authority of the Holy Office and moved it to post publicly throughout the realm an edict forbidding under the severest penalties the use of this "herb" [Leonard 1942:324].

Rätsch (2005:16) relates an Inquisition edict from 1620:

> As for the introduction of the use of a plant or root named peyote . . . for the purpose of uncovering thievery, divinations about other occurrences, and prophesizing future events, this is a superstition which is to be condemned because it is directed against the purity and integrity of our sacred Catholic faith. This is certain, for neither this named plant nor any other possesses the power or intrinsic property of being able to bring about the alleged effects, nor can anything produce the mental images, fantasies, or hallucinations that are the basis of the mentioned divinations. In the latter, the influences and workings of the devil, the real cause of this vice, are clear, who first makes use of the innate gullibility of the Indians and their idolatrous tendencies and then strike down many other people who do not sufficiently fear God and do not possess enough faith.

Part of this concern on the part of Spanish colonial authorities was due to assumptions that Native intoxicants altered the body's temperature and humors and were unhealthy and dangerous. Authorities also believed peyote was imbued with power by the devil and that users risked possession (e.g., Juan de Cardenas 1591). One priest equated peyote with cannibalism in severity (Anderson 1995:374). One of the names for peyote was *teonanacatl* or "flesh of the gods," which struck Christians as blasphemous (Emboden 1979a:xv; Hofmann 1971).

White concerns persisted after the establishment of the Western Territories and later states. Peyote was outlawed in New Mexico Territory in 1785. Missionaries among Native populations, most notably the Cheyenne, opposed the practice and lobbied for prohibition (La Barre 1960:47). Several states, particularly Colorado, passed laws prohibiting peyote use (Anderson 1996:189).

This was part of a program of suppression of Natives spurred by missionaries. In 1890 the BIA outlawed Native dances as well as the practices of medicine men and created Indian courts to prosecute violators. Punishments included fines, jail, and withholding food rations. Ironically many Natives charged were acquitted, since laws specified the erroneous "mescal bean" (Stewart 1980; Wiedman 2012:230). Natives attempted to prevent rephrasing this law once the error was discovered or denied that mescal bean was ever used. Despite these legal maneuvers, peyotists were subjected to surveillance, their freedom of travel restricted. While white authority was acting in reaction to unrest accompanying the Ghost Dance movement, the effect was to delegitimize Native religious practices for generations.

Wiedman (2012:223) summarizes BIA opinion at the turn of the nineteenth century:

> In order to suppress traditional religion and medical practitioners, an 1889 BIA policy specified arrest and jail time for those identified as practitioners. By 1890 Indian agents reported peyotism among so many western tribes that the BIA commissioner instructed agents that it was the government's duty to stop the use of the "mescal bean" [peyote]. It should be classified as an "intoxicating liquor," and its sale by traders should be prevented.

Proscription of peyotism and suppression of Native American religious freedom was central at the Oklahoma Constitutional Convention and first state legislature in 1908. Quanah Parker spoke at the convention, and the initial language of the state constitution, which guaranteed freedom of religion, seemed to favor peyote. But laws enacted at the first Oklahoma state legislature maintained the 1890 BIA ban. BIA persecution continued into the twentieth century after many state bans had been rescinded. The formation in 1918 of the Native American Church was an attempt to put Native peyote religion on par with Christian churches.

Objections to peyote were not solely a white concern; Native Americans were often divided on the issue as well. Some traditional healers opposed the practice as a threat to their influence. This was born out when peyote provided significant visions to those who failed to attain them in traditional vision quests (Radin 1920:430–449). Among some societies peyotism was driven to extinction by the mid-twentieth century due to the traditional opposition and personality conflicts within the community (Merriam and D'Azevedo 1957:616).

While some of the lifestyle adopted by peyotists was for the good, such as abstention from alcohol, other traditional aspects were potentially forbidden.

These could include feasting, offering tobacco to spirits, seeking guardian spirits, or any non-peyote-related rituals or dances. Such was the case for Winnebago peyotists, who found themselves pariahs within their society, causing fear and resentment on both sides. Stewart (1942) writes of Paiute families being torn apart as some converted to peyotism and others retained traditional lifeways or practiced Christianity.

Some perceived that peyotism advocates were using it to extract money from fellow Natives. There were also safety concerns, with some young or old individuals reportedly dying after taking peyote. While peyote is not toxic, it may contribute to cardiovascular stimulation that could worsen existing conditions. Also, there were concerns that peyote would exacerbate Native use of alcohol. Daiker (1914:67–68) cites a peyotist from Iowa in 1914:

> They say that if you eat this bean it will cure you from whiskey or other intoxicants, and it makes you a better worker. . . . I have been to Sioux City with many of the Mescal or peyote society and got drunk with them. . . . So when they say it keeps them from drinking I know that that is a lie. . . . I think maybe when they first start to use peyote they give up whiskey for a little while but they soon want it again. They are also spending a great deal of their money on these meetings and to make the Society grow. . . . I think the leaders spend much of the money themselves. . . . Another thing that is very bad is that when a baby is born they give it some of this mescal or peyote tea to drink and this kills them. There are many babies die from that cause.

There may have also been a class element, with peyotism embraced by poorer Natives and reviled by those better off. Peyotism was too white for traditionalists, yet too pagan for Christians.

Factionalism was significant among the Navajo, many of whom adopted Christianity or Mormonism in the early twentieth century (Aberle 1991:xliii; La Barre 1960:49). The Navajo weathered the contact period with less disruption than many groups and maintained traditional religion largely undisturbed. The spread of peyotism conflicted with the "conservative, esoteric and theocratical nature of pueblo religions" (Hultkrantz 1997:22), despite the fact that it also offered real benefits, such as alleviating fears of witchcraft and encouraging support of individuals. Since traditional Navajo religion and peyotism focused on healing, peyotism was deemed more of a threat than Christianity (Hultkrantz 1997:87). Peyotism conflicted with traditional tribal power structures. In addition, fundamental aspects of the two religions, such as the nature of prayer or human souls, were contradictory, making conflict inevitable.

By the 1930s, disruptions to Native society undercut traditional lifestyles and led to many Navajo adopting the peyote religion (Aberle 1991:3). Aberle attributed the growth of peyotism among the Navajo to the disruption of acculturation and diminishment of livestock, while Hultkrantz (1997:170) argues peyotism was only one religious reaction among several (many Navajo adopted evangelical Christian practices, and others reinforced Native religion): "No doubt deprivation paved the way for peyotism, but only in the sense that it made it possible for the Navajo to more generally adopt a religion which already existed among them." Peyote was banned by the Navajo from 1940 until 1967. By the middle of the twentieth century, many saw peyote as a violation of recently adopted Christianity; others perceived it as foreign, in contradiction to indigenous religion. While peyotism became widespread, it never achieved the pan-Indian appeal its originators had hoped.

Many anti-drug laws were passed from the 1950s through the 1970s; most were state level. This led to variation in penalties. Most laws that specifically addressed peyote allowed for its use (Anderson 1996:188). Amendments to the Food, Drug, and Cosmetics Act in 1965 banned hallucinogens, including peyote, as did the Comprehensive Drug Abuse Prevention and Control Act in 1970 (Anderson 1996:199). In the 1970 law, peyote was defined as a Schedule I "narcotic" along with LSD, marijuana, and heroin. Peyote was demonized in the popular press (Howard 1967:1), with peyote rituals described as drug-fueled orgies.

However, in 1978, the American Indian Religious Freedom Act was passed: "Notwithstanding any other provision of law, the use, possession, or transportation of peyote by an Indian for bona fide traditional ceremonial purposes in connection with the practice of a traditional Indian religion is lawful, and shall not be prohibited by the United States or any State." Peyote use was legal in Native religious practices through the 1980s, though a Supreme Court decision that employers could fire users, and that States could withhold unemployment benefits, cast peyote into a legal gray area.

Current Federal law permits peyote as long as it is used for religious purposes. State laws vary, and states have the right to restrict peyote, while some states, such as Utah (Utah v. Mooney 2004), have allowed its use. Native groups in Canada may use peyote, and some Canadian First Nations participate in the Native American Church. Under Mexican law it is illegal to harvest or possess peyote, but an exception is made for Native religious practices.

Ethnohistoric data exist for peyote among Native societies as early as the mid-1500s (Anderson 1996:5). Not all early references to peyote specifically refer to *L. williamsii*; some sixteenth- and seventeenth-century sources use the term to refer to any intoxicating substance (Slotkin 1955:202). What follows is a sample of early sources that most likely refer to peyote.

Friar Bernardino de Sahagún described Mexican hallucinogens in his *General History of the Things of New Spain* (1577), the "*Florentine Codex*":

> There is another herb like mountain prickly pear, named peiotl, which is white and can be found in the north. Those who eat or drink of it see terrifying or absurd visions; this inebriation lasts two or three days and then subsides. It is a delicacy often enjoyed by the Chichimeca, for it is sustaining and spurs them to fight with no thought of fear, thirst, or hunger, and they say that it protects them from all danger [quoted in Carod-Artal 2015:46].

Sahagún describes ceremonies associated with hallucinogen use, though confusion remains as to how to interpret his relations. Sahagún identifies a "*teonanácatl*" as a mushroom, leading many to associate it with psilocybin, while others believe he was misidentifying peyote, or conflating the two (Boyd 1998:236; Britten and Rose 1963:84). Whichever interpretation is correct, Sahagún's descriptions point to a central role of hallucinogenic plants and fungi among sixteenth-century Mexican Natives.

There are more detailed seventeenth-century descriptions of peyote from Mexico by Hernandez de Toledo. Hernandez addresses the supposed medical benefits of peyote, but also noted that it was supposed to have divinatory powers. Hernandez also refers to "*Peyote as Tepic*" but that probably pertains to *Senecio hartwegii*, alleged to have tranquilizing effects (Emboden 1979a:99).

Other seventeenth-century writers were more explicit. A Catholic priest described a peyote ceremony in 1626: "At dawn when a certain little breeze known to them begins to blow, they would gather the narcotic, attributing it to a deity, with the same properties as ololiuqui [morning glory] or *peyote*, since when eaten or drunk, they intoxicate those who partake of them, depriving them of their senses" (Safford 1915:309). A more detailed description of Mexican Native peyote use was published in 1649:

> The Indian men and women begin to dance in one or two circles around the fire . . . until the night is already dark, singing in their fashion whatever words they want, without having meaning, only harmony, and they sing them so harmoniously that one is not discordant from another, but it seems a single voice. Everyone who wants to joins in this group, sometimes a hundred, at other times more or less. They drink the peyote ground up and dissolved in water; this drink intoxicates in such a manner that it makes them lose consciousness and they remain, from the movement and the wine, on the ground like dead persons. They choose among two or three of such as these, and with some beaks from a fish called *aguja*

> ... they scratch them from shoulders to ankles and to the wrists, from whence flows a quantity of blood, and with it they smear it all over their bodies. They leave them in this condition until they are over their drunkenness [Troike 1962:954].

Another clergyman's 1690 observations highlight the organization of peyote rituals:

> Close to the musician was seated the leader of the singing whose business it was to mark the time. Each of these had his assistants to take his place when he should become fatigued. Nearby was placed a tray filled with peyote which is a diabolical root that is ground up and drunk by them so that they may not become weakened by so long a function, which they began by forming as large a circle of men and women as could occupy the space of ground that had been set aside for this purpose. One after the other went dancing in a ring or marked time with his feet, keeping in the middle the musician and the choirmaster whom they had invited, and singing in the same unmusical tune that he set them. They would dance all night from five o'clock in the evening to seven o'clock in the morning, without stopping nor leaving the circle. When the dance was ended, all stood who could hold themselves on their feet; for the majority, from the peyote and the wine which they drank, they were unable to utilize their legs to hold themselves upright [Safford 1917:402].

Several characteristics of Mexican peyotism can be extracted from these observations. Peyote rituals were collective and, at least in one case, were multi-gender. Some individuals were ritual leaders, but no mention is made of a specialist. Numerous substances played a role, including alcohol and psilocybin mushrooms, though peyote is emphasized. Dancing and music were major aspects. This may have occurred as part of other rituals, such as a maize harvesting ritual incorporating peyote and dancing observed in the mid-1700s (de Ortega 1754). It is no surprise that the Church attempted to suppress the practice, and also no surprise that they failed.

Spanish records begin to refer to peyote in northern Mexico and southern Texas in the seventeenth century, though archaeological evidence shows the practice predates that by millennia. A Spanish missionary near Laredo noted in 1700: "Only on the occasion of a *mitote*, or general dance, do they drink peyote and other herbs which causes a disturbance of sense, producing visions and apparitions" (Slotkin 1955:220). Observations from the early 1700s of the Caddo refer to "peyote, or some other herbs that affect their heads" and that "in their dances they have the Indian braves or the Indian women who get drunk on peyote or *frixolillo* [red bean], which they make for the occasion and the people believe everything these persons tell them they have seen" (Slotkin 1955:214–215). Trial records from Taos Pueblo refer to peyote among the Hopi as early as 1720. This was outside of the natural range of peyote, and it would have had to have been obtained via trade.

The most detailed accounts come from research on Native peoples of northern Mexico. Lumholtz (1900, 1902) conducted research among the Huichol, as did Furst in the 1960s (Furst 1972b). Peyote among the Huichol survived Spanish suppression due to the tribe's geographic isolation in northern Mexico and Huichol resistance to acculturation.

Huichol peyotism makes a useful analog for prehistoric evidence. Myerhoff (1974) analyzes the symbolic structure of Huichol life, focusing on maize, deer, and peyote, which are cultural equivalents to the Huichol. The deer is central; maize, peyote, and rain spring from the deer. Other studies corroborate these accounts. Huichol artwork shows the symbolic association of deer, maize, and peyote, and the Huichol deer god left peyote in its footprints when it first walked the world, with some of it being transformed into maize (Winter 2000d:279).

The study of Mexican peyote is contentious, with several works treading a line between fact and fiction. Among the least credible are the writings of Castaneda. In 1968 Castaneda wrote *The Teachings of Don Juan: A Yaqui Way of Knowledge*. In this book and 11 more to follow he wrote a supposedly autobiographical tale of his training in peyote shamanism. Castaneda's writings are controversial; some have argued them to be embellished (Fikes 1993; Rätsch 2005:330). Others have convincingly argued that Castaneda's writings are entirely an elaborate fabrication (De Mille 1980). The details of their critique of Castaneda's writing are complex. His accounts contain many contradictory elements. The culture from which he claims to have learned peyote shamanism did not habitually use peyote themselves. And many passages were shown to be clearly plagiarized from other anthropologists or even famed philosophers such as Wittgenstein.

Despite these clear red flags, some major figures in the anthropology of intoxicants maintained Castaneda's authenticity. The publisher of his early works continued to publish subsequent books as nonfiction. Castaneda himself withdrew from public life. A compromise argues that Castaneda's shaman character serves as a metaphorical figure (Bletzer 1976). However, his work was presented as factual, and is not, which renders it academically compromised, so it has not been consulted for this volume.

Myerhoff, while using peyote, sacrificing objectivity, was a student of Furst, so one might hope for greater accuracy in her research even if her coverage was limited. Myerhoff's (1976) interviews with a Huichol shaman provided a rich source of information about peyote's role in Huichol society. The consumption of peyote is central to Huichol religion, and peyote consumption during Huichol rituals even by elderly or pregnant women, or very young children, is not uncommon (Schaefer 1997). Equally significant is the process through which it is collected—the "peyote hunt." Only peyote that has been collected from a specific sacred landscape is suitable for ceremonies. This region is located 300 km from Huichol territory and is said to be the dwelling place of spirits, including the "principal deer" avatar of peyote (Furst 1976a:113). The peyote hunt involves personal purification, confession, and a sacrifice of peyote. Returning from the hunt, participants are symbolically reborn.

The term "hunt" is not metaphorical. Peyote is "tracked" with bow and arrow, and the first peyote found is shot with an arrow, and then shared by the group. Hunters only take as much as they need, lest peyote be withheld from future expeditions. An intriguing aspect of this collection, that it is closely tied to ritualized deer hunting (Lemaistre 1996; Schaefer and Furst 1996:19), would leave an archaeological signature, but one which could be misinterpreted as a "utilitarian" food-procurement practice.

The association of intoxicants with hunting is not limited to the Huichol, or to peyote. As discussed, hunting symbolism also factors into the use of red bean. Deer and deer hunting imagery play a prominent role in Pecos River rock art, which is influenced by hallucinatory imagery (see Chapter 2). Furst (1976a:168) notes the association of deer with tobacco and datura. These associations should not be surprising since shamanism is a feature in most hunting cultures, as are intoxicants. Associating deer with intoxicants completes a shaman-drug-prey triangle of symbolic associations. Furst notes that a connection between reindeer, shamans, and hallucinogens goes back thousands of years in West Asia and suggests that similar patterns in New World contexts derive from the same ancient associations.

Huichol spirituality references maize agriculture (La Barre 1975:33) and incorporates rain magic. Corn meal plays a role in the collection and consumption of peyote, and the ritual sequence is imperative to maintain individual and community health. Peyote rituals have evolved over time to include elements central to foraging (hunting), as well as to agricultural lifestyles. Given the age of farming in Mexico, this indicates significant antiquity to the practice.

While the ethnographic record documents peyote across the western Plains and northern Mexico, there are regional differences in how peyote is used and the overall function peyote rituals play in society (La Barre 1975:37). Examples of variation in peyote rituals include the importance of a central fire and of drumming in Plains rituals, which are absent in Mexican rituals. Drums were not background instruments; they were significant ritual objects with a key role in shaping the experience. A Washoe informant described the importance of drumming:

> The drum is the most important. The way the drummer handles himself can spoil the singing. The singer depends on the drum, it has to fit his way of singing. If the drummer is good-thinking, or knows his business, he can help the singer; he can sing real good.... Some ... say the drum is everything, that the drum is the way to the medicine. When you know that you know The Way [Merriam and D'Azevedo 1957:621].

An unpracticed, incompetent, or malicious drummer could make a positive, healing experience negative, even dangerous.

There are other differences between the Plains and Mexican traditions. Mexican peyote use ritualizes collection of the cactus as much as consumption; collection is not emphasized among Plains groups. Huichol ritual incorporates dancing, as well as racing and ball games, which are absent in Plains contexts. Mexican rituals are typically outdoors and involve entire communities, while Plains rituals are indoor, voluntary, and sectarian. Peyote rituals among Mexican groups emphasize healing and adequate rainfall. Among nomadic Plains groups, peyote aided in shamanistic conflicts as well as in predicting enemy actions (La Barre 1975:54). Among Plains farmers, the peyote ritual emphasizes community harmony. Peyote rituals in these contexts emphasize collective understandings of peyote visions (Calabrese 1994:497). There are regional variations in the consumption of the drug as well. Early observations in Mexico describe drinking peyote tea, while observations north of the Rio Grande refer to eating peyote buttons.

When Mexican practices were adopted in the Plains and Southwest, they were transformed to be more in keeping with local culture (Hultkrantz 1992:139):

> A tribal anniversary ceremony for the benefit of the vegetation and man, turned into a private ritual for man's wellbeing, and that the "shamanic" character of the proceedings gave way to a more democratic pattern. At the same time, Peyote itself became the center of ceremonies, and a heretical religion. The change was motivated by the new cultural situation on the Plains [Hultkrantz 1997:163].

In this way, the foreign was made familiar while still allowing an alternative religious expression. Peyote became a symbol among Plains cultures, in keeping with the tradition of physical bundles of sacred power embodied in particular objects associated with sacred societies.

While there is substantial recent evidence of peyote, the question remains as to the age of these practices. Slotkin (1955:210) argued that the geographic extent of peyote indicates considerable precontact history. Schultes (1938) has argued for an origin as early as 300 BCE. While this is plausible, physical evidence is limited. There are potential representations of peyote on pots from Central Mexico made between 100 BCE and 200 CE (Furst 1976a:109). These dates should be taken as minimal estimates. There are substantial challenges in recovering peyote evidence. Fleshy plants do not preserve well. Peyote requires no processing or paraphernalia to consume.

Most prehistoric peyote comes from dry caves. Two of the caves in the Pecos River region that provided evidence for red bean also contained peyote. The northern Mexican site CM 79 contained peyote dating between 1070 and 1280 CE fashioned into a necklace in a burial (Adovasio and Fry 1976:95; Terry 2005:30). Shumla Caves in Texas yielded three human effigies made from peyote that date between 4045 and 3960 BCE (El-Seedi et al. 2005; Terry et al. 2006). Terry (2005:27) reports finds from other caves in Texas, though no samples are available for analysis. Still, evidence points to peyote use in the region for over 6,000 years.

Ceramics from tombs in western Mexico feature effigies of people engaged in shamanistic activity, at least one of whom is consuming peyote (Furst 1965; Rätsch 2005:331). A first-century CE figure from Colima shows a child carrying peyote. A fifth-century BCE snuff pipe from Monte Albán is a deer effigy with peyote in its mouth (Furst 1976b:155; Ripinsky-Naxon 1993:168; Schultes and Hofmann 1987), evoking Huichol peyote/deer associations. There are no such effigies known from north of the Rio Grande, though there are possible rock art representations (See Chapter 2). Bird symbolism has become associated with the Native American Church, with drawings of bird silhouettes representing the "peyote bird," a "bringer of visions" (Rätsch 2005:322). However, despite the long history of Native bird symbolism, this particular association is of recent origin.

The Native American Church is alive and well in the twenty-first century. Membership estimates put the movement at over a quarter of a million participants across Canada, the United States, and Mexico. Conflict with local and federal government has continued despite the decriminalization of peyote for religious use, or the "turn-a-blind-eye" attitude of local authorities. A State Supreme Court case in Utah in 2004 ruled in favor of allowing peyote use. Further complicating matters have been attempts by non-church members attempting to emulate the legal cases brought by church lawyers, sullying the reputations of the church and peyotism.

Garrity (2000) writes of Native American Church attempts to use peyote to treat alcoholism by treating traumas instrumental in creating dependency. Natives have long been underserved by health care, and addiction is difficult to treat. Looking at the church role in combating modern Native alcoholism, several factors are at play. There is emphasis on family and social inclusion in church ideology. There is the proscription of alcohol, coupled with a supporting organization. Finally, there is the perceived value of peyote:

> Patients are cured by partaking of peyote and absorbing its "pure healing power." During NAC prayer meetings, the road man and other participants offer prayers to the "Merciful Creator" and the "Holy People," asking them to "bless this patient" and "fill him with the power that he needs." Peyote is said to have the ability to act as "a messenger between you [i.e., the patient] and the Creator" . . . Most importantly, peyote offers the opportunity for self-understanding through ritualized introspection and self-examination [Garrity 2000:529].

One should not advocate hallucinogens for anyone experiencing psychological disorders or substance abuse. Anthropologically speaking, context is everything. But, in the case described, we see how one intoxicant in a structured, socially supportive context can have therapeutic value.

We turn now to a substance that, while not as widespread in its use or social impact as peyote, has had a significant impact on the societies of Native America.

HALLUCINOGENIC MUSHROOMS

There are three groups of hallucinogenic fungi: *Psilocybe* mushrooms, *Amanitaceae* mushrooms, and Claviceps, or ergot fungus. Only the first two were used by Native American groups. There are over 200 species in the *Psilocybe* genus; in the Western Hemisphere, most of these are found in Central and South America. There is substantial artistic and some archaeological evidence that hallucinogenic mushrooms were widely used in Mesoamerica. As with peyote, mushrooms preserve poorly, and the Mesoamerican climate is not as favorable as that of northern Mexico and the Southwest. There are species whose range extends into Western North America for which there are ethnographic, ethnohistoric, and archaeological evidence.

The alkaloids psilocybin and psilocin were first extracted from Mexican *Psilocybe* mushrooms (Hofmann et al. 1959). While psilocybin is typically considered the active compound in *Psilocybe*, Schultes (1976:9; Schultes and Hofmann 1980) notes that this compound would break down rapidly once ingested, and that most of the effects are likely due to psilocin. Psilocybin and psilocin also

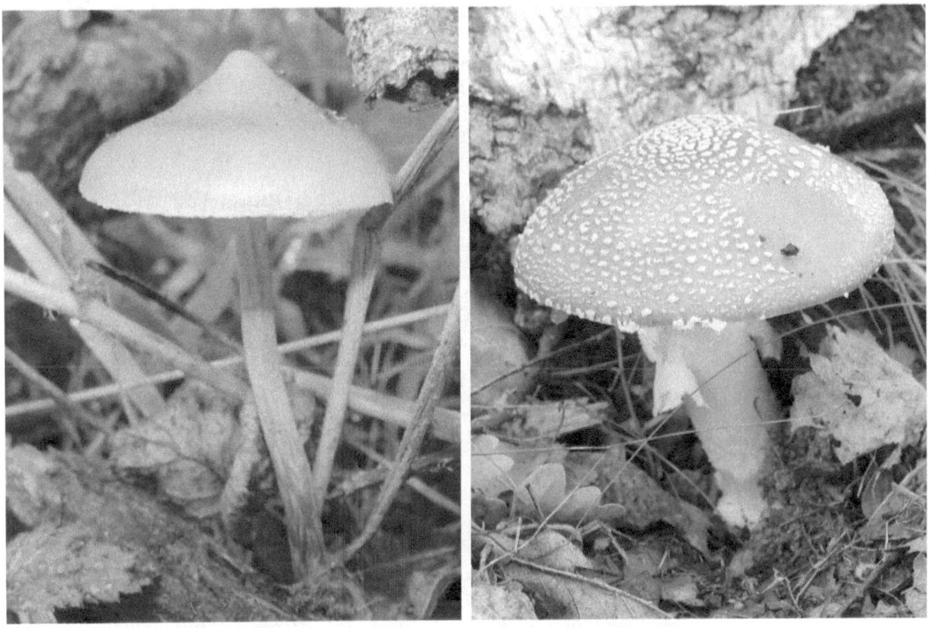

FIGURE 7 Left, *Psilocybe azurescens*. Right, *Amanita pantherina*.

occur in *Panaeolus* and *Conocybe* fungi. Psilocin intoxication includes euphoria and visual hallucinations lasting four to six hours. Psilocin is similar to serotonin, which regulates mood, and psilocin is thought to affect serotonin receptors in the brain. Lyons and Carhart-Harris (2018) investigated psilocybin for subjects with treatment-resistant depression. Subjects were administered with psilocybin and given psychological tests one week and one month afterwards. Subjects who were given psilocybin showed increased "nature relatedness" and a shift away from authoritarian political perspectives. If this result bears out, the implications are significant: "Lifetime psychedelic drug use in the general population positively predicted nature relatedness and negatively predicted authoritarian political views, in a manner that appeared to be mediated by acute and temporary 'ego-dissolution'" (Lyons and Carhart-Harris 2018). An increase in relating to the environment, and a decrease in authoritarian tendencies, would be adaptive in small-scale forager populations. Such groups are embedded in the natural environment and minimize social inequality. The use of an intoxicant with these properties would confer a potential selective advantage.

One North American species, the indigo psilocybe (*P. azurescens*), grows

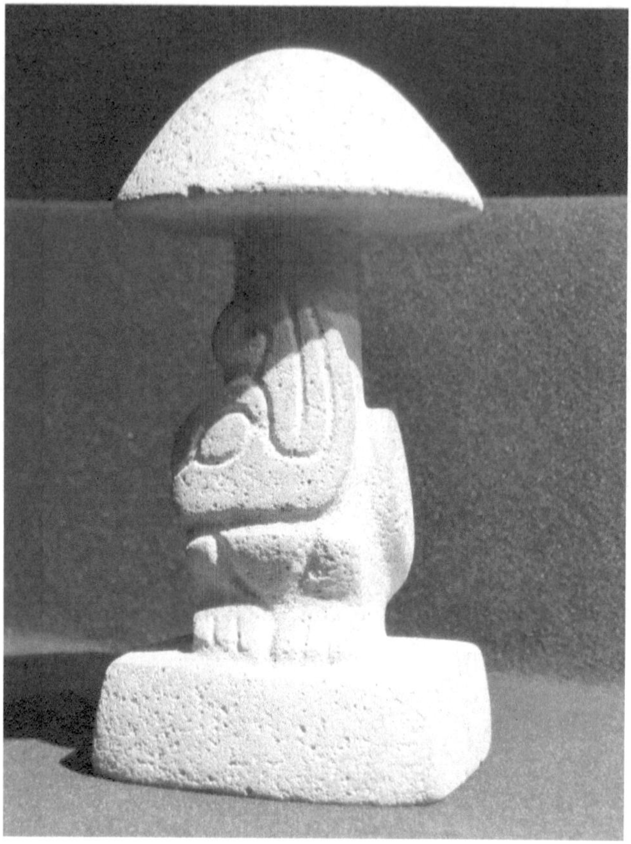

FIGURE 8 Maya "Mushroom Stone."

along the Pacific Northwest coast. These contain psilocybin but were only recently identified and little is known of their use by Natives. Two species of liberty caps (*P. semilanceata* and *P. pelliculosa*), also from the Pacific Northwest, are the most widespread intoxicating mushrooms in the region. In addition to liberty caps, there are a half dozen additional *Psilocybe* species, and five species of the related *Panaeolus* genus in the region (Guzmán et al. 1976). Liberty caps contain psilocybin, and most of the species identified have been used recreationally, though some (e.g., *P. baeocystis*) contain toxic alkaloids in addition to psilocybin (Weil 1977:139).

Details on prehistoric *Psilocybe* use is largely based on illustrations of the fungi. There are images of the mushrooms in stone and ceramic from the Mexican lowlands with dates as early as 1500 BCE (de Borhegyi 1961, 1963; Lowy 1971;

Ott 1977). These date to the Formative period, associated with the Olmec. There is evidence from Olmec sites of several intoxicants, including faunal-derived compounds such as bufotenine, discussed below.

The second group of hallucinogenic fungi are the *Amanitaceae*, specifically the fly agaric mushroom (*Amanita muscaria*). These are distinctive, with red, white-speckled caps (though other, potentially toxic, species can appear similar). Fly agaric has an Old and New World distribution and has been extensively observed in shamanistic practices among Native peoples of Northwest Asia.

Wasson (1968, 1971) hypothesized that fly agaric was the foundation of the beverage Soma mentioned in Sanskrit holy texts between 1500 and 1200 BCE. One passage is dedicated to consuming Soma:

> We have drunk Soma and become immortal; we have attained the light, the Gods discovered. Now what may foeman's malice do to harm us? What, O Immortal, mortal man's deception? Absorbed into the heart, be sweet, O Indu, as a kind father to his son, O Soma, As a wise Friend to friend: do thou, wide-ruler, O Soma, lengthen out our days for living (Griffith 1897:198).

This may refer to a hallucinogen, but other suggestions have been made. Others have speculated that the mushroom was used during the Western Europe Neolithic (Rätsch 2005:631).

Fly agaric contains two psychoactive compounds: ibotenic acid and its derivative muscimol (Weil 1977:141). Both are similar to specific neurotransmitters and decrease certain types of brain activity. Essentially, parts of the brain that regulate brain activity are suppressed, and activity in other areas increases, which is experienced as euphoria and hallucinations lasting up to 12 hours. Weil (1977) notes specimens from the eastern margins of their North American range are less potent than in the west, and their potency varies seasonally.

Allegedly, neither muscimol nor ibotenic acid are degraded by the kidneys and survive in high concentrations in urine. One can supposedly ingest an equivalent dosage by drinking the urine of a person (or animal) who had eaten fly agaric. Reportedly Native Siberians have been observed to drink the urine of reindeer who had eaten fly agaric. However, research did not find sufficient muscimol in the urine of intoxicated mice to intoxicate other mice (Ott et al. 1975). Furst (1989:112) describes the practice in Siberian Native populations:

> One shared trait not usually considered is a high regard for the transformational power of urine. In parts of Siberia, this was linked to a curious practice that first came to the attention of Europeans early in the eighteenth century and that was still very much alive when Jochelson and his colleague, Waldemar Bogoras, studied it in Siberia in 1900–1901. That

> phenomenon was the ritual consumption of urine suffused with the juice of the fly-agaric mushroom, *Amanita muscaria*. The object was to trigger ecstatic trance states.... Whatever it was that caused the effects of the mushroom to persist in the urine also accounted for communal shamanistic rites in which only the shaman himself consumed the fly-agaric, passing his intoxicating urine to a second individual, and he, in turn, to a third, until all had partaken and experienced their therapeutic vision.

As vivid as this description is, human subjects would be required to address this topic, and it will likely remain speculative.

Fly agaric is found along the West Coast and the Great Lakes (Guzmán et al. 1976). Reports exist of Native use in northwestern Canada and the Pacific Northwest (La Barre 1970; Schultes and Hofmann 1987). The distribution of the mushroom is limited by the distribution of symbiotic evergreens on which it depends. Furst (1989:113) states that there is no historic evidence of Northwest Coast Natives using fly agaric despite its regional ubiquity, speculating that the substance may have been forgotten after contact. While difficult to prove given the poor preservation environment, Furst argues it would be unusual for an aboriginal population not to take advantage of available intoxicants, and Northwest Coast Natives had a tradition of drinking urine as a symbolically charged practice. This could be a remnant of an earlier psychedelic practice.

Related fungi are found in Western North America. Panther caps (*Amanita pantherina*) appear similar but more yellow in color and are found in the Pacific Northwest. Panther caps contain the same alkaloids and induce drunken behavior, mania, stupor, and finally, deep sleep; the effects are believed to be more severe than for fly agaric (Buckskin and Benson 2005:88; Weil 1977). Extreme care must be taken in using panther caps as there are similar toxic species such as death caps (*Amanita phalloides*), which kill over half who ingest them.

Early research on Native use of fly agaric was conducted by Wasson (1979) on Natives of the Great Lakes. Ethnohistoric evidence is limited but intriguing. A 1626 Jesuit epistle from Quebec laments Native beliefs that they will dine on mushrooms in the afterlife and "hold intercourse with each other." Wasson argues this reference is the earliest observation of fly agaric over a century before it was observed in Siberia. He also references an 1888 BIA report regarding Great Lakes Natives which noted: "The ceremonial chants could be advantageously pronounced only under inspiration, which was of old obtained by a tedious form of intoxication, now expedited by alcohol." While ambiguous, Wasson interpreted it as evidence of hallucinogenic mushrooms. La Barre (1970:371) assigns shamanistic use of the mushroom to a Mesolithic complex of traits from northeastern Eurasia, including bear ceremonialism, soul flight, and bird symbolism.

Ethnographic data are similarly limited but intriguing. An Ojibwa myth may refer to *Amanita* sp. mushrooms (Keewaydinoquay 1979). Two brothers encounter a cave of giant mushrooms with bright red caps. The younger brother is transformed into a mushroom, and the elder brother turns him back, though he remains unusually happy and joyful. Later, the older brother sees the younger ministering to a crowd, singing: "Because of my supernatural experience in the land of Miskwedo, I have a cure to alleviate your ills, to take away all your unhappiness. If you only will come to my penis and take the quickening waters flowing from it you, too, can be happy forever." They then drink his urine, and: "Throughout the fullness of time these people sing their happy songs, their hearts are strong, and each one does the work of ten" (Keewaydinoquay 1979:31). The mushroom's description, and the potency of the user's urine, are congruent with fly agaric. The transformation and ministrations of the brother evoke shamanistic tropes (Navet 1988).

Navet (1988) speculates on the lack of information for North American Native hallucinogenic mushroom use. He suggests either knowledge was lost, or the practice was ignored by Europeans. He also identifies an ambivalent attitude on the part of the Ojibwa/Chippewa regarding fly agaric. It was the food of the dead, as they grow from rotten matter, but was a phallic symbol of life and source of knowledge. Some Ojibwa myths paint mushrooms in an ominous light, with the knowledge and power they bring being potentially dangerous.

Prehistoric evidence of fly agaric suffers from the problem of fungi preservation. There is iconographic evidence that has been interpreted as hallucinogenic imagery. Red ocher pictographs along the north shore of Lake Superior depict images of supernatural underwater monsters. While these are common motifs in the Northeast, some depict images that are congruent with shamanistic traditions. Human figures exhibiting priapism have been interpreted as the magico-sexual potency of the shamanic, and priapism can accompany mushroom intoxication (Whitley 1994:21). A figure with radiating lines from its head near Scotia Lake in Ontario could represent a shaman experiencing hallucinatory enlightenment (Conway and Conway 1990:71). Regrettably these figures are not well dated.

There are more explicit representations of fungi in Native American material culture. Among objects from the Hopewell site in Ohio is a wooden staff carved into a mushroom. While Rätsch (2005:678) identifies it as a *Psilocybe* specimen,

Romain (2009:183) describes it as *Amanita muscaria*. The artifact appears consistent with *Psilocybe* species, with a long, narrow stem and small cap, but *Amanita* sp. would make more sense by geographic location. Whichever species, it is reasonable to assume the object represents a hallucinogenic fungus, given Hopewellian propensity for ASCs using other substances, notably tobacco.

Buckskin and Benson (2005) describe fly agaric and panther cap use by Ajumawi in Northern California. They describe hunting for mushrooms by singing songs prior to collecting them, and how collecting mushrooms was a household activity. They describe prehistoric use of the mushrooms for divination and healing, portraying a shamanistic practice, but they do not cite data that lead them to project contemporary activity into the past. Their primary focus is on the contemporary use of fly agaric in Native Californian society.

Native symbology associates fly agaric with pileated woodpeckers. Fly agaric and the woodpecker have similar names in several languages. Woodpecker feathers are prized by Ajumawi shamans (Buckskin and Benson 2005:90), perhaps due to the bright red color of both the fly agaric cap and woodpecker's scalp. As discussed previously, birds are common symbols of soul transportation in many shamanistic traditions along with intoxicating drugs. A woodpecker may seem an odd association, but other non-predatory birds are seen as symbolically powerful, such as waterfowl symbolized in smoking pipes.

Ethnographic data exist for Native use of lesser-known hallucinogenic fungi. Several genera within the *Polyporaceae* family, known as "polypores," are known or suspected to contain hallucinogenic compounds. The most famous example of polypores was found on the Tyrolean Iceman, nicknamed "Ötzi." Fungi identified as either larch polypore (*Laricifomes officinalis*) or birch polypore (*Piptoporus betulinus*) were found among items on the body. While initially thought to be tinder, these fungi are now referred to as "medicinal" and by some as an intoxicating drug. Related species are found in North America. Rätsch (2005:661) cites polypores used as hallucinogenic snuff in the Pacific Northwest. There is iconographic evidence of mushrooms consistent with polypores in nineteenth-century Pacific Northwest burials (Blanchette et al. 1992).

Looking to early observations of hallucinogenic fungi, Sahagún refers to sixteenth-century Native Mexican use of *Psilocybin mexicana*:

> The little mushrooms that grow in this land are named teonanácatl. They grow beneath the hay in the fields and plains. They are round, and their stems are tall and round and slender. Their taste is unpleasant; they cause sore throat and drunkenness. They are used as medicine for fever and gout. No more than two or three should be eaten. Those who eat

> them see visions and feel fluttering of the heart; the visions they see are sometimes frightening and sometimes humorous. Those few who eat them in excess are driven to lust. Silly and naughty boys are told that they have eaten nanácatl [quoted in Carod-Artal 2015:45].

Sahagún goes on to provide additional descriptions of the teonanacatl's effect:

> At a banquet the first thing the Indians ate, was a black mushroom which they called nanacátl. These mushrooms caused them to become intoxicated, to see visions and also to be provoked to lust. They ate the mushrooms before dawn when they also drank cacao. They ate the mushrooms with honey and when they began to feel excited due to the effect of the mushrooms, the Indians started dancing, while some were singing and others weeping. Thus was the intoxication produced by the mushrooms. Some Indians who did not care to sing, sat down in their rooms, remaining there as if to think. Others, however, saw in a vision that they had died and thus cried; others saw themselves being eaten by a wild beast; others imagined that they were capturing prisoners of war; others that they were rich or that they possessed many slaves; others that they committed adultery and had their heads crushed for this offence; others that they had stolen some articles for which they had to be killed, and many other visions. When this mushroom intoxication had passed, the Indians talked over amongst themselves the visions they had seen.

This collective hallucinogen use is reminiscent of peyote in the Native American Church and differs from hallucinogen use by shamans as a tool to achieve specific goals.

A less pleasant experience was related by Motolinía Toribio de Benavente in the 1520s (1914:21):

> They had another way of becoming intoxicated which made them even more cruel. This the Indians did with some fungi or small mushrooms native both to this country and found in Castile . . . they eat and drink them together with some honey . . . and shortly afterwards they see a thousand visions, usually of snakes. But being completely out of their mind, the Indians imagined to have their legs and bodies covered with worms which were eating them alive.

Some would beg others to kill them, or hang themselves, to end their suffering. The vivid hallucinations described are not actually consistent with *Psilocybe*, but with datura intoxication. Also, Toribio de Benavente may have exaggerated to demonize Native religious practices.

There has been speculation that hallucinogenic mushrooms were traded from as early as the Formative period in Mesoamerica (McGuire 1982). This is plausible as trade in intoxicants is common in economies with luxury items. Tobacco was widely traded throughout the New World, and opium was an Old World trade item as early as the Bronze Age.

Taking all the data into account, prehistoric use of hallucinogenic fungi is probable but largely unsubstantiated. Several species with intoxicating properties are found in North America. It is unlikely Native populations would not have been familiar with these or would not have taken advantage of them, which is supported by ethnographic research. However, physical archaeological evidence beyond iconography is absent due to poor preservation. Systematic use of hallucinogenic fungi would appear to have been a largely Mesoamerican and South American phenomenon. The absence of large-scale use of hallucinogenic fungi in North America, despite their availability, is likely due to tobacco's dominance in North America (see Chapter 5).

ANIMAL-DERIVED INTOXICANTS

Few intoxicants have acquired the notoriety of the secretions of toads of the genus *Bufo*. Toad secretions have been reputed to have hallucinogenic effects in many regions across the globe. These substances have been reported in associations with various contexts, from European witch ointments to Haitian zombie powder. Part of this notoriety has to do with their macabre origin. It is

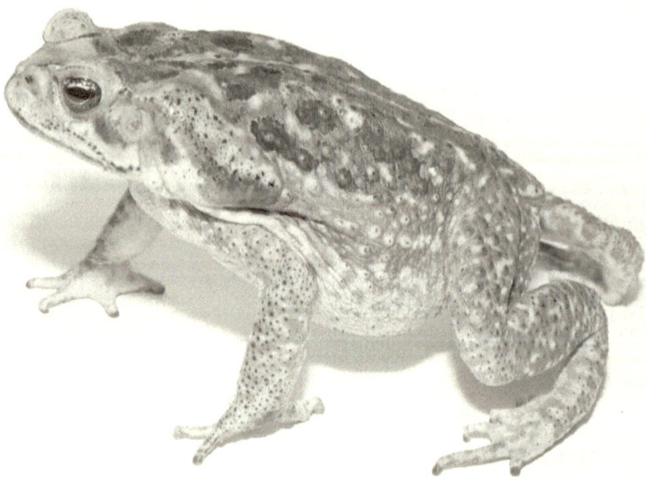

FIGURE 9 The Cane Toad (*Bufo marinus*).

also true that these animals generate substances that rival the plant and fungi kingdoms for their psychoactive potency.

There are approximately 150 species in the *Bufo* genus, but the species most often considered is the cane toad, typically referred to as *Bufo marinus*, properly known as *Rhinella marina*. These have an extensive natural range, including Amazonia and northern South America, Mesoamerica, and southern Texas. There is a substantial history of their use throughout their range, though it is difficult to separate food consumption from psychoactive exploitation.

The psychoactive properties of toad secretions are attributed to the alkaloid compound bufotenine. This compound is related to other hallucinogenic compounds, including psilocybin. Bufotenine is found in several plants and fungi, including *Banisteriopsis* sp., *Anadenanthera peregrina*, and species of *Amanita* mushrooms. There is some debate as to bufotenine's psychoactive effects. Rätsch (2005:817) cites studies of bufotenine's effects, and while toxicity was common, ASCs were not reported. One other study (Fabing and Hawkins 1956) reported hallucinogenic effects, but also severe toxicity. These were poorly constructed studies often conducted on unwilling subjects, leaving the properties of the compound ambiguous. Recent research indicates bufotenine does have hallucinogenic properties but does not readily cross the blood-brain barrier, limiting its effect (McBride 2000). Toxicity has been reported in dogs that ate *Bufo* toads, and while it is difficult to assess a dog's mental state, "neurological abnormalities" were reported (Roberts et al. 2000).

Bufotenine is only one compound found in *Bufo* secretions, which contain dopamine, adrenaline, serotonin, and a range of other toxic compounds. The Colorado River toad (*Bufo alvarius*) is even more pharmacologically endowed (Davis and Weil 1992; Weil and Davis 1994). These toads, native to the American Southwest, secrete highly hallucinogenic DMT and related compounds (Erspamer et al. 1967; McClean et al. 2002). When DMT is smoked or snuffed the compound is a fast-acting, short-lived, extremely potent hallucinogen. DMT occurs in a variety of other hallucinogenic plants, most notably *Anadenanthera peregrina* used by the Natives of Amazonia and the Caribbean. Colorado River toads do not secrete as many toxins, though smoking the dried secretions is best, as heating destroys many toxic compounds while DMT is preserved. Oral consumption is not advisable, as toxic effects are likely to overwhelm psychoactive effects, and some toxins have dangerous cardiovascular effects.

While there are populations of hallucinogenic toads in Western North America, there are few ethnographic observations of their use as intoxicants, and the archaeological record is ambiguous. Wihr (1995:52) cites an 1890 census which relates the use of toads by Tlingit shamans:

> In illness the Tlingit sent for his shaman or medicine-man, who, continuing his fasts in the forest throughout life, continued to receive inspiration from his guardian and familiar animal spirits. In frantic parades and dances about a village, a shaman bit live dogs and ate the heads and tongues of frogs, which contained a potent medicine. He performed his miraculous cures under the spell of his special totemic spirit, and an emetic of dried frogs and sea-water gave him a vision to perceive the soul leaving a man's body, ability to catch and replace it, and cast out the evil spirits which had possessed the patient.

Winter (2000d:280) cites a Huichol shaman who refers to the hallucinogenic potential for toads: "When the Deer Person looked at the [tobacco] plant, he noticed a little animal eating it. When the animal left, he followed it into its cave, where he saw that it was a toad. When he hit the toad, seeds came out of its skin, which produced a powerful medicine for visions." Such observations are rare, and we are left with archaeological evidence and iconography.

We are limited archaeologically in that it is difficult to discern whether animals were used as intoxicants or as food. Finding remains in contexts with a probable ritual function can indicate psychoactive usage. Colorado River toads are common in faunal assemblages of sites in Arizona. One recovered from the fourteenth-century Grasshopper Ruin (Olsen and Olsen 1970:42) was probably used as an intoxicant. However, toad remains are often written off as intrusive or as food (e.g., Shaffer and Neely 1992:349). They are more often recognized as intoxicants when recovered from Mesoamerican contexts, either alone (e.g., Hamblin 1981; Kennedy 1982) or as additives for alcoholic beverages (Hammond and Miksicek 1981:269). In North American literature, one comes across references to *Bufo* remains, but they are relegated to tables of faunal specimens with little discussion of what cultural role they may have played.

The symbolic significance of *Bufo* toads in the Pacific Northwest is hard to dispute when considering iconography. Effigy bowls representing spotted toads (*Bufo boreas boreas*) have been found in coastal British Columbia and on Vancouver Island; examples are depicted from burials dating between 1000 and 2600 BP (Hickok et al. 2010:252). Several of these include objects associated with shamanistic burials (red ocher, crystals, etc.); one individual is buried with a carved antler figurine of a human with a giant spotted toad on its back. Wihr (1995:52) writes:

> It is interesting or highly suspicious, then, that there seems a high incidence of frogs or toads in the shamanistic art of the northern Northwest Coast. Any suggestion of a dan-

> gerous side to shamanism is uncertain and not argued here. However, these depictions in shamanistic art of toad-kissing, licking, or swallowing might very well be an indication of the use by shamans of bufotenine in order to produce the "ecstatic" state so often associated with the profession.

Several Tlingit shaman masks recorded by the Museum of the American Indian depict a frog emerging from their mouths (Dockstader 1961; Jonaitis 1988).

Northwest Coast shaman rattles also depict toads. Wihr (1995) describes Tlingit and Haida rattles that incorporate human figures kissing or sucking on toads, which he argues is a representation of toad-induced intoxication. He describes a Tlingit wooden helmet in the form of a shark sucking on a toad and speculates toad hallucinogen use by warriors as a performance-enhancing drug. He describes accounts of shamans having images of toads painted on their bodies during ceremonies. The presence of hallucinogenic toads along the Northwest Coast, as well as this remarkable iconography, is sufficient evidence that Natives were at least aware of the animal's properties, and likely availed themselves of them.

There is an additional factor why toads might be accorded symbolic power. Emboden (1979b:52) notes that the amphibian life cycle is congruent to shamanistic beliefs. For most animals, the immature form is a smaller version of the adult, but in amphibians, they appear to be a totally different animal, which is transformed into the adult form. This transformation mirrors that of shamans, who transform themselves from human into spirit/animal and back. Such an example can be seen in one Olmec figurine of a human with a toad incorporated into its head (Klein et al. 2002:391). This could indicate a person transforming into the toad or containing the toad within them. There have been discoveries of *Bufo* toad remains from Olmec sites, suggesting the Olmec used them for their psychoactive properties (Coe and Diehl 1980), though others have argued these discoveries are secondary intrusions (Cyphers et al. 2005).

Toads fulfill other characteristics for animals sacralized in shamanistic cultures. Such animals are typically dangerous, being predatory or venomous, or are ambiguous, falling between or outside typical categories. Ambiguous animals are often accorded spiritual power (VanPool 2009:182; Whitley 1994:25). *Bufo* toads are toxic, and toads are seemingly neither fish nor reptile, aquatic nor terrestrial, but incorporate elements of all these categories. This makes them attractive as symbols in shamanistic worldviews.

Historic references to animal-based intoxicants are rare, but one can be found in the writings of José de Acosta. Acosta was a Jesuit scholar who spent

1570 through 1586 in Mexico, Panama, and Peru. He was also an ardent naturalist, and among his many achievements was the correct intuition that Native Americans were of Asian origin, opposing the views of the time. He was a keen observer and less blinded by ideology and dogma than his peers. In 1590 Acosta made the following observations in Peru:

> The priests of the idolles in *Mexico* were annoynted in this sort, they anointed the body from the foote to the head.... This unction was made with diverse little venomous beastes, as spiders, scorpions, palmers, salamanders, and vipers ... to make an ointment of these beastes they took them all together, and burnt them upon the harth of the Temple ... untill they were consumed to ashes; they did they put them in morters with much Tobacco or *Petum* (being an herbe that Nation useth much to benumme the flesh that they may not feel their travel) ... they did likewise mingle with these ashes scorpions, spiders and palmers alive, mingling all together; they did they put to it a certain seede being grownd, which they call Ololuchqui, whereof the Indians make a drinke to see visions, for the virtue of the herbe is to deprive man of sence.... By means of this ointment they became witches, and did see and speake with the Divell [Acosta 1880:364-365].

He states how those anointed with this mixture lost all fear, committed human sacrifice, and walked alone at night not fearing beasts or humans.

Acosta describes an ointment made of numerous potentially venomous animals, including arthropods, worms, amphibians, and snakes, adding to that Native tobacco, and ololiuqui, or morning glory. Nicotine in high doses has an intoxicating effect and is absorbed by the skin (the power of South American tobacco is discussed in Chapter 5). Morning glories can contain LSD-related compounds. We are left with a substance that could cause intoxication without the inclusion of various animals. While the lack of distinct species makes it difficult to assay its composition, it is included to give a historic example of the use of animals in intoxicants.

While there is popular awareness of toad intoxicants, few are aware of the practice of ingesting insects to experience hallucinations. Groark (1996, 2001) has presented substantial ethnographic and historical evidence that shows the use of ants for experiencing hallucinations by California Natives. Groark analyzed early twentieth-century ethnographies and found evidence of ant eating for 17 groups from Central/Southern California. While the original accounts left the ant species ambiguous, Groark (2001) makes a case for the California harvester ant (*Pogonomyrmex californicus*). These ants possess one of the most painful insect stings:

> *Pogonomyrmex* stings are exceptionally intense and piercing—often maintaining this high level for up to several hours—and have been characterized as approximating "ripping

> muscles or tendons" or "turning a screw in the flesh around the sting site. . . ." The venom is also reported to cause a nervous, chilling sensation to sweep upward from the sting site [Groark 1996:3].

Groark places the venom of *Pogonomyrmex* within the "sacred trinity" of Californian intoxicants, with tobacco and datura. Regrettably much information on the practice of consuming ants was lost during the contact period. Fortunately, Harrington was able to identify Natives in the early twentieth century with memory of the practice, and there are ethnohistoric documents from early nineteenth-century Mission San Juan Capistrano.

Of the Southern Californian Native groups for which ant consumption data exist, only seven engaged in the practice for intoxicating effects; the remainder used ants only for medical purposes. The groups that used ants as ritual intoxicants were all Shoshonean speakers, including Chumash and Yakut (Groark 1996:6). Ant eating was a means to acquire "dream helpers" and shamanic power.

Groark (1996:7) quotes Harrington's observations of Chumash ant consumption:

> [These] are the ants that you take if you wish to become an hechicero [curing or bewitching shaman]. . . . You take ants again the following summer and so on every summer till they tell you [that you have had] enough. . . . They give you power to injure or cure people and help you to escape when in peril . . . you always have these powers if you take the ants successfully. Toloache [datura] also gives you the power of escaping from danger, but only 2 or 3 times, and pespibata [green tobacco powder] gives it only once.

Ants gave spiritual power and were preventative medicine more potent than tobacco or datura.

Harrington's informants describe a process where a person makes an informed choice to take part. Unlike datura or tobacco, ant ingestion is not associated with any rite of passage, nor is there any change in social status. It is done for acquiring a dream helper. The ritual takes place away from the village, and ants clinging to eagle feather fluff are administered by an older woman. Large numbers are eaten, up to 400 in cases (Groark 2001:134). Following consumption, the attendant would startle the subject, which incites the consumed ants to sting, dropping the subject into a coma-like sleep. Visions are experienced which identify dream helpers ("*suertes*") who have attached themselves to the subject. Sometimes hallucinations are experienced while conscious; one informant, for example, after ingesting red ants, claimed to see the stars at midday as if it were night (Whitley 2006a:302). This process may be repeated several times over up to five days. The animal spirit identity determines what powers will be conferred. Many are pragmatic, such as avoiding gunfire, or agility. The most venomous spirits could confer "highly specialized shamanic powers that enabled the recipient to cure, bewitch, make rain, or transform into an animal" (Groark 1996:10).

Other tribes would use the ants applied externally in male puberty ordeals in addition to flogging with nettles. Those who completed these rituals were deemed protected from harm. It is unclear whether visions were experienced in these examples, though there was loss of consciousness. The use of ants was abandoned by the early twentieth century, but vestiges remain. Horned toad lizards, for example, who consume harvester ants, are still seen as spiritually powerful animals associated with shamans (Whitley 1994:27).

It is not surprising that such an ordeal might induce a hallucinatory ASC; the fasting, trauma, and sleep deprivation alone might suffice. Groark (1996) discusses how deep unconsciousness is symbolic and necessary to the shamanistic process, so we must question to what degree the ASC described was physiologically induced. There are two possibilities to explain the purported hallucinogenic properties of Californian harvester ants. First, ants might contain psychoactive substances. There is little evidence of such compounds in arthropods, but also little research on the topic. Animal venoms are notoriously complex, and identifying every component is laborious. Numerous alkaloids have been identified from ants, including anabasine, also found in tobacco. Groark (1996:19) aptly summarizes the state of our knowledge: "Given the extreme plasticity of the ant's venom gland and the preliminary state of our knowledge concerning the chemicals it synthesizes, the possibility remains that a directly psychoactive compound awaits our discovery." Whitley (2006a:302) ascribes the effect of ant ingestion to injection of formic acid into the stomach lining, but there are not any known intoxicating properties for that compound, nor does that interpretation agree with reports of ASCs induced through external biting.

Despite the potential psychoactive compounds in ant venom, Groark suggests that the effect described in the ethnographies are side effects of the toxic venom. At an estimated 10 times the toxicity of the honeybee, these ants have a powerful sting, and their venom includes neurotoxic compounds. Groark (2001:137) estimates that the amount of venom injected was up to 35% of the fatal dose. Victims of other venoms have reported hallucinations, so it is not surprising such side effects might occur. In addition, the venom of these ants contains compounds that can disrupt the blood-brain barrier, allowing compounds to have a neurological effect they otherwise would not.

While limited geographically, this practice shows the extreme ends to which humans will go to achieve ASCs. It is striking that Southern Californian Natives were choosing this method when other potent intoxicants, datura and tobacco, were available. Different intoxicants have different effects, so perhaps there are qualities of ant venom intoxication that made it a viable alternative despite the trauma. Or, trauma could have been a desired effect.

This is a difficult intoxicant to investigate archaeologically. There is no material culture needed to ingest ants and finding them on Californian archaeological sites would only indicate that the ants were present in the environment. The only evidence would be identification of ant remains in paleofecal samples, and one would have to make a case that they were not simply food.

There is evidence for the significance of ants in Southwestern mythology. Ants, or "ant-men," play a role in the myths of the Hopi, for example. In these myths, the ant-men prevent the first humans from sinking into the primordial sea. In the myth, a series of worlds are created and then destroyed. During the destruction of the first world, humanity hid by dwelling underground with the Ant People and remerged. This could be an example of attributing an intoxicant with agency and mythological history, as is the case with tobacco, peyote, and datura.

Evidence from Native iconography is equivocal. Insect-like figures feature in Californian rock art, in the form of human-insect hybrids or actual insects, though identification is difficult. In the Chumash area, rock art features dots or figures that have been interpreted as ants (Lee and Heider 1991:19). These forms are found with elements attributable to the neuropsychological model where portions of Native artwork are influenced by, or represent, intoxicant-induced hallucinations (see Chapter 2).

DATURA (*DATURA* SP.)

Another significant plant hallucinogen used by Native Americans are several species from the genus *Datura*. Datura species are found on nearly every continent (excepting Australia and Antarctica) (Emboden 1979a:65; Rudgley 1999:76). Schultes (1979:139) writes: "Undoubtedly Datura represents the most important group of solanaceous hallucinogens—at least, insofar as its widespread use is concerned. Many species have been employed from earliest times in both the Old and the New World." Some argue for a New World origin of datura and a spread to the Old World only postcontact. This assumes Old

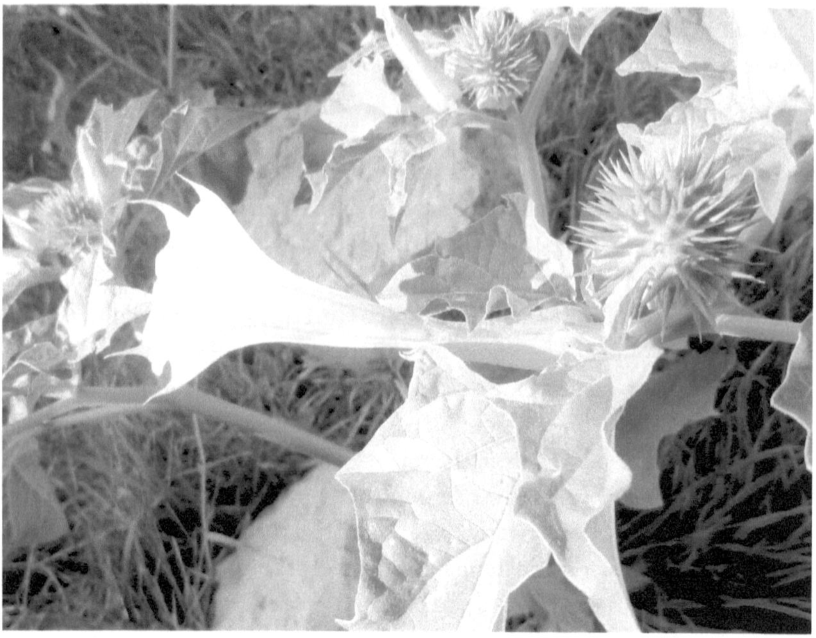

FIGURE 10 Jimson Weed (*Datura stramonium*).

World datura identifications have been based on misreading historical documents. Others have argued that Old World datura was of recent, but precolumbian, age (Geeta and Gharaibeh 2007). This would require precolumbian transatlantic contact, which has yet to be demonstrated and lacks plausibility. There are similar genetic sequences found in New World and Old World species (Baker 1994:263), indicating recent common ancestry. However, New World species, such as *D. stramonium*, are genetically distinct, indicating lengthy independent development, predating human use.

Datura is generally used as an intoxicant wherever it occurs in the natural environment. *D. metel* has been associated with Hindu deities in India, was ingested along with opium in Malaysia, and was used for numerous purposes in Africa (Rätsch 2005:204–205). Datura includes many species, but most share similar intoxicating properties. The most widely used North American species is *D. stramonium*, common name jimsonweed or thorn apple. *D. stramonium* or *D. innoxia* (also referred to as *D. meteloides*) grows throughout the southern latitudes of North America, while *D. wrightii* grows in Southern California. It has been supposed that *D. stramonium* is of postcolonial introduction and not

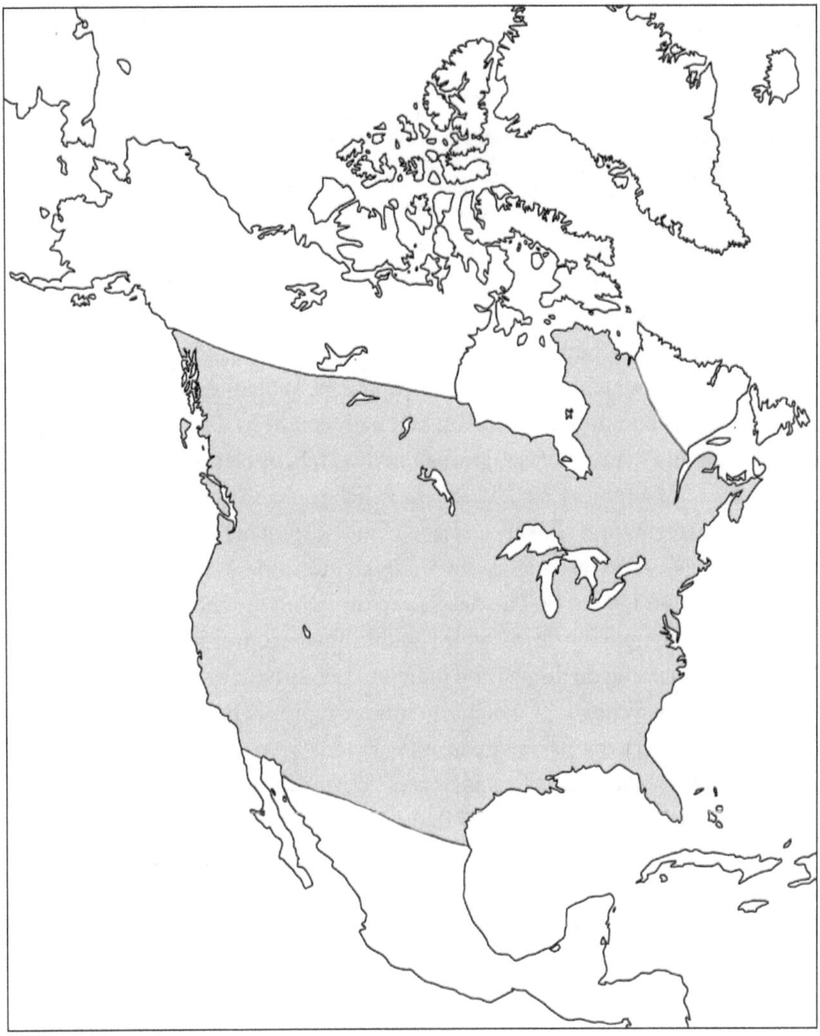

FIGURE 11 Approximate distribution of *Datura* sp. in North America. (Author's map.)

native to the Americas, unlike *D. innoxia* and *D. wrightii*; others have argued all have a New World origin (Rätsch 2005:209). For ease of discussion here they are all referred to simply as "datura."

The *Datura* belong to the nightshade, or Solanaceae family, which includes 90 genera and over 2400 species, including tobacco, as well as Old World plants such as deadly nightshade or belladonna (*Atropa belladonna*), mandrake

(*Mandragora autumnalis*), and black henbane (*Hyoscyamus niger*). Of all Solanaceae, datura have the most potent effect (Jacobs 1995:342–343). Psychoactive Solanaceae get their properties from three alkaloids: scopolamine, atropine, and hyoscyamine. These compounds occur in differing concentrations among species; *D. stramonium* has among the highest (Schultes and Farnsworth 1980:165), and this may increase over the season. Some groups ban its use late in the season or take season into account for dosage (Jacobs 1995:343).

Atropine causes agitation, repetitive movements, talkativeness, loss of emotional control, drying mucus membranes, muscle spasms, and heart arrhythmia. It has uses to dilate pupils or to counteract nerve toxins. Atropine is related to hyoscyamine, which converts into atropine. Scopolamine has hypnotic and narcotic effects and induces delirium and hallucinations. In low doses, scopolamine is an anti-nausea drug (Jacobs 1995:342). Scopolamine can cause light sensitivity and temporary farsightedness, which could be interpreted as a supernatural transformation (Baker 1994:271). Since datura includes scopolamine, it can also act as a sedative, the subject rendered motionless, apparently in a deep sleep (Emboden 1979a:15). The deep sleep of datura intoxication could be associated with temporary death, which could allow one to enter the spirit world. However, depending on dosage and individual sensitivity, these compounds can induce violent psychosis, of which the subject typically has no memory.

Datura inhibits the parasympathetic nervous system, which governs resting processes in the brain. This increases activity in the sympathetic nervous system, which governs the fight or flight response. Sufficiently high doses are potentially lethal, causing paralysis, convulsions, seizures, respiratory arrest, and sudden cardiac death. Studies have found that datura's effects are exacerbated in sleep-deprived subjects, which has implications for the application of datura in ritual contexts. These are not drugs that one indulges in lightly and require expert knowledge. Datura can induce a powerful dissociative and delusional consciousness, more intense and realistic than with other intoxicants. The nature, intensity, and duration of the hallucinations can vary. The lethal toxic dose is only slightly more than the effective dose, so fatal overdoses are a strong possibility. Schultes (1963:22) describes datura intoxication: "The intoxication, fraught with grave dangers because of the extreme toxicity of the alkaloids, is marked by an initial state of violence so furious that the partaker must be restrained until a deep, disturbed sleep overtakes him. Visual hallucinations, interpreted as spirit visitations, are experienced." Datura intoxication can also cause retrograde amnesia, and its consumers are often unable to remember any of the experiences they had under the drug's influence.

Datura can be ingested by nearly any method. Ethnographic references typically mention teas, in water or a fermented beverage (Ball 1962:67; Rätsch 2005:215). Sometimes it is simply eaten. Datura can be used as incense, or smoked, alone or mixed with tobacco or other plants. Other methods, such as enema, have been reported. Datura compounds can be absorbed through the skin; groups in Mexico mix datura into an ointment to rub on their bodies (Rätsch 2005:197).

The Huichol, who glorify peyote, are more reticent with datura. Huichol shamans will recite the story of *Kiéri Tewíyari*, a "dangerous sorcerer." *Kiéri* can transform into datura and entices travelers to ingest his plant form, leading to insanity and death:

> The plant *Kieri* [sic] has white, funnel-shaped flowers and a spine-covered fruit. It lures the careless, enticing them to taste its leaves, flowers, roots and seeds. Those who succumb either die or suffer insanity through its bewitching powers, and believing themselves to be birds, jump to their destruction from cliffs. If they do not kill themselves, they eat more and enter an eternal sleep. Only the shaman can handle such a malevolent spirit, offering prayers and gifts [Schultes 1979:150].

Kiéri is respected and feared by the Huichol. Ethnologists have argued he is the personification of datura (Furst 1976:134–135; Zingg 1938), though some research has shown the related species *Solandra* is a more likely candidate (Furst 1995:43–44; Schultes 1979:150). Huichol use the same term for datura, solandra, and brugmansia. All are related species with potent alkaloids.

The Huichol have another mythic figure, *Kauyumarie*, associated with peyote. When *Kauyumarie* learns of *Kiéri's* evil, they battle, and *Kiéri* is relegated to his plant form. Furst (1976:137) interprets this story as evidence of a past replacement of one intoxicant by another as Huichol migrated from regions where datura was plentiful to areas where peyote was available. "[The] narrative framed in the language and imagery of myth a religious reform, during which a solanaceous species with tropane alkaloids that trigger visionary states but also pose physiological dangers, came to be replaced by the far more benign native of the north-central desert, the peyote cactus" (Furst 1995:55). There are other examples of intoxicants being replaced by less toxic plants, such as peyote supplanting red bean in the Southwest, or tobacco replacing datura in the Eastern Woodlands.

The earliest documentation of datura are sixteenth-century accounts from New Spain. Sahagún's *Florentine Codex* refers to datura only as a treatment for pain and fever. Sahagún does acknowledge the plant's psychological effects:

> It paralyzes one, closes one's eyes, constricts one's throat, holds back the voice, makes one thirsty, deadens the testicles, splits the tongue. It cannot be noticed when it has been drunk. Those whom it paralyzes—when that person's eyes are closed, he remains behind with closed eyes for all time. That which he looks at, he looks at forever. One becomes stiff, dumb. This can be relieved a little with wine [Sahagún 1963:11:7].

Sahagún also discusses Aztec use of the more geographically limited species *D. ceratocaula*: "It causes one harm, takes away the appetite, makes one mad, inebriates one. He who eats of it will not want any other food until he dies. And if he eats it regularly, he will always be confused, mad; he will always be possessed, never again calm" (Sahagún 1963:11:7). Sahagún notes that datura seeds "if eaten, will intoxicate and cause permanent madness."

Several accounts of datura are summarized in an early twentieth-century Smithsonian report (Safford 1922). The most comprehensive is a 1615 compilation of notes by Francisco Hernandez de Toledo, who traveled in Mexico in the 1570s compiling information on medicinal plants. The volume contains numerous references to what is most likely *D. meteloides*, though Hernandez misidentifies it as morning glory (Safford 1922:550). Hernandez states datura treats conditions from venereal disease to broken bones. He notes its use by Native priests who "when they wished to hold converse with spirits and receive responses from them ate of it in order to throw themselves into a frenzy and to see a thousand phantasms revealed and presented to them . . . if it were taken somewhat abundantly, it would cause madness [and] alienation of the mind, visions and deliriums" (quoted in Safford 1922:551).

Jacinto de la Serna, a contemporary of Hernandez, wrote of Aztec datura as follows:

> For in drinking these herbs they consult them like oracles regarding whatsoever maladies they may attempt to cure and whatsoever objects they wish to know about whether lost or stolen and those things which are beyond human knowledge such as the origin of infirmities especially if they are chronic and of long standing and are attributed to witchcraft. In order to dispel doubts regarding this and also for other purposes they have recourse to these herbs through the medium of their impostor medicine men who after drinking reply to all their questions. The person who practices this office is called *payni* which signifies the drinker of a purge or sirup. They also pay these persons very well and if the medicine man is not very skillful in his office or if he wishes to excuse himself from the trouble which the drinking of these philters would cause they advise the sick to drink them or those in quest of lost objects who seek to discover where those things are or in whose possession they may be [quoted in Safford 1922:551].

Jacinto de la Serna also discusses the veneration given to the plant, its storage in specialized vessels, and the maintenance of altars dedicated to it. These accounts point to institutionalized datura use for religious purposes during the sixteenth to seventeenth century.

A 1653 source by Bernabé Cobo in Peru relates the effects of datura (termed *chamico*):

> If a person drinks a decoction of these seeds, his senses will be benumbed. The Indians use this drink of intoxication, but he who takes too much of this brew will so much be deprived of his reason that, though he has his eyes open, he cannot see or comprehend anything. The Indians formerly wrought great harm with the brew. Not long ago, it happened in the Kingdom that a man who I knew was walking with a companion, who, having plans to rob my friend, gave him a *chamico* drink. This caused the man to lose his mind and to become so enraged that, naked for his shirt, he started to throw himself into the river. He was seized like a mad man and restrained. For two days, he remained in this condition without regaining consciousness [Cobo 1890–1893:IV:chap. C].

Datura's sedating effect was so severe there are reports of it used to stupefy Chibcha sacrificial victims in sixteenth-century Columbia (Gayton 1928:19). Victims buried alive with a deceased chief were given a mix of corn beer and datura to ensure compliance (de Castellanos 1886–1887):

> Before being brought to this [tomb] that they will not suffer any fright or pangs of death, the women and slaves are given by the chiefs a certain potion mixed into their ordinary beverage. This potion is prepared from intoxicating tobacco and from other leaves of a tree which they call *borrachero* [*D. candida*]. And this their senses become so benumbed that they will not feel any pain.

There have been reports of Aztec priests administering datura-infused pulque to sacrificial victims (Rätsch 2005:46), but what was used may have been solandra (Furst 1976:136). There are observations of datura use by South American Natives during the nineteenth century, ironically to divine the location of antiquities from tombs to trade with foreign tourists (Gayton 1928).

Europeans avoided consuming datura. The plant's effects were obviously dangerous even to a naïve observer, and most would have been familiar with similar Old World plants such as deadly nightshade (*Atropa belladonna*) (Furst 1976:216). Beverley describes accidental ingestion by soldiers at Jamestown:

> [T]he Effect of which was a very pleasant Comedy; for they turn'd natural Fools upon it for several Days: One would blow up a Feather in the Air; another wou'd dart Straws at it

> with much Fury; another, stark naked, was sitting up—in a Corner, like a Monkey, grinning and making Mows at them; a Fourth would fondly kiss and paw his Companions, and snear in their Faces with a Countenance more antick than any in a Dutch Droll.... A thousand such simple Tricks they play'd, and after Eleven Days, return'd to themselves again, not remembering anything that had pass'd [Beverley 1947:139].

Furst (1995:45) opines the English were using the drug intentionally. In any event, the name jimsonweed is a contraction of "Jamestown weed" due to this incident.

In Native rituals using datura, the desired effect was the suspension of consciousness and memory. Beverley describes at length huskanaw initiation ceremonies in Virginia:

> The choicest and briskest young men of the town and such only as have some treasure by their travels and hunting are chosen out by the rulers to be huskanawed and whoever refuses to undergo this process dares not remain among them. Several of those odd preparatory fopperies are in the beginning which have been before related but the principal of the business is to carry them into the woods and there keep them confinement and destitute of all society for several months giving them other sustenance but the infusion or decoction of some poisonous intoxicating roots by virtue of which physic and by the severity of the discipline they undergo they become stark staring mad in which raving they are kept eighteen or twenty days. During these extremities they are shut up night and day in a strong inclosure.... In this cage thirteen young men had been huskanawed had not been a month set at liberty when I saw it. Upon this occasion it pretended that these poor creatures drink so much of that water of Lethe they perfectly lose the remembrance of all former things even of their treasure and their language ... before they are perfectly well they bring them into their towns they are still wild and crazy through the violence of the medicine.... Thus they must pretend to have forgot the very use of their tongues so as not to be able to speak nor understand anything that is spoken till they learn it again.... Thus they unlive their former lives and commence men by forgetting that they ever have been boys [Beverley 1947:207].

Children, Natives reasoned, were irrational beings governed by family ties. After the ritual, childhood ties were severed, and the adult Natives could exercise reason free of obligation.

Lawson's eighteenth-century observation of the North Carolina Tuscarora is consistent with datura intoxication (Johnson 1967:I:240). Lawson (1903) in 1714 notes an "abominable custom" called "*husquenaugh*" where boys are initiated in the same way as observed in Virginia:

> Besides they give them Pellitory Bark and several intoxicating Plants, that make them go raving Mad as ever were any People in this World; and you may hear them make the most dismal and Hellish cries, and Howlings, that ever Human Creatures ever expressed; all

> which continues about five or six weeks. The boys were traumatized and took months to re-accustom themselves to society. Deaths were not uncommon. Girls had their own version, and many children ran away to avoid the ordeal.

A 1612 document by John Smith of Jamestown describes a similar ritual (Gardner 1907:112), though with no specific mention of datura. Smith describes boys selected at random, forcefully taken from their village, and then "cast on a heape in a valley, as dead: where they made a great feast for all the company." It is then claimed the boys were not really dead, that most lived and were excluded for months, after which they could rejoin their village. While ambiguous, this account overlaps with later observations and probably indicates use of datura.

Beverley's account uses the terms "infusion" and "decoction" which indicate datura was drunk. Some have suggested keeping subjects in a prolonged state of intoxication would be easier via enema (de Smet 1985:35; Emboden 1979a). While intoxicant enemas of datura tea have been documented (Furst 1976:27–29; Robicsek 1978:38), references are from Mesoamerica or South America, not North America. While enema use has advantages, such as avoiding nausea, rapid absorption, and bypassing the liver (Diamond 2001), it is likely that if European observers had witnessed the practice, they would have noted it.

This initiation used datura to induce temporary psychosis, suppressing past memories and leaving subjects free to start new adult lives. This corresponds with anthropological theory on initiatory rituals, where individuals must be separated from society, in this case by removing them from normal reality. The amnesia associated with datura facilitates social reintegration after the ordeal (Jacobs 1995). If an initiate could still remember his childhood, stronger doses would be given until amnesia was achieved, or the individual died (Furst 1976:142). Beverley acknowledges there is a possibility of "counterfeit" in their amnesiac behavior. A child would likely be highly motivated to play along with expectations rather than endure the procedure more than once.

A range of seventeenth- and early eighteenth-century documents from Canada provide evidence of hallucinogenic infusions, possibly datura, though their exact nature is ambiguous. Von Gernet (1992:174) cites these as evidence of Iroquoian hallucinogenic beverages, citing *Amanita muscaria* and datura as possibilities. Datura seems the more likely candidate. Fly agaric are distinctive in appearance, and European observers would have been aware of mushrooms' possible physiological effects. Datura is less obvious. While descriptions of symptoms are vague, they are more compatible with datura intoxication. Also, these references are of beverages, while mushrooms are usually eaten.

In 1619, Samuel de Champlain, describing Huron sweat lodge rituals, observed (quoted in Biggar 1929:154): "There are also women who go into these rages, but they do not do so much harm; they walk on all fours like beasts. Seeing this the magician called the Oqui begins to sing, then with some grimaces blows upon her, ordering her to drink certain waters." The term "certain waters" as opposed to "water" argues for a special quality, and the subjects are clearly in an ASC.

In the early 1700s, describing a Native shaman, Charlevoix (1923:152) writes:

> An Indian accompanied bearing a vase filled with I know not what liquor, of which he gave him to drink from time to time; the quack had no sooner put it to his lips than he thrust it from him again, blowing on his hands and staff, and at each time divining all such riddles as were proposed to him.

Charlevoix also describes Native sweat baths (164–165):

> There are some who, before they enter the sweat-box, take a draught of a composition very proper, say they, for disposing them to receive the divine impulse. . . . Then full of his pretended divinity, and more like a person possessed by the devil than one inspired of heaven, he pronounces in a positive tone of voice on the state of the patient, and sometimes guesses tolerably just.

Charlevoix incorporated older accounts in his writing, so it is difficult to date this observation, but it seems to depict an intoxicating tea in a shamanic healing practice, again most likely datura.

The Jesuit Relations include references to beverages taken by Native shamans. In 1636 Brébeuf describes a Huron healing dance during which participants "give poison to one another" to achieve hallucinations (Thwaites 1959:10:205). He makes his feelings on the practice clear: "The greatest evil is, that these wretches, under pretext of charity, often avenge their injuries, and purposely give poison to their patients, instead of medicine." During a 1637 epidemic among the Huron, there are observations of Native rituals involving such decoctions. When one young woman is afflicted, the Jesuits blamed her declining health and unsuitability for conversion on such an intervention (Thwaites 1959:13:137): "Therefore God, who often employs the sins of men as instruments to punish them, permitted that, on account of a medicine man blowing upon her and giving her some potion, she should not be effectively urged to accept Baptism." In another passage (Thwaites 1959:13:227), a Huron shaman, after fasting and drinking a beverage, experiences "demons" who give him cures, but the passage describes the drink as "warm water." This could be misidentified psychoactive tea, or simply hallucination after fasting. Other examples have shamans pouring "mysterious water" over individuals (Thwaites 1959:13:241, 19:243) but no indication of consumption or physiological effects. Jesuits witnessed a shaman adding powder to a broth being fed to the sick (Thwaites 1959:13:257). In 1640, a Huron has a vision of a Christ-like figure, who exhorts him administer an unspecified potion to the sick, after which all the men should act like animals or madmen. Jesuits noted: "They were six of the Elders who bore in silence a great kettle full of that diabolical water, whereof they made all the sick people drink." Again, it is unclear what is drunk, or if the ASCs described are simply theatrics.

The clearest observation of a hallucinogenic tea in New France was published in 1664 by Du Creux based on the Jesuit Relations. A Christianized Algonquian resident of Tadoussac fell ill, and Natives and French thought him close to death. Du Creux writes (1969:2:686):

> As having no hope in man he turned to God and told them to steep a piece of some kind of bark along with the buds of a twig of fir tree in warm water . . . scarcely had he drunk the infusion when suddenly the life-giving liquid pervaded all parts of his afflicted body, and somehow or another gave strength to his limbs; at the same time he seemed to see about him cherubs which were more beautiful he said, than the holy angels to be seen in Christian pictures, and these cherubs with the bright faces encouraged him by telling him that his disease would go no farther.

The man recovered, which Du Creux attributes to God. Of all references to intoxicating beverages used in the Northeast, this one makes the most explicit link between drinking an infusion and an ASC. The plant is not identified, but datura would be the most likely.

Von Gernet (1992:174) notes Huron mythology includes depictions of plants that induce trances and visions to facilitate contact with spirits, and also (174–175) an Iroquois tradition "little water medicine" applied externally and drunk, which could induce ASCs, but the ingredients of which are no longer known. This indicates that plants producing symptoms consistent with datura are sufficiently present in Iroquoian cultures to become embedded in mythology.

There has been little research in the Northeast on medicinal or psychoactive plants. This contrasts with volumes of research on Western or Southwestern cultures. Working from accounts of Native informants, as well as ethnographic accounts, Herrick (1983, 1995:92–93) listed over 100 "powerful medicinal species." Seven (including datura) are listed as used to "bring about insanity," the only symptom listed that corresponds to those described in seventeenth- and eighteenth-century accounts. The remaining six include tall thimbleweed (*Anemone virginiana*), water hemlock (*Cicuta maculata*), liverleaf/liverwort (*Hepatica nobilis*), early meadow rue (*Thalictrum dioicum*), white clover (*Trifolium repens*), and violets/pansies (*Viola* sp.). Water hemlock, also known as "the suicide root," contains a neurotoxin. While water hemlock poisoning does cause amnesia like datura, it is more likely to kill or cause brain damage. The remaining plants do not have known intoxicating properties.

Von Gernet (1992:174) lists 11 Northeast species or genera allegedly having psychoactive properties. These include sweet flag (*Acorus calamus*), Queen Anne's lace (*Daucus carota*), field horsetail (*Equisetum arvense*), eastern teaberry (*Gaultheria procumbens*), catnip (*Nepeta cataria*), common buttercup (*Ranunculus acris*), pokeweeds (*Phytolacca* sp.), bulrush (*Scirpus* sp.), lettuces (*Lactuca* sp.), species of the genus *Lobelia*, and morning glories (*Ipomoea* sp.). Sweet flag may have hallucinogenic properties and has been recovered from Mammoth Cave. Queen Anne's lace contains compounds that may cause intoxication, but only in large quantities. Field horsetail contains bioactive compounds including nicotine and is toxic to horses. Buttercup has been used to treat headache. Pokeweeds contain toxic alkaloids. *Lobelia* sp. contain compounds similar to nicotine and can be toxic. Some species of morning glory contain alkaloids with hallucinogenic effects, but the genus is largely confined to tropical and subtropical ranges. Examples with hallucinogenic effect are found in Mesoamerica. One species, the man-of-the-earth (*I. pandurata*), does have a northeastern range, and is listed as an edible plant with mild analgesic properties, but no intoxicating properties.

These data indicate that datura (specifically *D. stramonium*) is the most plausible candidate for intoxicants documented from French colonies in North America. Other candidates do not have intoxicating properties, are dangerously toxic, or are too mild to account for the symptoms documented. Datura is common, consistent with the evidence, and likely played a role in Northeastern rituals similar to Southeastern contexts.

Additional accounts of datura are found in early ethnographies from the West and Southwest. Datura has been ethnographically observed in a number of Western cultures, usually drunk as tea or smoked. Datura was especially prevalent among Southwestern, Californian, and Great Basin tribes, used during vision quests (Emboden 1979a:80; Winter 2000b), rites of passage (Safford 1922:555), or shamanic rituals (Gamble et al. 2001:192; Safford 1922:553). Gayton (1928:24–38) cites datura among the Akimel O'odham (Pima), Hualapai (Walapai), and White Mountain Apache for hunting success or prophesizing. Californian or Southwestern tribes consumed datura either alone or mixed into alcoholic beverages. Some tribes, such as the Havasupai, used the drug sparingly for hedonistic purposes.

Gayton (1928) defines three patterns for shamanic datura use in Southern California. In southwestern California, datura was used in male initiations. In the San Juaquin basin and Sierra foothills, datura was used in visionary ceremonies by all adults. Outside of these areas, datura use was for divination or influencing events.

Rogers and Evernham (1983) describe shamanic datura use among the Diegueño of Southern California. They describe the spiritual complexity of the Diegueño, whose shamans contend with powerful spiritual forces. Whereas Natives of the Eastern Woodlands tended to navigate such dangers through individual invocation and sacrifice, the Diegueño: "sought aid for their ills not through appealing to divinities but through power manipulation, and this was the province of the shaman" (Rogers and Evernham 1983:104). Neophyte shamans were mentored by older shamans, who would impart the necessary knowledge to fulfill their role. But knowledge was useless without assistance from spirits, and for that datura was necessary (Rogers and Evernham 1983:105–106):

> Before his initiation, the student shaman was required to go through a period of fasting, and during this time he was told by his instructor the significance and character of the dreams that he would experience during his final initiation rite. On sundown of the appointed day the neophyte was given a decoction of Datura to drink; this induced a series of hallucinatory dream experiences that included seeing mythological beings and mythic animals . . . after he awakened, the shaman initiate had the sense of beginning a new life, enhanced with the power that he had just received, as evidenced by the dreams of entities and states that were beyond normal experience and sensation.

Reading this description, one is struck by a difference from the East. In Californian examples, the process is controlled and mentored by experts, and the resulting experience, while disorienting and hallucinatory, is relatively benign. Compare this to the traumatic rituals of the Eastern Algonquian, where young people are repeatedly dosed and left largely unsupervised, temporary psychosis being the best outcome. Given that datura compounds also cause suggestibility, coaching a subject would have an effect on the outcome. This need for supervision with datura to mitigate its danger is likely a cause behind its being overshadowed by tobacco.

In addition to shamanistic use, there are references to datura use for medicinal purposes. The Apache used datura-based salves for a range of ailments, such as sores, while the Akimel O'odham would use it for ear troubles (Curtin

1984:85). However, use of the plant for healing was a matter of dire consequences: "Old Mary [Pima informant] further stated that if a man was hopelessly ill with 'bad disease,' he had to choose between suicide and the following treatment: He chewed the fresh root of *Datura* and went crazy for a day and a half, and when he recovered from that, he was cured of his sickness" (Curtin 1984:86). Southwestern healers used it as an anesthetic (Parsons 1996:414), and the Apache used it as a panacea for a range of afflictions (Curtin 1984:85–86). Datura played a role in Southwestern Native weather magic; uprooting the plant was believed to cause wind (Parsons 1996:136).

Datura use in initiations is documented for California tribes such as the Yakut (Emboden 1979a:81; Schultes 1979:140), where both sexes must consume the drug as adolescents to ensure prosperity and health. Yakut shamans would take the drug throughout their life to maintain their abilities. In Western contexts, datura (and other hallucinogens) often involved the ritualistic creation of rock art (see Chapter 2).

The use of datura in California was described by Havard:

> In Lower California the Indians, says the same author [H. H. Bancroft], found drunkenness in the fumes of a certain herb smoked through a stone tube and used chiefly during festivals. This herb was doubtless a species of Datura . . . the California, Colorado River and Payute Indians prepare a beverage from the leaves and seeds of *Datura meteloides* [*D. innoxia*] which excites, intoxicates, and then stupefies them. It was also added to alcoholic drinks to render them more effective [Havard 1896:39].

Kroeber (1925) details initiatory datura use by Southern California groups. The rituals are similar to those of Eastern Natives. Male children are separated, given datura, and made to dance until falling unconscious. Females are not subjected to the process though there are reports of female datura use in Northern California. Separation, intoxication, and reintegration mirrors Algonquian groups. The length and severity of the ritual does not seem as extreme, though fatalities were not uncommon (Furst 1976:144). Kroeber relates datura use by the Chumash, for whom it was fundamental in mythology and religion (Baker 1994). Kroeber hypothesized datura played a role in the creation of rock art in Chumash territory (Wellmann 1978:1524).

Chumash shamans were called "causer of intoxication" or "giver of datura." The production of datura was replete with sexual imagery, with the pestle symbolically phallic, the mortar symbolically a vulva, and grinding symbolically intercourse. This correlates with priapism that often accompanies datura intoxication and with perceived sexual potency of shamans (Whitley 1994:23).

These were members of a special society who were also tasked with: "naming children, interpreting astrology, curing with herbs, making rain, collecting information for the *wot* [chief] and acting as symbolic or actual executioner" (Holliman 2000:187). People in charge of administering datura were powerful in Chumash society, and the right to administer the drug was "owned" by individuals who could hand down that right to their descendants.

Datura was seen as a female spirit (Applegate 1975:10; Rätsch 2005:214) whose role in Chumash culture was to provide prophetic dreams. One of the first people, an old woman, was transformed into datura after a great flood, when all the first people were turned into plants and animals (Baker 1994:260). Timbrook (1987:174) writes "In the sense that Native American medicine is integrally involved with religious beliefs and practice, Datura . . . probably was the single most important medicinal plant of the Chumash." Datura was primarily used by the Chumash to acquire guardian spirits or to experience visions. Datura was also used in medicinal contexts, particularly for snakebite.

One aspect of Californian rituals absent in the East is the significance of particular visions. Kroeber (1925:669) writes:

> This vision is usually an animal, and at least at times they learn from it a song with they keep as their own. It seems also that they will not kill any individual of the species. It is clear that the concept of the vision corresponds exactly with what among certain primitive tribes has been unfortunately denominated the "personal totem." It is certain that a special and individual relation of a supernatural kind is believed to exist forever after between the dreamer and the dream.

Kroeber's description of the Luiseño initiation ceremony notes datura is never consumed again after the initiation. This is a distinction when compared with other intoxicants that are more likely to be used periodically throughout one's life.

Applegate (1975) describes how young Chumash males fast, smoke copious tobacco, and drink datura prepared by their grandmother. The boys are sequestered and experience visions interpreted in context of their future plans. This compares to research into using datura alkaloids in psychotherapeutic settings, where the period of twilight awareness following a datura coma was ideal for therapeutic interventions (Baker 1994:269).

The Chumash have three uses for datura: acquiring a guardian spirit, contacting the dead, and as a medicinal panacea. Unlike other Californian tribes, where datura was limited to males or specific rituals, it was open to all Chumash at any time (Applegate 1975; Baker 1994:260). Chumash women might take datura for protection during childbirth, and any adult might use the drug to reveal their true name, enhancing their social position. Some would take it repeatedly to collect as many spirit guardians as possible to become a shaman. These individuals were viewed as separate from society, potentially threatening, and often lived alone. In addition to medical uses, Chumash would also use datura when illness was perceived as due to loss of soul.

Kroeber's Chumash observations mirror earlier work by Gayton (1928:29), who relates observations of a physician of the Mountain Cahuilla:

> The ceremony was called *manet* and was performed every few years when needed as a "prayer" against shortage of food or water, or an epidemic of sickness, or when there were several boys to be initiated. The southern clans gave *manet* to boys of 18–20 in connection with a 3–6 day ceremony in which boys of 6–10 years were taught their clan and "enemy" songs by their fathers. . . . The boys practiced songs in a secluded place away from the village. Then occurred the esoteric part of the ceremony called *kikawel*, the "the drinking," which occurred inside the ceremonial dance house. No women or children were permitted to see this. The *manet*-dancer whirled a bull-roarer and warned the uninitiated to stay away. The clan chief prepared the Datura which was dried and pounded in a ceremonial mortar. Water was added, and the liquid was put in a pottery bowl. The *paha* gave each boy a swallow. The men in the enclosure then took each boy by the waist, and led by the *manet* dancer they all danced around the fire. Some fell into the fire in the excitement but none were burned. The unconscious boys remained in the house all night. The following afternoon they were removed to a secluded cañon by the *paha*, where they remained for a week, learning songs and dances every night. . . . On the last afternoon of the week a ground-painting was made, and its symbolism explained to the boys.

This prepared boys for growing from adolescents into men by securing supernatural aid.

Datura was less used for initiation rituals in Northern Californian societies such as the Western Mono. As opposed to the once-in-a-lifetime, male-only rite of passage, datura use was open to men and women of all ages and could be repeated as desired, similar to the Chumash. Participants were those who were ill or had sick children, who were secluded prior to the ritual. After five nights of conversing with spirit helpers and the dead, they would drink datura, dance, and sing until they collapsed. The subsequent visions would reveal the source of their illness, which would then be dispelled. Those seeking lost items would have their locations revealed, and those seeking revenge for a dead relative would learn the identity of the killer.

While there are differences in datura between the Southern and Northern Californian patterns, there are some similarities. Participants are separated from society prior, during, and immediately after their consumption of the drug. And, the ritual's goal is to experience visions of spirits who provide information: "In California as elsewhere the narcotic was employed primarily for the purpose of communicating with supernatural power" (Gayton 1928:48). The use of datura is shamanistic, even if it is not used by full-time shamans.

Gayton also refers to datura used to influence games of chance. One might debate whether this is ceremonial use as an individual activity. But individuals do engage in ceremonial activities, notably prayer. This still involves using intoxicants to achieve ASCs to influence real events.

While Beverley, Gayton, and Kroeber describe shamanistic practices, they do not mention datura being used by actual shamans. Datura is generally taken for a particular purpose at a particular stage in a person's life and never again. However, that does not preclude datura-using shamans alongside such specific use. Ethnologies of other Southern Californian cultures, notably the Cahuilla, show true shamans who habitually ingest datura. Furst (1976:145) summarizes:

> Datura afforded the *puul* (shaman) a means of transcending ordinary reality and coming into contact with specific guardian spirits, as well as enabling him to go on magical flights to Otherworlds or transform himself into certain animals, such as the mountain lion or eagle. Such flights and transformations in the Datura trance were a necessary and routine activity of shamans, for such purposes as bringing back information about the Upper- and Underworld, visiting the dead, or retrieving lost or strayed souls.

These examples of datura shamanism are likely holdovers from prior to the adoption of tobacco, though Cahuilla shamans also use native tobacco species.

Southwestern tribes such as the Hopi, Zuni, or Navajo used *D. innoxia* for healers to make diagnoses, as a poison, or as a narcotic (Keur 1941:12; Vestal 1945; Whiting 1939). Zuni use is well documented (Yarnell 1959:177). Yarnell (1965:667–668) noted that *D. meteloides* grew near Hopi villages and that seeds had been recovered from many nearby caves. He also notes the recovery of datura from Chaco Canyon and states (1965:671): "Among the genera of plants utilized for their drugs in the New World, Datura attained a pre-Columbian distribution of aboriginal utilization exceeded only by *Nicotiana*, and *D. meteloides* was the most widely used species of the genus in North America." Yarnell notes depictions of datura blossoms on Zuni headdresses. Protohistoric murals depict moth-human hybrids that resemble moths which drink datura nectar, and who carry datura (VanPool 2009:186).

Late nineteenth-century Zuni research has implications for Southwest use (Stevenson 1915): "A minute quantity of the powdered root is put into the eyes, ears, and mouth of each of the *A'shiwanni* (rain priests) when they go at night to ask the birds to sing for rain" (Stevenson 1915:89). Datura is divine to Zuni, and only rain priests gather it (Schultes 1979:140). Rain priests use datura to find lost or stolen belongings, allegedly derived from Navajo practices (Keur 1941:12; Parsons 1996:196). Zuni priests would administer datura as a sedative or anesthetic (Stevenson 1915:41), to treat injuries (Stevenson 1915:46–47), or to identify a witch (Bunzel 1929:863).

This research described other Zuni uses of datura, all medicinal:

> The Zuñi priests administer *Datura meteloides*, that one may become a seer, and the Zuñi "doctor" gives the root of the plant to render his patient unconscious while he performs simple operations, setting fractured limbs, treating dislocations, making incisions for removing pus, eradicating diseases of the uterus, and the like. The narcotic is seldom employed by the Zuñi for the extraction of bullets, as men, they say, are not like women, and they must be *men* [Stevenson 1915:41].

Rain priests told fortunes and were clairvoyant. However, they often did not eat datura, giving it to a supplicant; nor is there evidence of ASCs attained by the rain priest (Stevenson 1915:90–91).

Contemporary Hopi research also shows shamanistic reliance on datura. There has been debate whether it was adopted from the Zuni, but Malotki (1999:109) argues for indigenous roots. *D. meteloides* would be chewed by healers to diagnose (Whiting 1978:31), and datura intoxication was a part of rituals where foreign objects were "removed" from the sick (Beaglehole and Beaglehole 1935:9). As described by Loftin (1991:138):

> Hopi shamans and Magicians belonged to curing societies, the *poswinkya* and the *Yaya't*, respectively. The former, typical of many shamans, cured by sucking a foreign object from the body of the patient. Hopi shamans also gazed into crystals to diagnose illness. They were also the only Hopis to induce trance, which they did by ingesting datura.

Unpleasant individuals could be held over burning datura to improve their disposition (Whiting 1978:37). Datura flowers could be included in burials or in facilities associated with Kachina dances (Whiting 1978:41) and could adorn kachina masks (Malotki 1999:109). One particular kachina was named "Jimsonweed Girl" (Malotki and Lomatuway'ma 1987:133–138).

The Hopi used datura medically despite its potential toxicity:

> A Hopi doctor at Sichomovi administered doses of Datura to two children who were brought to him from Shungopovi. One of the patients, a child of three months, afterward suffered from a succession of convulsive fits, with loss of muscular control and did not fully

> recover or acquire the power of speech; the other, a girl of about three years of age, lost muscular control and died about a month later [Robbins et al. 1916:55].

This account shows use of datura as a medical intervention for even very young children or infants, even in the face of the risk of death or permanent brain injury.

Similar observations can be found in accounts of the Navajo, where datura "is used only as a last resort to control excessive pain and only by those who possess the proper knowledge. The average person is much afraid of this plant and its effects" (Vestal 1945:59). Hill (1938:19) details Navajo reticence regarding datura:

> The Navajo, like the majority of Southwestern tribes, used jimsonweed (*Datura meteloides*) [*D. innoxia*] only to a limited extent. They feared narcotic effects and avoided it except in certain ceremonial capacities. These included its utilization as an aid in locating thieves and lost or stolen property, for diagnostic and curative purposes, and for revenging unrequited advances. It seems never to have been taken except one individual at a time and no ritual of the magnitude of the California *toloache* rite existed.

Despite this proscription, the literature shows numerous instances of Navajo datura use by specialists. The plant is harvested with ritual gestures and incantations, then ingested by shamans to induce visions (Brugge 1982; Hill 1938). Datura can be ingested for protection from witches, or for love magic, where one slips one's intended a small amount of the drug (Rätsch 2005:198). In the Navajo ritual "the excess way" a man ingests datura, symbolically becomes the plant, and its aphrodisiac effects are meant to attract a woman. The ritual is similar to rituals used to attract game. Hill (1938:21) summarizes the ritual, though the datura is not actually ingested:

> If a girl repulsed a man who wished to have intercourse with her he might get revenge in the following manner. He went to the place where the girl lived and watched until he could get some of her saliva or dirt from the bottom of her moccasins. He took either the dirt or the saliva to a jimsonweed and while singing, tied it to a plant. Then he sang some more songs. The girl would go crazy right away. She would take off her dress and run around naked and everyone would laugh at her. The man would be angry at the girl and would want everyone to know it. The man would call the girl's name as he tied the material to the plant.

Misogynistic as this may be, it shows the power represented by datura in Navajo society.

Eastern Iroquois or Algonquians used datura (Emboden 1979a:97; Herrick 1995:200), though it is poorly understood in Eastern North America. Some opined there was no evidence of datura in the East (e.g., Driver and Massey 1957:273), despite ethnohistoric evidence of the huskanaw ritual already recounted. Other references point to datura used medicinally: "The Rappahannock Indians from Virginia used seeds and leaves of thorn apple, mixed with fat, as hot compresses, placed on snake-bitten areas in turn, the Algonquian and Shawnee tribes stupefied themselves with thorn apple included in a tobacco mixture, the so-called 'kinnikinnick'" (Herbert et al. 2006:7). Rätsch (2005:211) also refers to datura in kinnikinnick smoking mixtures (see Chapter 5).

Prehistoric datura use is poorly understood, and botanical evidence is scant. Gayton (1928:39) reasons that the geographic extent of historic datura consumption indicates considerable age. He argued datura consumption diffused from Mesoamerica to the Southwest and then to California. This was based on the belief of the time that significant cultural developments in the Americas had Mesoamerican origins. Gayton also argued datura use began more recently than that of tobacco based on pure speculation.

While there are botanical discoveries of datura, much evidence is iconography in rock art or ceramics. A kiva wall painting dating to 1300–1550 CE in New Mexico shows a female bearing a datura flower (Wellmann 1981:92). VanPool (2009:187) notes Southwestern kiva art: "[is] dominated by entoptic images with vortexes, liminal creatures such as horned serpents, winged anthropomorphs including "hawkmoth" men, ghost-like birdmen, lots of birds . . . and colour symbolism that is consistent with both datura and tobacco induced visions." Pecos River rock art has themes consistent with hallucinogens, including datura (see Chapter 2).

We see Southwest vessel iconography associated with datura. Prehistoric vessels sometimes indicate their contents, such as opium containers of the Levantine Bronze Age, whose shape is evocative of the opium poppy (Merrilles 1962). Litzinger (1981) identified a rare pottery style in the Southwestern United States and northern Mexico. Vessels featured noded appliques, giving them exteriors evocative of datura fruit. Litzinger interprets these as datura effigies. Such vessels have been recovered from Snaketown in Arizona. Gladwin and others (1938) reported noded pottery at Snaketown as early as 1000 CE, while Haury (1976) identified similar artifacts as early as 500 CE. Malotki (1999:110) cites noded ware from Basketmaker III (ca. 600 CE), Pueblo III/IV (1150–1600 CE), and Hohokam (1050–1450 CE) contexts.

A recent survey of artifact collections from the region identified over 150 of these vessels ranging in age from 500 CE to the historic period (Huckell and

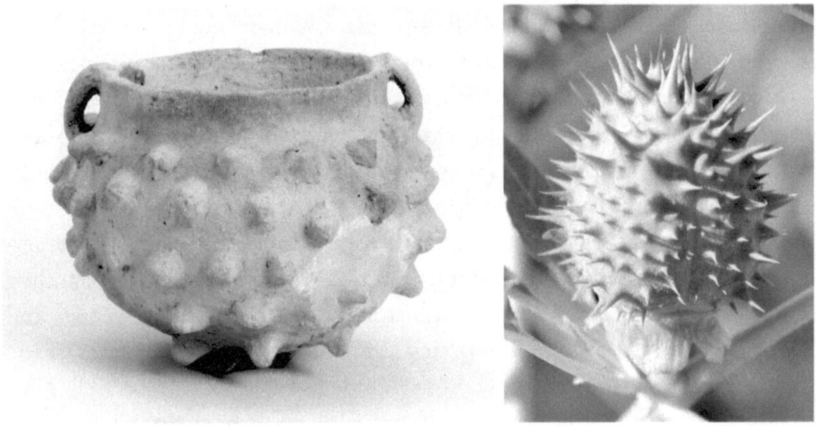

FIGURE 12 Left, Noded Mississippian vessel. Right, Jimsonweed Fruit. (Left, peachstatearchaeologysociety.org.)

VanPool 2006). Lankford (2012) shows very similar noded pots in contemporary contexts to the east in Plains sites and Mississippi Valley sites. Kan and others (1989:129, 201) record examples throughout Mexico. These vessels represent a repeated stylistic element evocative of datura in several ceramic traditions that overlap datura's distribution. In another iconographic tradition, Native art generally thought to depict squash blossoms have been interpreted by some as datura fruit. These include Hopi female hair styles (Furst and Furst 1982:56), Hopi pictographs (Patterson 1992:189), Zuni head ornaments, and Navajo squash blossom necklaces (Rätsch 2005:199).

Litzinger's hypothesis is plausible. These vessels likely represent a widespread pattern of datura use. Lankford's analysis points toward a wider distribution than Litzinger had envisioned. Huckell and VanPool, and Lankford interpret these vessels as evidence of shamans ingesting and/or storing datura in effigy vessels. What is lacking so far is an association between the vessels and datura, or residue evidence of datura compounds on the vessels. Since methods by which datura is consumed do not require processing, and only small amounts of the plant would be required to elicit its effects, preservation of botanical remains is comparatively unlikely. If noded pots were used only for storage, transfer of active compounds from the contents to the pottery fabric is also not likely. If they were used to drink datura tea, the vessels may hold residue encapsulated in the pottery fabric. Future research might yield such data. There is some residue evidence for datura from pipes in the Southeast (see below).

Hohokam cremations or caches occasionally include stone pallets (Bayman 2001:279). Lowell (1990), noting similarity between these pallets and South American snuff trays, proposes they were also tools for drug ingestion. Snuffing hallucinogens is common in South America (Schultes 1967). Lowell notes similarities between Hohokam tablets and pallets from Chile. These are numerous in both areas between 800 and 1150 CE, after which they decline. Snuffing is also known from prehistoric and historic Costa Rica (Wassén 1967) and Mexico (Furst 1974). Often interpreted as pigment processing artifacts (many show pigment residue), this need not preclude use as snuff trays as well. They could have multiple uses, and pigments are often applied to give symbolic power to objects. Also, some pigments, which include heavy metals such as manganese, can be neurotoxic, causing hallucinations themselves (Greer and Greer 2003:115).

Datura and tobacco are the most likely candidates for Hohokam snuff. Both could be powdered and inhaled; both have hallucinogenic effects. Hohokam and Chilean specimens have a decorated rim around a flat interior. Animal or human effigies sometimes decorate the rim. Some include handles, which may also be decorated. Decorations often evoke hallucinogenic form constants (see Chapter 2). Bone tubes through which snuff would be inhaled are also decorated with form constants, as are small vessels that could have been storage containers. Some of these were formed as human or animal effigies (Lowell 1990:338).

There have been some prehistoric identifications of datura in the Southwest. Yarnell (1959) noted six pueblo sites with *D. meteloides* seeds, all postdating 1000 CE. Botanical evidence for datura has also been recovered from cave sites in Arizona. Richard Caves, near the twelfth-century pueblo Montezuma Palace, produced a *D. meteloides* seed pod (Cutler and Kaplan 1956). This probably indicates these caves were the site of datura-fueled rituals undertaken by shamans from the pueblo. Seed pods were recovered from the Late Archaic O'Haco Rockshelter and undated White Mana Cave (Malotki 1999:110). A Basketmaker III village on Hopi reservation territory contains datura remains as well as seeds of *Nicotiana attenuata* "coyote" tobacco (see Chapter 5; Sebastian 1985:172). In addition, numerous pipes were recovered. Winter (2000c:114) notes this comprises the earliest evidence of datura used with tobacco.

Prehistoric datura in Eastern North America is less documented than in the west due to poor preservation and less surviving iconographic data. Ceremonial contexts in the Midwest dating to the Mississippian period (ca. 800–1550 CE) are exceptions. A structure at the BBB Motor site in Illinois contained pottery with datura residues (Emerson 1989:48–49, 2003:143; Wagner 2000:196; Whalley 1984). These were found with remains of red cedar (*Juniperus virginiana*), often found in Native ceremonial structures (Wagner 2000:196). The structure was a pithouse with posts supporting internal structures. It was re-excavated in several stages, with radiocarbon dates converging around 1200 CE. The structure is interpreted as associated with shamanistic activities involving ingestion of datura. BBB Motor is located near the periphery of Cahokia and could have been the locus of rituals engaged in by elite members of Cahokian society.

Datura was recovered at Cahokia itself from a cluster of pits containing plant remains, including tobacco (Collins 1990; Lopinot 1991:141–142). While the datura was initially discounted as intrusive, Emerson (2003:143) notes other colonizing plants are not found, and datura does not appear in any other features. Also, the seeds were burned and contained in sealed, intact features in association with tobacco, a known ritual plant, arguing for human agency. Researchers described the features and structures as "domestic," which seems to write off any ritual context; however in chiefdom societies such as Cahokia, not all domesticities are created equal. In Emerson's (2003:143) estimation: "Given their location, within a short distance of several mounds and just outside Cahokia's Grand Plaza, there is reason to suspect that these were not just the residences or the debris of simple farmers." The distinction between domestic and ritual contexts is a false dichotomy in such societies, which include ritual practices in their daily lives, in what might be labeled "domestic" contexts.

Other intoxicants have been recovered from Cahokia and Mississippian sites of similar age. Tobacco pipes and tobacco seeds are ubiquitous, including not only large effigy pipes (see Chapter 5) but also more numerous simple, small clay pipes. Evidence of "black drink" ilex (discussed in Chapter 3) is also found on Mississippian sites. From Cahokia, there is evidence of morning glory (*Ipomoea* sp.; Emerson 2003:143). Morning glory has been recovered at other Mississippian sites such as the Olszewski site in Illinois (Wagner 2000:197).

Excavations at Cahokia have recovered a species of nightshade (*Solanum americanum*). No intoxicating properties are known for American nightshade, but the plant has featured in Native American medicinal traditions and has been recovered at other Mississippian sites such as the Sponemann site in association with tobacco and exotic artifacts (Wagner 2000:196). Another nightshade specimen from Sponemann was recovered from a "busk pit" associated with the corn-harvesting busk ceremony. The pit also contained tobacco and red cedar. The Spencer site in Tennessee produced a smoking pipe that tested positive for atropine, evidence of smoking datura (Carmody, Caffrey, et al. 2017). This confirms speculation that datura was smoked in pipes in addition to tobacco. Spencer is a Mississippian site, so this pipe could not date earlier than 800 CE.

These discoveries show datura was used as far back as the late prehistoric chiefdoms in Eastern North America, in combination with other intoxicants. The fact that contemporary occurrences of datura have been documented in the Mississippi Valley and the Southwest attests to a geographically widespread practice. Datura's toxicity likely means not much was used at one time, so botanical evidence is likely to remain rare. Efforts should be made to subject noded-ware vessels to residue analysis to see whether they were used to contain or process datura.

One such study has recently been conducted. A recent analysis of 31 sherds dating between 1400 and 1700 CE and 18 shell vessels dating between 1250 and 1400 CE from the Gilcrease Museum used residue analysis to identify the composition of organic residues (King et al. 2017). Seven shell vessels and 14 ceramic vessels tested positive for atropine, indicating they were used to drink datura. The shell vessels included specimens from the Craig Mound and the Spiro site, both discussed in Chapter 3 in reference to ilex "black drink." These results do not rule out ilex, but they do present a more complex picture of late prehistoric ritual drinking.

Comparisons of datura residues could show whether the datura use documented historically had significant prehistoric roots prior to late prehistory. Are only high-status vessels associated with datura, such as the remains from BBB Motor site, or was it widespread within Mississippian society? Was intoxication monopolized by social elites, by members of chiefly lineages, or by priests or shamans? The evidence so far indicates the latter, a controlled and restricted use, but evidence is lacking for earlier societies with less marked social ranking, where unrestricted access is more likely. We also know relatively little about how datura was ingested, by eating, drinking, or smoking, or by numerous methods? Evidence from vessels indicates drinking datura "tea," but there was also at least some datura smoking. As discussed in Chapter 5, plants other than tobacco were smoked historically, and there is ethnohistoric evidence datura and tobacco were used together, possibly mixed in a beverage (Winter 2000a:3).

As for other hallucinogens discussed in this chapter, there is much research to be done, and much direct evidence to be explored. Hallucinogens have clearly played a major role in Native American ritual practices throughout the period documented by direct or indirect observations and, depending on the specific substance, well back into the archaeological record. The next chapter investigates hallucinatory intoxicants using the indirect evidence of Native iconography.

2

ROCK ART AND HALLUCINATORY INTOXICANTS

THE INTERPRETATION OF PREHISTORIC ART HAS GONE THROUGH several phases which correlate with developments in archaeology theories. Several theoretical approaches to prehistoric art are relevant to the use of intoxicants by Native Americans. Early research largely attempted to grapple with the meaning of Upper Paleolithic cave paintings in Europe. Opinions in the late nineteenth century were that these images were isolated renderings devoid of meaning. In the early 1900s, Breuil interpreted depictions of ice age megafauna in caves such as Lascaux or Altamira as sympathetic hunting magic, attempts to influence the physical world by depicting desired outcomes (Lewis-Williams 2002:47). Leroi-Gourhan (1967) developed an elaborate explanation for European cave art, arguing that animals depicted, and their locations within a cave and relative to each other, were a structural model of past society, expressed through binary oppositions such as male:female or nature:culture. Early explanations in New World locations were similarly functionalist, for example, that they were territorial or directional markers (Whitley 2011:307), or that repeated marks were "tally marks" for counting (Loendorf 1994).

None of these interpretations have been shown to have sufficient explanatory potential. The symbols in rock art traditions clearly have meaning, and to argue otherwise infantilizes the artists. They depict animals that are not game animals, few animals in the images seem to have been wounded or killed, there are few correlations of humans with hunting weapons and animals, and there are images that are clearly supernatural, as well as numerous abstract shapes. The hunting magic hypothesis is thus insufficient. Structural interpretations are subjective and do not explain symbolic associations of elements; what makes one animal "male" and another "female"? Territorial marking explanations have been discredited (e.g., Kroeber 1925:939) as based on Western biases about landscape that do not fit with indigenous worldviews. Assumption that repetition of elements was the result of counting records does not address what was counted or why such a medium was chosen.

The most promising interpretation of prehistoric art is cognitive and addresses mental and ideological aspects of past society while remaining empirically grounded. The basis of this approach is that all humans share the same neurology, and all artistic renderings are created using that neurology; so one can derive meaning from art by seeking patterns with probable biological causes. The best-known example was undertaken by Lewis-Williams and Dowson (1988), though a similar model was presented by Reichel-Dolmatoff (1978, 1987) and Blackburn (1977). The Chumash, for example, use designs consistent with datura-induced hallucinations:

> Typical images seen under the influence of Datura are mandala forms (i.e., elaborate circular designs) and tiny dots that surround objects. These forms are ubiquitous in Chumash rock paintings and possibly were inspired by drug-induced phenomena [Lee and Heider 1991:15].

Lewis-Williams and Dowson's neuropsychological model posits all humans will experience the same visual experiences under the effects of hallucinatory stimuli, regardless of how those stimuli are induced. Their argument is that ASCs can be sorted into three categories (Clottes and Lewis Williams 1996:15-19). The first category is the perception of: "form constants which include abstract geometric forms such as '(a) grating, lattice, fretwork, filigree, honeycomb, or chessboard; (b) cobweb; (c) tunnel, funnel, alley, cone, or vessel; (d) spiral' [Klüver 1966:66]. There is a limited range of simple geometric forms that can be perceived by the human brain. These are neurological phenomena and do not require stimulation of the retina (Siegel and Jarvik 1975). Such perceptions are also referred to as "phosphenes" (Oster 1970), though this includes only simple, point-like images, while form constants include more complex patterns. The term "entoptic" ("within the eye") includes phosphenes and form constants (Lewis-Williams 2001:339). In practice the three terms are used interchangeably. These images occur in normal consciousness, interrupted consciousness (loss of consciousness), or intermediate consciousness, such as the hypnogogic experience of moving into or out of sleep.

Knoll and colleagues (1963) demonstrated form constants could be stimulated electrically and also through hallucinogens. In extreme ASCs, form constants are more intrusive and may persist for days or weeks (Blackburn 1977:91). Hedges (1982:5) noted similarities in experimentally induced phosphenes and images found in North American rock art, indicating a hallucinatory origin. This contrasted with Willcox (1973:30) who placed the North American art in a "young child" level of development, which smacks of significant researcher bias. In a later article, Hedges (1994) details a widespread phosphene, the "pipette" design, in artistic traditions in North and South America. This battlement-like pattern is present in Hohokam contexts, where datura and tobacco have been established. Datura, as mentioned in the previous chapter, is prone to instilling form constants. South American Jivaro, ingesting *Datura arborea*, often perceive a *tsentsak* or invisible arrow, depicted as a snake-like effigy with crosshatched triangles that directly correspond with another category of form constant (Clottes and Lewis Williams 1996:22).

The second category of ASC proceeds when form constants combine into patterns that elaborate a single pattern or combine multiple patterns, making a complex abstract image. The third category includes complex, realistic hallucinations, such as animals, objects, or people not present, or creatures combining elements of different animals. These may grow out of first or second category hallucinations, or they can appear alone. While category one and two are culturally independent, category three is culturally mediated (Whitley 1996:13). A wavy line might become a snake in one culture or a rope in another. The association of form constants and complex depictions strengthens the argument that ASCs were a factor in the art's creation:

> How can one determine if geometric images reflect entoptics that are part of SSC [shamanic state of consciousness]? Because shamans are defined as religious practitioners who interact directly with the spirit world, entoptic imagery should ideally be embedded with aspects of the spirit world. Thus, entoptic images should not occur in isolation but will instead be combined into cosmologically significant beings [VanPool 2009:182].

Lewis-Williams's hypothesis is that most prehistoric art records images experienced under an ASC, and thus the art should incorporate elements from the three categories of imagery. This hypothesis was evaluated by comparing three different rock art traditions: Upper Paleolithic Europe, the San of the

Kalahari Desert, and the Shoshone of the Great Basin. In all three contexts, rock art conformed to the three categories. Whitley (1998b:27–31) proposes that trance-inspired imagery was not recorded to preserve the images, but to recreate the emotional state associated with them. Memory is impaired during ASCs, thus the imperative to create a record.

This neuropsychological model has been applied to rock art from several North American contexts (Greer and Greer 2003; Hedges 1994; Loendorf 1994; Schaafsma 1994; Turpin 1994; Whitley 1994, 1996, 1998a, 2011). Kroeber (1925:938) argued that pictographic art of prehistoric California was connected to datura (Whitley 1998b:23–24). Discussing Archaic period rock art of the Colorado Plateau, Schaafsma (1994:48) argues: "In addition to spirit helpers, transmogrification, and other somatic as well as aural trance symbolism, what may be entoptic (neuropsychological) phenomena appear to be represented in these art styles, raising the question of the use of hallucinogens." Schaafsma refers to humanoids experiencing bodily distortion and symbolic death, associating the exaggeration of physical features with bodily hallucinations and the death of the figures with the symbolic death of the shaman. Lines emanating from some figures' ears represent aural hallucinations associated with many hallucinogens. Schaafsma is less successful at identifying what substances were used, citing accounts of the use of tobacco and datura by shamans in the region, as well as the presence of *Amanita muscaria* fungi.

One must not assume that all prehistoric art is hallucinatory. Some researchers have argued that prehistoric art of Australia is a poor fit for the model and is more consistent with totemic associations, for example (David 2002). Others have argued that the hallucinatory interpretation for Australia holds, at least for the earliest examples (Chippindale et al. 2000). However, in at least some circumstances, it is plausible that the subject matter of art is inspired by hallucinations experienced in ASCs induced by intoxicants.

This leaves the question of the art's creation. Lewis-Williams and others (Pearson 2002; Stahl 1985, 1986; Winkelman 2002) argue that hallucinatory art was the work of shamans during or following trances. Hedges (1994:103) summarizes:

> While it seldom is possible to provide precise interpretations of particular rock art examples, a wide range of comparative data provide support for the use of shamanic concepts to construct a broadly conceived interpretive framework for many rock art subjects. The importance of the shamanic trance as the mechanism for contact with the supernatural realm presents us with the opportunity to construct an explanatory model for sources of imagery associated with ASCs.

Whitley (2011:308–309) distinguishes between shamanic rock art, created by shamans, and shamanistic, created by non-shamans but still in ASCs. In either case art represents visions attained in an ASC.

Quinlan (2000) argues since there are informants from California and the Great Basin who deny shamanistic origins for rock art, Whitley's arguments are suspect. However, Whitley points out that not all art can be plausibly argued to be "visionary," and that some motifs, such as vulva-forms, or rock alignments, while ritual in nature (fertility rituals, pilgrimages, or meetings of secret societies), were not likely created in an ASC. Hedges (1982), analyzing anthropomorphic/geometric traditions of the Great Basin, argues interpretations of hallucinatory origins should be applied only when they are the most plausible explanation. In seeking plausible explanations for phosphenes, particularly when superimposed over anthropomorphic or zoomorphic figures with distorted or mixed body forms:

> If we interpret the body patterns as representations of supernatural power manifested in visions of the spirit world, then the figures might be anthropomorphizations of that power as embodied in deities, spirit beings, or the shamans who control power . . . one would be hard pressed to find an explanation for them couched in terms of ordinary reality [Hedges 1982:6].

Having discussed what we think these art traditions represent, we must now turn to who created them and why. First, we must consider what was important to the artists: the art or the process of making it?

A modern, Western mindset is focused on a final artistic product, a painting for example. However, it is possible the final product in Native traditions was secondary, that it is the process that is significant. This approach has been applied in the context of historic rock art in California, which cannot be understood without understanding its shamanistic context, and shamanism cannot be understood without its association with hallucinogen-induced ASCs (Whitley 1996).

Lewis-Williams [2002] argues that a neuropsychological explanation is more parsimonious than other explanations. It explains difficult to access locations, as borders between the natural and spirit world. Caves and other inaccessible locations are liminal contexts, the occupation of which takes people out of their daily existence to a place ideal for rituals using ASCs (Crothers 2012:530). Winkelman (2002:77) hypothesizes that the difficulty of access associated with caves is symbolic of birth and correlates that symbolism with spiritual rebirth in shamanic traditions.

Also, when we think of rock art our minds evoke cave sites of Europe such as Lascaux or Chauvet Cave, with extensive panels of art with numerous figures. Most rock art sites are less extensive, and analysts can have difficulty locating images. This is another indication that it is not the final image that is significant, since there might not be a substantial image left to enthrall future viewers. It is the act of creation that mattered: "Once created, pictographs and petroglyphs are symbolic manifestations and powerful things in themselves; they are not mere reflections of either natural or supernatural phenomena" (Hampson 2016:220).

The model explains part human, part animal figures, a common shamanistic trait:

> Imagery used by shamans typically contains patterned geometric shapes (entoptics) associated with images of tutelary creatures (especially birds or powerful creatures such as bear), supernatural non-naturalistic entities reflecting liminality . . . and anthropomorphs that combine the attributes of humans and animals [VanPool 2009:182].

The model explains musical instruments at some cave sites, particularly flutes and drums, which contribute to ASCs (Winkelman 2002:76). It explains art's purpose, not as a passive product but an active tool used in the mediation of human-spirit relations. Finally, this model is empirically grounded, based on shared neurological reactions to known stimuli.

The model has not been without critics. See for example Helvenston and Bahn (2003) who, while not denying the possibility of prehistoric shamans achieving trances, are critical of the connection between trances and art. The abstract nature of much rock art allows criticism of the medium depicting whatever the interpreter is predisposed to see (Quinlan 2000). This argues for caution but does not invalidate the approach. Wallis (2013) argues that the "Western" materialist paradigm underpinning the model ignores the ontological and epistemological context of prehistoric shamans, what was real to them and what comprised knowledge to them. However, acknowledging that experiences of shamans are influenced by predictable neurologic stimuli takes nothing away from their subjective experiences or belief systems.

Marshack (1989) criticized the model as seeking to explain all art as hallucinatory and ignoring the possibility of motifs persisting due to tradition. For a detailed and convincing refutation of this critique, the reader is referred to Lewis-Williams and Dowson's (1989) response, as well as to Hedges (1994:117–120). To summarize, the model parsimoniously accounts for the repetition of specific forms as well as patterns in context of the art and is ethnographically supported. Also, the critique that it tries to explain all art is a straw man; applicants of the model argue it accounts for a notable subset of art, but that there are other sources of rock art as well. Finally, the critique that artistic motifs can be retained due to tradition does not account for potentially hallucinatory origins of those motifs. Despite criticisms, while some may consider this a "dated" model, a neuropsychological approach to Native American art is plausible and corroborates what we already know about Native intoxicant use.

We can now turn to North American art traditions and their relation to intoxicants, but with several caveats. Interpretation of rock art faces problems of dating (Beck et al. 1998; Chippindale and Taçon 1998:6). Rock art, by definition, is not in a depositional context, so it is difficult to date by association. Even if art occurs at a dated site, we still must make an argument of association between vertical art and the horizontal site. Direct dating of pigments is possible in cases where organic substances are used; but many pigments are mineral, and petroglyphs where images are pecked into the rock use no pigments.

Also, art requires interpretation and is only an indirect indicator of any specific intoxicant. One must often rely on correlation—that a given body of art incorporates probable hallucinatory images, and certain intoxicants are known to have been used in that area; and so the two may be connected. This is simpler where the art incorporates images of the plant or of people ingesting it, and more complicated when there are multiple intoxicant candidates.

The idea that North American rock art is associated with ASCs was proposed by Kroeber (1925) and Steward (1929). And as Whitley argued, not all North American art is the product of ASCs. Greer and Greer (2003:107) note that a third of the rock art they identified in Montana was ceremonial. The rest were "markers" whose function is "announcing a message to those who see [the art]" or "event records." Whitley (2011:308–314) divides rock art into visionary (shamanistic) and nonvisionary. Kitchell (2010) analyzes anthropomorphic rock art from Utah and Arizona and argues that they are not hallucinatory images but representations of shamans.

There are two types of motifs that can shed light on intoxicant use: depictions of intoxicant pants, and images that possibly depict hallucinations. Depictions of intoxicant plants, or of their use, is most direct. Sometimes depictions are clear. An anthropomorphic figure from Utah holds a mask in one hand and mushroom in the other; *Psilocybin* mushrooms grow in the area (Rätsch 2005:624). Medio period (1200–1450 CE) Casas Grandes pottery in the Southwest has images of males smoking pipes while transforming into bird-humanoids. VanPool (2009:184) interprets this as evidence of tobacco-shamanism. In most cases representations are more ambiguous. An image interpreted as peyote could also be a flower. Much art corresponds with themes drawn from ASCs but do not depict any particular intoxicant. Sometimes the best one can say is an intoxicant was likely used but not which specific example.

The following North American art traditions are some of the best examples for connections between art and hallucinogenic intoxicants. This is not an exhaustive list, only the clearest examples where researchers have made plausible arguments about the use of particular intoxicants.

SOUTHERN CALIFORNIA AND GREAT BASIN ROCK ART

A survey of Californian and Great Basin ethnographies shows a pattern of rock art sites associated with visions experienced by shamans in ASCs influenced by hallucinogens (Whitley 1992). Rocks and caves were seen as portals to the supernatural world, and painting or entering them was central to shamanistic rituals. Great Basin Native words for shaman translate as "one who writes [on rocks]" and terms for rock art relate to shamanism, poison, death, and trance:

> "To have died" was "to have hallucinated/dreamed," and this was also "to have been [in the] supernatural" and "to have painted." Rock art, in other words, was perceived—and linguistically encoded—as some function of the shamans' dreams of hallucinations [Whitley 1992:97].

Blackburn (1977), citing Applegate (1975), speculates that Southern Californian art was associated with shamanistic or initiatory rituals, influenced by *Datura innoxia*.

Whitley (1996:25–26) describes a late nineteenth-century female puberty ritual:

> The girls' puberty ceremony in southwestern California . . . is particularly well known. The girls were isolated for a number of days, ritually enacting the procedures and carefully following the taboos of women during childbirth. The isolation, sensory deprivation, and fasting the girls experienced could result in hallucinations, but to ensure that end the girls also ingested tobacco. At the culmination of the ceremony, the girls ran a ritual race to a special rock . . . the high point of the race was the girl's arrival at [the rock] to paint the spirit helpers they saw during their visions. In the majority of cases, the girls' spirit helper was a rattlesnake, a symbol closely associated with women through the Far West.

Rattlesnake drawings were red zigzag/diamond shapes consistent with form constants and also with scale patterns of local snakes. Quinlan (2000:97) notes the ceremony is not intended to produce visions, only induce an ordeal, and that in many cases those producing art were not involved in the initiatory ordeal. This does not deny rock art was produced by people who ingested intoxicants and that elements of the art would have been influenced. Whitley (2006a:306) notes Native girls painted rock faces while under the influence of intoxicants.

The creation of art associated with datura for initiation rituals was documented by DuBois (1908). The boys' initiation was similar to the girls', but instead of tobacco they were given datura. Regrettably we lack detailed information of the boys' ceremony, but Whitley (2006a) describes isolation, instruction, datura ingestion, ordeal/race (of up to 60 miles), and finally rock art creation. The boys experienced spirit visions and recorded them on the rock face (Wellmann 1981:92). There is variation in accounts of female rituals, with some describing young women being given datura and having intercourse with shamans (Whitley 1994:21). Shamans are often ascribed sexual as well as spiritual potency (Dowson 2007:56).

Whitley (2006a:301) presents a Spanish account of the Luiseño from 1822:

> A kind of drink was administered to [the children] made from a plant called *pibat* [tobacco], which was reduced to a powder and mixed with other intoxicating ingredients. Soon after taking this preparation, they became insensible, and for three days were deprived of any sustenance whatever. During this period they were attended by some old men or women, who were continually exhorting them to be on the alert and not sleep.

The combination of nicotine, other intoxicants (likely datura), sleep deprivation, and physical stress would have caused ASCs. Several interpretations of the nineteenth-century accounts agree that these rituals were undertaken to acquire spirit guardians. Yuman male puberty rituals focused on ordeals, including nasal piercings, required to enter the land of the dead, but given that: "[the ritual] involved nasal piercing without anesthesia and a 10–15 mile run across the Colorado Desert during summer, followed by four days without sleep, with sustenance limited to a single bowl of watery gruel," hallucinations would have been likely, and the paintings reflect that (Whitley 2006a:309).

Another study from Southern California links shamanism, hallucinogens, and rock art:

> A man was sick. He tried various ways to get well, but nothing worked. Finally, he realized that he must visit [Yahwera] [a powerful spirit]. He went to a rock and took tobacco.

> The rock opened; he went inside. He crossed a large rattlesnake, then he passed a grizzly bear. He heard strange noises, and deer. He met [Yahwera], who was dressed in mountain quail feathers, and was surrounded by gifts from proper hunters. [Yahwera] fed him and gave him songs, dances and cures. The man then left, passing once again the bear and the snake, and exited through a spring, though without getting wet. After following [Yahwera's] instructions, the man got well [Whitley 1992:102].

Kawaiisu narratives speak of attempts to contact Yahwera through intoxicants or ordeal:

> Long ago there was a man. . . . The man was sick or perhaps he just wanted luck. So to cure himself or to get that luck he took jimsonweed (alternatively fasted, swallowed tobacco, walked naked through stinging nettles, or ingested ants wrapped in eagle down). He then went to a place in Back Canyon (or another cave) and found the opening to the animal underworld, Yahwera's home. At that hole, that goes down into the mountain, was a rock that opened and closed [Garfinkel et al. 2009:186–187].

The story tells how the man entered the rock, met the spirits of animals and ultimately Yahwera, who gives him luck and medicine.

Loendorf (1994) makes a similar interpretation of Pacific Northwest Salish rock art as hallucinations from vision quests. These accounts place much rock art from Southern California and the Great Basin in the realm of hallucinogenic rituals, provide explanation of the rituals in which art was created, and provide insight into the meaning of artistic motifs.

Whitley (1994:4) dismisses alternative hypotheses for North American rock art as unsupported ethnographically. Most North American art does not portray game animals, and when it does, it is abstracted and non-naturalistic, arguing against hunting magic (Willcox 1973:29). Garfinkel and colleagues (2009) interpret anthropomorphic figures from the Coso Range in eastern California mythologically, not shamanistically. Whitley (1998b) and Hedges (2007) note the supposed Coso Range mythological figures are decorated with imagery identical to phosphenes of the neuropsychological model and that their creation was likely influenced by intoxicant-related ASCs.

The two hypotheses are not mutually exclusive, and a mythic image could be envisioned in a drug-induced ASC. Another issue with Coso Range petroglyphs is whether they are shamanic—the product of, or representations of, shamans—or if they are shamanistic—representing shaman-like behavior by nonspecialists. Garfinkel and colleagues (2009:184) argue for the latter: "In Southern California, jimsonweed or toloache (*Datura* sp.) use was also correlated with dreaming as a personal means for ordinary people to acquire life-long spirit helpers." Images of feathers, supposedly quail, are suggested as evidence for datura, as they were documented to be used exclusively to decorate datura containers. Overall, these figures fit the neuropsychological model and are likely evidence of hallucinogen use, probably datura, specific users and context of use notwithstanding.

Whitley notes an exception to the shamanistic pattern at a site in Southern California that depicts a myth; but the myth is of the origin of shaman spirit helpers, so it fits with the model (Whitley 2006b:252). He describes puberty-related rock art traditions in California (2006a), the Great Basin, and the Columbia Plateau. Petroglyphic cupule traditions from central California/western Great Basin and a Columbia Plateau vision-questing tradition were also examined; the cupule tradition is associated with female puberty rituals, the cupules possible containers for quids of tobacco and datura (Sutton et al. 2011). Several quids were found in cupules at Pinwheel Cave in Southern California. The Columbia Plateau tradition shows a pattern of male and female rock art recording including dreams and hallucinations (Whitley 2006a:316).

Quinlan (2000) questions the degree to which postcontact ethnographies can be applied to precontact cultures. This is something ethnoarchaeologists have been grappling with for decades. The consensus is that the approach works best with close historical correspondence between the archaeological and ethnographic data and where one is dealing with aspects of culture that are resistant to acculturation, such as religion. One should be cautious, should use rock art data to corroborate intoxicant use, and avoid specific identifications except in obvious cases.

There is corroborating linguistic evidence as well. The rocks where ritual races concluded were referred to as "shaman's houses" or "shaman's caches" (Driver 1937; Whitley 1994:4). In Numic languages, the root of the term for "shaman" is the same as the word for "to paint" (Zigmond et al. 1990), which supports the association of rock art with shamans. The translation of place names for some rock art sites, such as "place to go below," "place to drown," or "place of the whirlwind" are evocative of shamanistic ideas of transcending worlds, metaphorical death, or shamanistic flight (Whitley 2006b:244–250). So, linguistic evidence supports ethnographic evidence that some Californian rock art sites were associated with shamanistic activity.

These sites were also viewed as places where spirits lived:

> Some rock art sites are considered by Native peoples to be entrances to the supernatural world.... In fact, some indigenous peoples believed that spirits actually lived inside the

> rocks and cliff faces, and these beliefs sometimes appear to have influenced the location for rock art sites. . . . Kawaiisu rock paintings at their cave of creation in Sand Canyon in the Tehachapi Mountains were believed to lead to a subterranean world inhabited by supernatural animals [Garfinkel and Waller 2012:37–39].

The locations of some rock art sites were likely influenced by acoustical properties. Rock faces decorated with rock art in the region have pronounced echoes. This would have been exaggerated during an ASC, contributing to a place's supernatural identity. Some Californian rock art sites are believed to represent a single shaman recording images experienced in ASCs.

In terms of iconographic analysis, the diamond patterns which form a primary form constant are interpreted by subjects as diamond patterns of rattlesnake and as significant female figures guarding rock art sites, as well as symbolizing the vagina (Whitley 1992:94). The grizzly bear is a male equivalent (Whitley 2006b:248). In either case, rock art creation is recording spirit helpers (Whitley 2006a:312). Intoxicants, including tobacco and datura, are prominent in both examples. Summing up the evidence, Whitley (1992:107) writes:

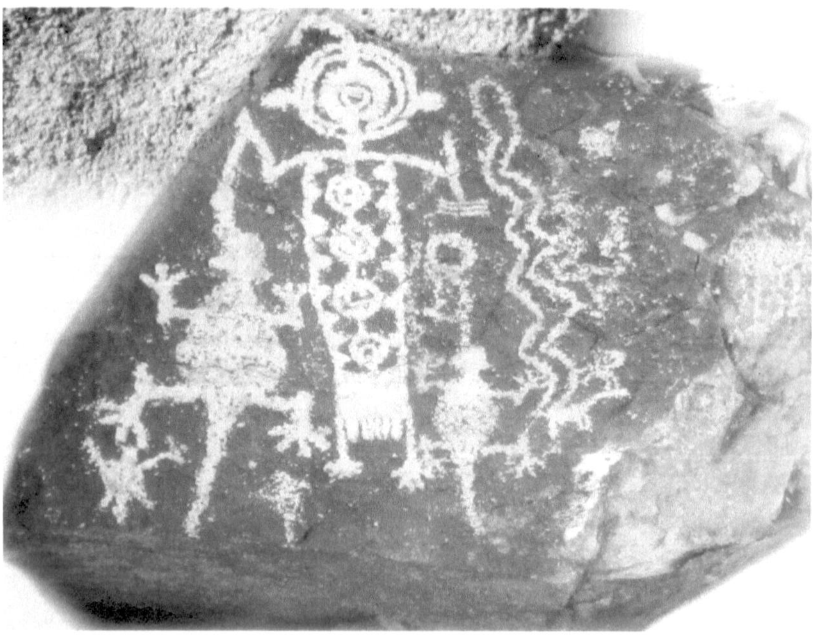

FIGURE 13 Coso Range Rock Art.

> Even in the most divergent case, the initiatory art of southern California, the creation of the paintings occurred after the ingestion of known hallucinogens and following periods of ritual deprivation and stress, all of which involved careful supervision by shamans, while the paintings themselves incorporated motifs known to represent important "guardians" of the supernatural world.

In Southern California, a pipe and pestle were found near a panel depicting a spirit-being shown as a chimera of animal and human, a common shamanistic theme (Garfinkel and Waller 2012:42). The panel includes phosphenes, including spirals and concentric circles. Ethnographic accounts, the shamanistic figures, phosphenes, and the smoking pipe and pestle taken together are evidence of the consumption of intoxicants in association with rock art. Taking all of this evidence together shows rock art traditions of California and the Great Basin were influenced by datura and tobacco, and in some cases their consumption was fundamental to the art's creation.

THE PECOS RIVER TRADITION

Southern Texas and northern Mexico, within the range of both red bean and peyote, feature the Southern Pecos River rock art style. This tradition dates between 2000 and 1000 BCE (Turpin 1994). Southern Pecos pictographs include anthropomorphic figures referred to as shamans (Campbell 1958; Kirkland and Newcomb 1967). The preponderance of evidence supports that characterization. These figures are shown dancing and hunting. Many carry medicine bags, staffs, or weapons (Wellmann 1981:96). They show bodily transformations—absence of or excess heads/limbs, exaggeration of bodily features, skeletonization, piloerection, the isolation or singular depiction of female genitalia—and incorporate animal elements, particularly from birds and mountain lions. Hampson (2016) places all these traits within the framework of shamanism, observing that all are consistent with ASCs. Piloerection has symbolized spiritual power (Hollman 2002). Skeleton imagery is central to shamanistic iconography (Eliade 2004). Campbell (1958) noted that the depicted garb and possessions corresponded with those observed among red-bean-using shamans.

The Southern Pecos tradition also features geometric figures, and deer and sheep (Sneader 2005:9). The co-occurrence of animals, anthropomorphs, and geometrics is consistent with shamanistic practices. The Southern Pecos pictographs correlate with red bean evidence from caves (Willcox 1973:27). Campbell (1958) and Newcomb (1967) attributed the art to red bean. Campbell's case hinges on similarities in dress and material culture worn or carried by the figures depicted with documented red bean users (Boyd 2003:89). Turpin (1990:270) argues that the homogeneity of the style argues for a set of symbolic forms expressed in the creation of art. While acknowledging that red bean is not as hallucinogenic as other drugs, the "dreamlike" state associated with it "prepared the seeker for reception of culturally informed visions" (Turpin 1990:271).

Turpin (1994) suggests that images of birds, bird/human hybrids, humans with birds perched upon them or accompanying them in flight, and anthropomorphic figures seeming to fly/fall should be interpreted as flight representations. Flight in shamanic contexts should be interpreted as "soul flight," out-of-body experiences (Clottes and Lewis Williams 1996:26). The departure of the soul is a common motif in shamanistic traditions; a cross-cultural survey by Bourguignon (1973:11) found that some form of institutionalized, depersonalized trance was ubiquitous among Native North American cultures. The sensation of flying and bodily dissociation is associated with numerous intoxicants. Turpin (1994:80) joins flight symbolism with intoxicant use:

> Extravagant claims aside, voluminous literature leads to the inescapable conclusion that ordinary people do spontaneously experience the sensation of leaving their bodies and floating, levitating, or flying with or without the aid of drugs.

The use of tobacco, red bean, and of peyote, all readily available, could induce depersonalization symptoms recorded in the South Pecos Tradition rock art.

The creation of shamanistic rock art and consumption of intoxicants allowed ritual specialists to reduce stress in Trans-Pecos Archaic cultures induced by growing populations in a challenging environment. Other archaeologists (e.g., Boyd 1998) attribute this hallucinogenic imagery to peyote, rather than red bean. Boyd and Dering (1996) argue that the use of red bean was more likely associated with ritual purification:

> Throughout North America, ritual cleansing through the use of purgatives and emetics was considered a necessary preparatory activity prior to the acquisition of an altered state of consciousness. The consumption of mescal bean decoctions is likely to have been part of a pan–North American approach to achieving an altered state of consciousness.

It may be impossible to distinguish the two substances based on abstract, indirect evidence, though the themes in this tradition point to the significance of psychoactive drug use.

Since peyote has poor preservation characteristics, much evidence for its prehistoric use is rock art. Symbolic motifs featured in north Mexican/

south Texan rock art are similar to images drawn on the faces of participants in Huichol peyote rituals (Mountjoy 1982:118). Boyd (1998, 2003; Boyd and Dering 1996) interprets the Pecos River rock art tradition and correlates it with Huichol peyotism. One panel at the White Shaman site in Texas depicts figures identical in number and orientation to Huichol participants in the peyote hunt. Skeletal figures depicted correspond with native depictions of shamans overseeing the hunt. The panel depicts arrows being shot into deer with motifs representing peyote buttons. Boyd and Dering (1996) state:

> The deer is commonly depicted with dots or flowers that represent the peyote button. It is important to remember that to the Huichol the deer is peyote and peyote is the deer. Images of impaled deer within the Lower Pecos rock-art, such as the one identified at the White Shaman site, are metaphors for peyote when found in association with impaled dot motifs or antlered anthropomorphs.

These motifs are common in the Southern Pecos style. Boyd and Dering (1996) identify additional sites that include peyote button motifs, deer hunting, and figures in similar arrangements as the White Shaman site. The correspondence between twentieth-century peyote rituals and petroglyphs over 3,000 years

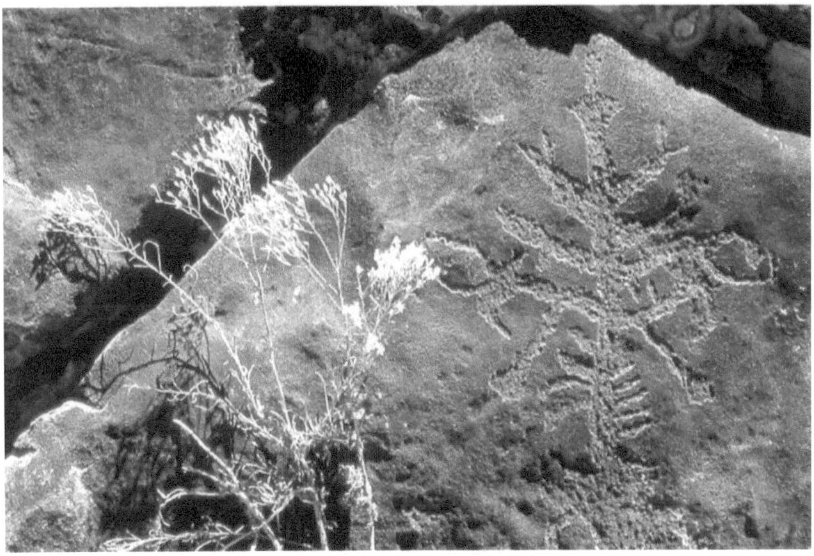

FIGURE 14 Southern Pecos River Style Petroglyphs, Panther Cave, Texas.

old is compelling. These art panels have been estimated to date between 4200 and 2750 radiocarbon years BP (e.g., Rowe 2001; Rowe and Steelman 2002).

Boyd identified elements in the Pecos tradition, "enlarged distal end of staff-like objects with spinescent protrusions (Boyd 2003:91)," as datura effigies. Boyd and Dering (1996) state:

> Over 50% of the Pecos River Style shaman figures are associated with the motif we have identified as Datura. The Datura seed-pod motif is located at the end of a staff-like object that typically extends from the right hand of the shaman. In only one instance, so far identified, is the motif found extending from the left hand. In some cases the thorny Datura fruit is realistically depicted, including stem and calyx. Other images of the Datura fruit are more stylized.

Datura was available in the region, and the motifs are similar to datura effigies in Southern California. Gonzalez Davila (2012) argues, based on interviews with Apache and Huichol, that the Trans-Pecos art was not related to datura or peyote at all. Instead, the colors and artistic motifs agree with Campbell's and Turpin's interpretations of red bean; the supposed datura effigies are explained as representing prickly pear, a partner of red bean in Native world view.

It is probable that Native artists used numerous intoxicants at times or in different contexts (i.e., for different types of rituals). The hallucinogenic diversity of the Trans-Pecos region makes the rock art ambiguous as to specific intoxicants but still speaks to the central role intoxicants must have played.

PALAVAYU ANTHROPOMORPHIC STYLE

Another example is Archaic Basketmaker sites in the Palavayu region of northern Arizona (Malotki 1999). Some 235 sites feature over 2,000 anthropomorphic images, as well as numerous depictions of animals and geometric elements (McCreery and Malotki 1994). The Palavayu Tradition predates farming in the region at around 1500 BCE, perhaps as early as the Middle Archaic, ca. 4500 BCE (Malotki 1999:103). The images can be incorporated with the neuropsychological model and include:

> Depictions of hardwired phosphenes and other endogenous phenomena such as monsters and grotesques; the recurring and consistent mix of iconic and entoptic elements that convey the coherent concept of the ecstatic shaman, shamanic flight, animal familiars, and transformational themes; humans and animals portrayed in skeletonized fashion; animal metaphors for the idea of liminality; anthropomorphs with features of distortion and attenuation, possibly as a result of somatic hallucination; pictorial clues for the

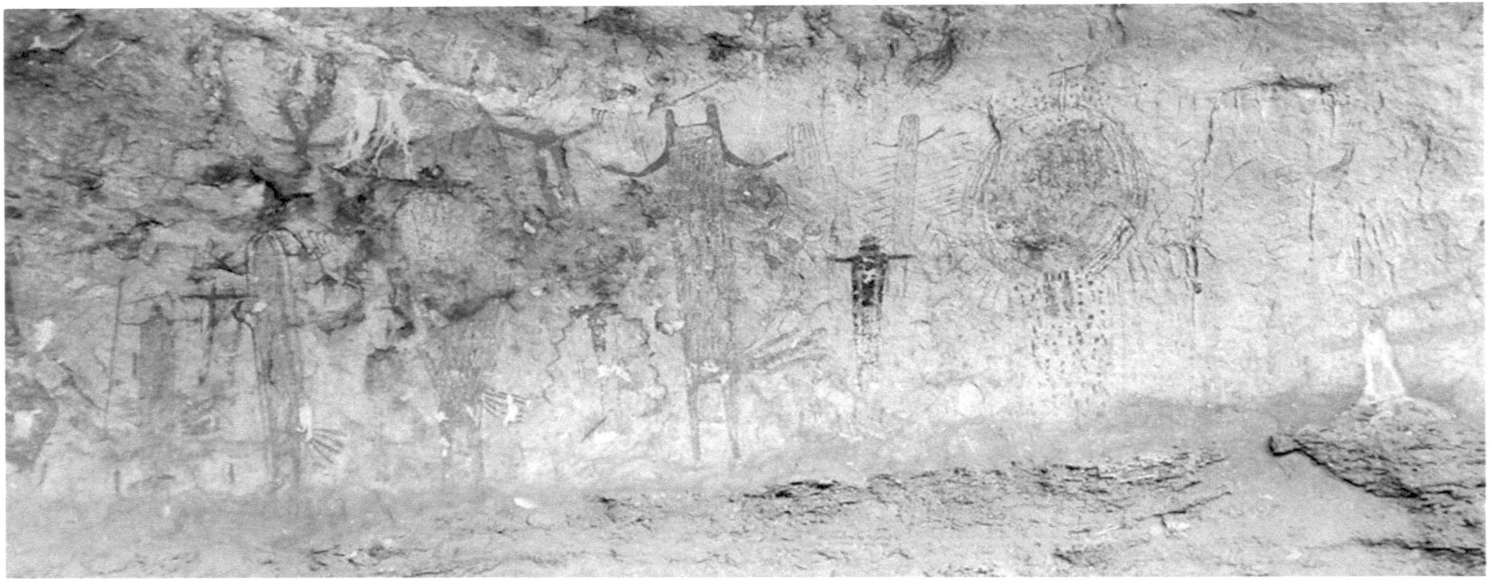

FIGURE 15 Palavayu Tradition Rock Art Depicting Datura. (Courtesy of Ekkehart Malotki.)

> trans-experienced sensations of macropsia and micropsia, polymelia, piloerection, and other tactile hallucinations [Malotki 1999:107].

The hypothesis again is that images were drawn by shamans under the influence of datura (Malotki 1999:108) similar to the Chumash and Yokuts of California (Latta 1977:600; Willcox 1973:27).

Palavayu art includes humanoids carrying linear objects with lines radiating from one end. Many of these figures have lines radiating from their heads. Researchers argue that these represent the spines of datura fruit. Pecked dots commonly occur, representing datura seeds, though dots are a primary form constant in general. Many figures exhibit traits consistent with biological responses to datura, such as large eyes (pupillary dilation), wings (sense of flying), or erections (priapism; Whitley 1994:21). Most significantly, Palavayu art includes depictions of the plant itself. A petroglyph from the Tsimona site shows the plant's stem, leaves, fruit, and roots. Tobacco likely also played a role in Basketmaker rock art, as smoking pipes became significant in the ritual panoply in the region at that time (Hays-Gilpen 2006:606), though the vibrancy of Palavayu Tradition art argues for datura providing the main influence.

MIMBRES POTTERY

Mimbres pottery from the Southwest features a variety of decorations similar to pottery styles linked to hallucinogen use (e.g. Stahl 1985). Mimbres art is an expression of Mogollon culture between ca. 1000 and 1130 CE, in southern Arizona, New Mexico, and northern Mexico. Mimbres Black-on-white pottery includes patterns derived from form constants (dots, lines, grids, zigzags, etc.). There are numerous animals, humans, and human-animal hybrids, consistent with a shamanistic worldview (Huckell and VanPool 2006:155). Datura grows locally throughout the area, though peyote is also a potential candidate.

While Mimbres imagery does not feature particular intoxicants, elements lead researches to favor datura. Circles with exterior ticks have been interpreted as datura fruit much as noded pots (for an example, see Brody 1977:Figure 150). Some pots feature zoomorphs of moths known to be pollinators of datura, similar to Zuni images discussed in the previous chapter (Kay 2005). Datura seeds have been identified at Mimbres pueblo sites (e.g., Anyon and LeBlanc 1984). Other intoxicants may also be represented, such as tobacco. Fewkes (1914:27) records a Mimbres pot depicting human figures smoking tubular

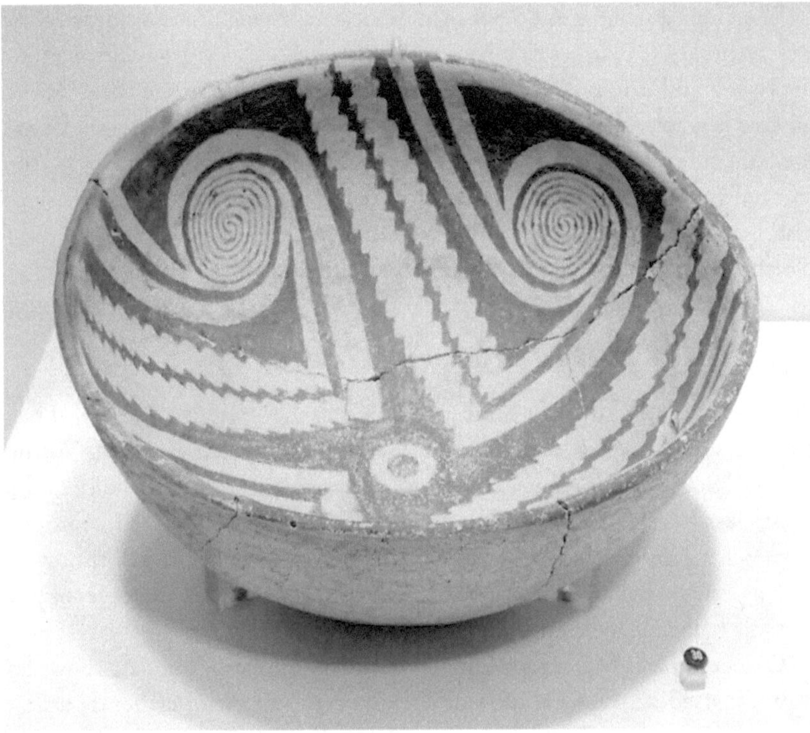

FIGURE 16 Mimbres Bowl Depicting Phosphene Patterns.

pipes. Several species of wild tobacco are available in the region, though it is possible that datura was smoked in pipes as well.

ARCHAIC AND FORMATIVE PERIOD ROCK ART IN NEW MEXICO

Rock art from the Doña Ana Mountains in New Mexico appears to have been influenced by hallucinogens, particularly petroglyphs of "circles, concentric circles, nucleated circles, tailed circles, spirals, and curvilinear meandering forms" (Loendorf et al. 2015:102). These are hallucinogenic form constants, probably over 5,000 years old (Loendorf et al. 2015:104; Schaafsma 1994). There are also painted images incorporating form constants, as well as plants and humans. These likely date to later in time, during the Formative period.

The Doña Ana images do not include clear representations of intoxicants. Researchers note that "desert tobacco" (*Nicotiana obtusifolia*) grows throughout the region and is found adjacent to some rock art panels in the area. Desert tobacco is among the most potent tobacco species (Winter 2000e:321). Given the hallucinogenic properties of tobacco in large doses (see Chapter 5), the co-occurrence of the plant at these sites is compelling evidence of its use in instilling ASCs in the artists. This would be some of the oldest evidence of North American tobacco use, albeit of an indirect sort.

ROCK ART IN EASTERN NORTH AMERICA

Rock art in North America is most common in the West, with several thousand sites in the region, and mere hundreds east of the Mississippi (Willcox 1973:27). Some of this may be due to greater preservation and visibility in the West's less forested terrain and more arid climate. Also, given the hypothesis that rock art correlates with intoxicants, the West is home to hallucinogens such as peyote that are absent in the East. However, there are examples of potentially hallucinogenic art in Eastern North America.

One example is Mammoth Cave, in Kentucky. Radiocarbon data show the cave was used between ca. 1000 BCE and 200 CE, a time of elaborate burial rituals in the region (Crothers et al. 2002). Crothers (2012) argues the cave was used for rites of passage, as a liminal space and source of medicinal mineral deposits ingested during rituals. The cave contains several panels that include geometric and human images consistent with the neuropsychological model. Several intoxicants may have been used based on paleofecal evidence, including sweet flag (*Acorus americanus*), which may contain hallucinogenic essential oils (Motley 1994; Schultes and Hofmann 1980), or alcoholic beverages brewed from maygrass (Schoenwetter 2001).

Sweet flag contains an oil called "asarone" which is similar to mescaline and amphetamine (Motley 1994:399) and has been reported as similar to LSD in its effects (Hoffer and Osmond 1967), making one feel they are "walking a foot off the ground" (Schultes and Hofmann 1980). Others have been unable to substantiate psychoactive effects for the plant (Rätsch 2005:39). Sweet flag has a long history in the Old World and was mentioned in the Bible, by Hippocrates, and in ancient Chinese texts, and was found in the tomb of King Tutankhamun. During the Middle Ages it was suspected of being used in witch's "flying ointment." There is botanical evidence sweet flag was used by Native Americans as a medicine (Motley 1994:404). The Cree and Cheyenne used sweet flag as an additive to the kinnikinnick smoking mixture (see Chapter 5) or as a ritual incense. Datura also grows wild in the local environment and could easily have induced the hallucinatory images found in the cave.

There are other examples of Eastern caves which could represent the influence of ASCs. Faulkner (1988) describes caves in Tennessee with etchings in the mud-covered walls. In Williams Cave, spirals and lattices are potential form constants. Faulkner argues for a Mississippian age (800–1500 CE) for most Tennessee cave art, and we have evidence for intoxicants, including datura, used during that time. Examples of form constants from Zarathustra Cave may date to the Late Archaic period. Images of bird/human hybrids are present in the Tennessee caves, a common shamanistic theme.

ANIMAL FIGURES AND SHAMANISTIC ART

As discussed in Chapter 1, there are rare instances of animals that produce hallucinogenic compounds. In areas with rock art traditions and evidence of animal intoxicants, is there a relationship between the two? Within Southwestern rock art, there are motifs that are interpreted as red ants (Patterson 1992:11). These are vertical lines with small radiating lines for legs and/or embellishments at the end for antennae. Insect-like designs feature in many Western rock art traditions. Insect designs have been identified in Californian art, near areas where ant consumption was observed (see Whitley 1987:172). The distribution of these motifs is congruent with *Pogonomyrmex* ants, endemic throughout the Southwest and California. Also discussed in Chapter 1 was the tradition of anthropomorphic figures incorporating insect attributes, such as the "ant people" of the Hopi. Figures that may depict ant people are included in many Southwestern rock art traditions and typically take the form of human figures with polygonal heads with what appear to be antennae.

These representations indicate that, in the Southwest, ants were symbolically significant and played a role in shamanistic ideologies. They are not necessarily indicative of ant consumption. Stinging insects feature prominently in many rock art traditions worldwide. So, while the depiction of ants in Native rock art contributes to the circumstantial evidence of their cultural significance, additional evidence of their consumption must await future research.

Depictions of animals including toads, while not common, exist in North American rock art. As noted, toad iconography is more common in Native

American portable art. At the Hohokam Johnson Camp site in Arizona, there is a panel exhibiting possible hallucinatory images, including spiral and pipette form constants. Also, there is a large toad or frog. Bostwick (2002:49) argues the toad is depicted due to its hallucinogenic properties. He argues the toad is associated in Hopi mythology with shamans, rain, or water. As with red ants, evidence for hallucinogenic toads from rock art is limited but not inconsistent with the neuropsychological model.

SUMMARY

Based on a perspective that views much aboriginal art as shamanistic and on specific examples presented, we can say the following. There is a correlation between elaboration of rock art and powerful hallucinogens in the local environment. The most elaborate rock art in North America is in the Southwest, in the natural range of peyote, red bean, datura, and several tobacco species. The evidence supports arguments of Lewis-Williams, Winkelman, and others that rock art is a representation of visions experienced by individuals experiencing ASCs.

In some circumstances, such as the Palavayu rock art tradition, we can identify representations of specific plants. In other situations, we can look at geographic propinquity, with specific plants occurring in association with rock art, as is the case for the New Mexican Doña Ana pecked petroglyphs or the Mammoth Cave art. In most cases, we are left with the argument that a range of possible intoxicants contributed to art in a particular region, as is the case for the Pecos River tradition. In all cases, elaborate prehistoric art should be included as evidence to support the often-ephemeral material remains of intoxicant use.

3 STIMULANTS

STIMULANTS CAUSE PHYSICAL AND/OR MENTAL STIMULATION. OTHER symptoms typically include increased heart rate, suppressed appetite, increased stamina and energy, euphoria, and mania. Stimulants can be arbitrarily divided into strong and weak categories. Strong stimulants include cocaine and amphetamines. While cocaine occurs naturally in South American coca leaf, amphetamines are synthetic derivations of ephedrine, itself a mild stimulant (Wadley 2016). Strong stimulants are not found in North America.

CAFFEINE

The most common stimulant used in prehistoric America is caffeine, which increases overall brain activity and stimulates adrenaline (Weckerle et al. 2012:262). Caffeine also stimulates the brain's pleasure center. Caffeine is soluble in water and alcohol and is ideal for drinking in a liquid infusion. Caffeine is found in several plants such as coffee (*Coffea arabica*), tea (*Camellia sinensis*), and cacao (*Theobroma cacao*) but is also found in plants no longer popularly consumed that played a large role historically and prehistorically.

Caffeine, like nicotine, is addictive and loses efficacy with continued use.

The fact that caffeine affects the reward pathway can lead to compulsive consumption. The stimulatory effect is short-lived, and the body rapidly builds up tolerance with withdrawal symptoms such as fatigue and headache. The "jolt" experienced by the "first cup of the day" is actually the abatement of withdrawal. While caffeine withdrawal is benign in contrast to other addictive compounds, these properties contributed to the degree of caffeine consumption today and in the prehistoric past.

The effects of caffeine may go beyond stimulation. Jones and Fernyhough (2009) analyzed caffeine intake, stress, and tendency toward hallucination on 219 adults. Individuals reporting highest levels of caffeine intake also reported a significant increase in hallucinations. Other researchers have shown correlation between caffeine and auditory hallucinations (Crowe et al. 2011). This supports accounts, among the Cherokee for example (Moerman 1998:232), of caffeine-induced hallucinations. The possibility that caffeine contributes to ASCs is intriguing, since, in aboriginal cultures, the amount of caffeine ingested is far more than for modern populations, and caffeine was also used with more potent intoxicants. We turn to discussing what caffeine-containing substances were likely used by Native North Americans.

CACAO

Cacao (*Theobroma cacao*) is native to South America and was a garden crop in Mesoamerica. Linguistic analyses indicate cacao use by 1500 BCE (Coe and Coe 2007). The earliest physical evidence of cacao use in Mesoamerica dates to the Maya Preclassic. Hurst and others (1989, 2002) conducted high performance liquid chromatography (HPLC) on vessels dating between 600 BCE and 250 CE. They identified caffeine and related theobromine, indicating the vessels were used with a cacao-based beverage. Such vessels are found in elite burials, so the practice of drinking cacao was probably socially restricted.

Cacao is usually discussed with regard to its stimulatory caffeine and theobromine. Less discussed are references that it may have hallucinogenic properties in extreme concentrations. Sahagún's sixteenth-century observations in Mesoamerica noted: "Cacahuacuahuitl . . . its name is cacao . . . when the cacao is drunk in too large quantities, especially when it is young, makes people drunk . . . makes them lose their heart, and makes them mad" (Elferink 1988:431). It is unclear whether it is the quantity consumed, other added substances, or whether it was allowed to ferment, that may have led to this effect. We should

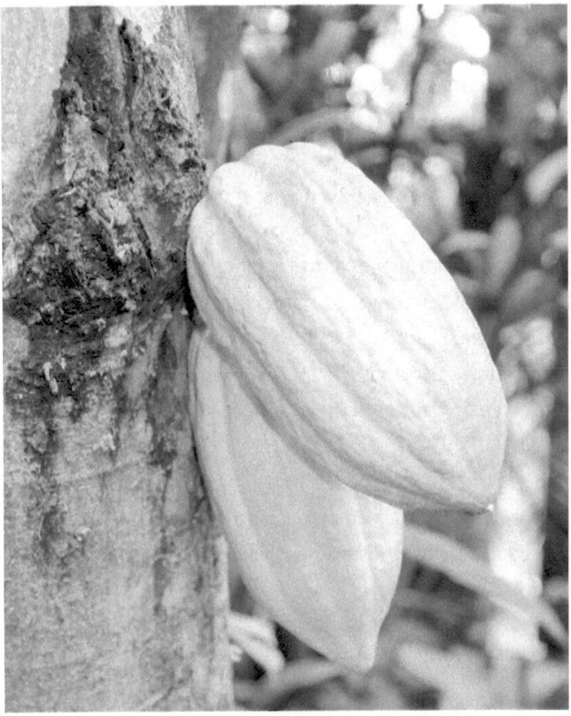

FIGURE 17 *Theobroma cacao.*

be aware that more than a caffeine high may have been involved in cacao or that significant ingestion may have had hallucinogenic effects.

While there is ample Mesoamerican evidence of cacao, the practice extended into the Southwest. Ancestral Puebloan sites from the 900s CE contain nonlocal vessel styles used for cacao. Theobromine was identified in sherds from Chaco Canyon (Crown and Hurst 2009). This shows trade between Mesoamerica and the Southwest. A study on the Four Corners region identified theobromine in 50 specimens using liquid chromatography-mass spectroscopy/mass spectroscopy (LC-MS/MS) (Washburn et al. 2011). These were recovered from elite and non-elite sites, and cacao may have been payment for craft labor (Washburn et al. 2011:1639). Similar results were found for eighth-century CE vessels from Utah (Washburn et al. 2012). Nielsen-Grimm and colleagues (2017) used HPLC-MS to identify cacao at Ancestral Pueblo sites in Utah. These results contribute to our understanding of the cacao trade after 800 CE.

ILEX

While most know chocolate contains caffeine, it is also found in holly plants, genus *Ilex*. Three species contain caffeine (Hu 1979). The species most commonly used are *I. vomitoria* and *I. cassine*, native to the Southeast (Merrill 1979:40). Ilex was used by the Cherokee or Creek to make "black drink," "cassina" (from Timucuan), or "yaupon" (Catawban; Hudson 1976). The plant is called "ássi" in Creek (Gatschet 1884 Vol 1:173), though they added other psychoactive plants including tobacco (Driver and Massey 1957:262). It is simplest to refer to such beverages as "ilex." Drinking it was widespread in Spanish sixteenth-century colonies and in the English colonies through the 1700s (Sturtevant 1979). After it was largely replaced by tea, coffee, and chocolate, it was still used historically in the Carolinas and Florida.

One ilex species, *I. paraguariensis*, or "yerba mate," is cultivated today in South America, particularly in Paraguay and Argentina, and used to make a beverage termed "mate" (Hudson 1979:6–7; Sturtevant 1979). Yerba mate,

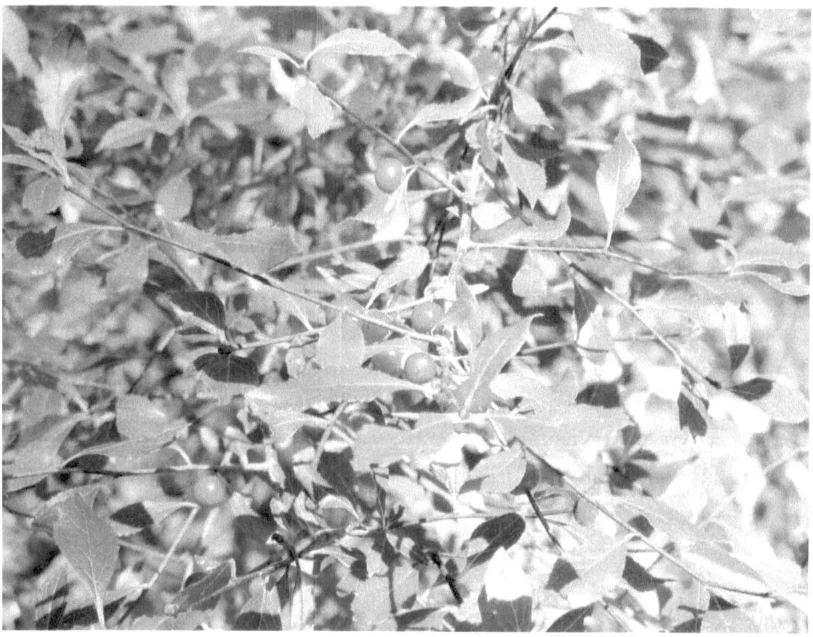

FIGURE 18 *Ilex cassine.*

exported from South America, is also popular among Druze communities in Syria and Lebanon. Yerba mate contains the alkaloids caffeine, theobromine, and theophylline, but in lower concentrations than North American ilex species, as well as in other modern alternatives such as tea or coffee. Mate is drunk as a stimulating beverage much as coffee or tea, and yerba mate is also included as an ingredient in some modern energy drinks.

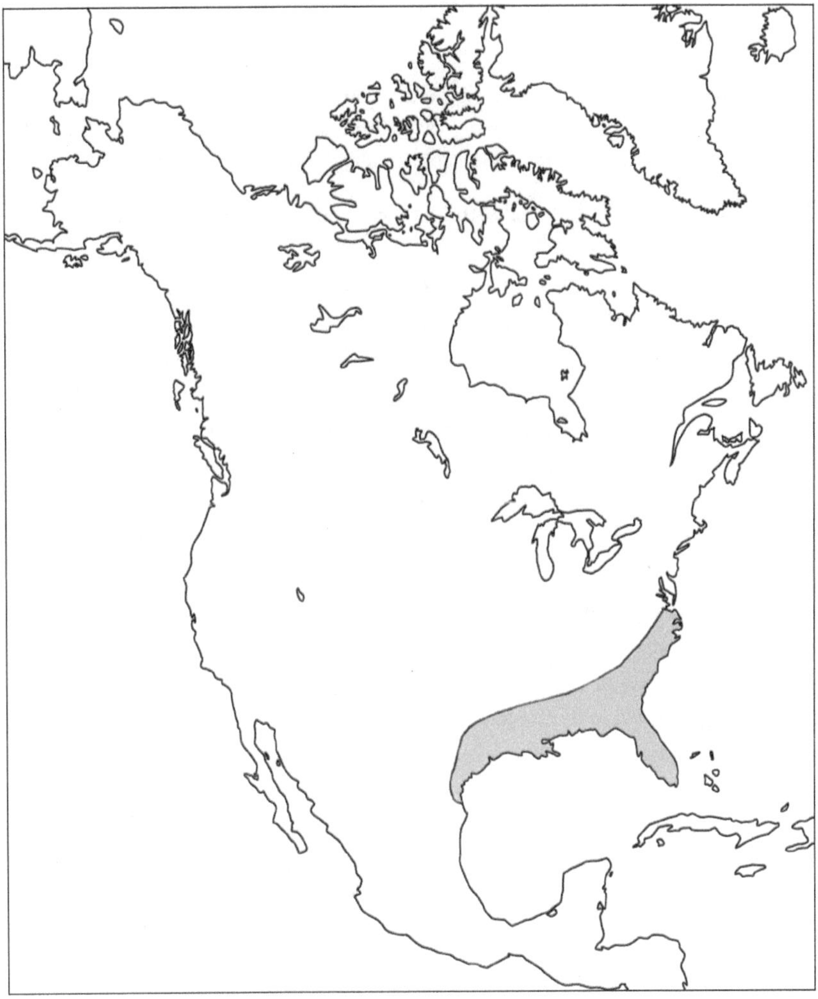

FIGURE 19 Range of Ilex species. (Author's map.)

Historically and prehistorically ilex was mostly drunk in ritual settings requiring purification. "Black drink" was so associated with purity that some referred to it as "white drink" (Hudson 1979:2). In some contexts, it was used only by male warriors, while in others it was restricted to high-rank males and females. Some accounts show ilex used to facilitate interaction between hostile tribes, like sharing tobacco. Drinking ilex was generally formalized; it was not a secular beverage (Merrill 1979). There are material correlates, and accounts describe shell cups, as is discussed below.

A description of ilex comes from the North Carolina Tuscarora (Johnson 1967:180–181):

> The Indians of eastern North Carolina drank vast quantities of the tea from the yaupon bush, which was found along the coast and the great tidewater rivers. They dosed themselves every second morning or oftener when they could get the drink and vomited it up again.

This account offers little social significance, instead focusing on health benefits against malaria.

Ilex has physiological effects. Aside from stimulatory and diuretic caffeine, the beverage is an emetic, causing vomiting, as well as a diaphoretic, causing sweating, both seen as purifying. Caffeine effects do not explain these symptoms. Anecdotal evidence indicates other plants were added such as button snakeroot (*Eryngium aquaticum*), blue flag (*Iris versicolor*), or Indian tobacco (*Lobelia inflata*), also known as "puke weed" (Havard 1896:41). Some accounts say some effects were due to adding seawater or to drinking a large volume (Swanton 1946). Trace amounts of compounds similar to turpentine in ilex could also be a cause (Hudson 1979:4).

The emetic effect is called into question by accounts of a Seminole drink infusion that caused vomiting but which did not contain ilex (Sturtevant 1954). There are accounts of ilex drinking that do not include vomiting; it may have been brewed in various concentrations depending on the context (Havard 1896:41). Hudson (1979:4) suggested that vomiting was a regular practice of many Southeastern Natives for purification, and the correlation with ilex is due to confusing the correlation of ilex drinking and regurgitation with causation.

Ilex tea is among the earliest Native intoxicants observed by Europeans. Cabeza de Vaca observed ilex in Texas in the 1530s (Varnum 2014:140). He described ilex consumption as a male activity. Women interrupting the ritual were subject to harsh sanctions:

> When the women hear these shouts [inviting men to drink], they stand motionless, fearing to move. Even if heavily laden, they dare not budge. Should a woman make a motion,

> they dishonor her, beat her with sticks, and in great vexation throw out the liquor that is prepared. Those that have drunk any of it regurgitate, which they do readily and painlessly. They say they do this because a woman's movement when she hears the shout causes the tea to carry something pernicious into the drinker's body which will presently kill him [Cabeza de Vaca 1983 [1542]:99].

Cabeza de Vaca's description of a male practice is consistent with later accounts (Millspaugh 1974:416). Nineteenth-century accounts from Texas attest to ritual use of ilex along the Gulf Coast (Gatschet 1891:134). One must maintain some reservations regarding Cabeza de Vaca's observations as he described smoking peyote when tobacco is far more plausible.

There are accounts of ilex from the Timucua of sixteenth-century Florida (Merrill 1979:45). Observations by Le Moyne in 1564 were among the first European accounts, including impressive (but often inaccurate) illustrations by de Bry. Le Moyne (Swanton 1922:375) describes daily use of ilex, exclusively by high-ranking males, centering on the Timucuan chief:

> The chief and his nobles are accustomed during certain days of the year to meet early every morning for this express purpose in a public place . . . the chief orders the women to boil some cassine, which is a drink prepared from the leaves from a certain root, and which they afterwards pass through a strainer. The chief and his councilors being now seated in their places, one stands before him, and spreading forth his hands wide open, asks a blessing upon the chief and the others, who are to drink. Then the cupbearer brings the hot drink in a capacious shell, first to the chief, and then, as the chief directs, to the rest in their order in the same shell. They esteem this drink so highly that no one is allowed to drink it in council unless he has proved himself a brave warrior. Moreover this drink has the quality of at once throwing into a sweat whoever drinks it. On this account those who can not keep it down, but whose stomachs reject it are not intrusted with any difficult commission or any military responsibility being considered unfit, for they often have to go three or four days without food; but one who can drink this liquor can go for 24 hours afterward without eating or drinking. In military expeditions also the only supplies which they carry consist of gourd bottles or wooden vessels full of this drink. It strengthens and nourishes the body and yet does not fly to the head as we have observed on occasion of these feasts of theirs.

Le Moyne's relation is interesting as it shows the effects of ilex and its significance in social organization and rituals, as well as its use as a performance-enhancing drug during war.

In 1567, de Gourges led a punitive expedition against the Spanish in Florida. During the expedition, the French interacted with Natives:

> Before leaving there the savages made a beverage they are accustomed to take at all times and when they go to fight and there is danger. This beverage made of a certain plant and

> drunk kept them from being hungry or thirsty for 24 hours. They presented it to Gourges who pretended to drink it and swallowed none of it [Hale 1891:16].

Following de Gourges' tactful avoidance, the Natives all drank according to their rank.

Lescarbot made a 1614 account, based on sixteenth-century accounts (Lescarbot 1914:177):

> The Floridians have a sort of drink called casinê , which they drink hot, made of certain leaves of trees. But it is not lawful for every one to drink of it, but only for the [chief], and those who have made proof of their valour in war. And this drink has such virtue, that as soon as they have drunk it, they are all in a sweat, and after this is over they have no need of food for twenty-four hours, such is its nourishing force.

Lescarbot's secondhand account is still useful in pointing to socially restricted access to ilex.

Adair, during the mid-eighteenth century, recorded Creek use of ilex:

> When this beloved liquid or supposed drink offering is fully prepared and fit to be drank one of the magi brings two old consecrated large conch shells out of a place appropriate for containing the holy things and delivers them into the hands of two religious attendants who after a wild ceremony fill them with the supposed sanctifying bitter liquid then they approach near to the two central red and white seats which the leaders call the war and beloved cabins stooping with their heads and bodies pretty low. Advancing a few steps in this posture they carry their shells with both hands at an instant to one of the most principal men on those red and white seats. The favored persons whom the religious attendants are invoking the divine essence to bless hold up their shells with both hands to their mouths during the awful sacred invocation and retain a mouthful of the drink to spurt out upon the ground as a supposed drink offering to the great self existing giver which they offer at the end of their draft. If any of the traders who at those times are invited to drink with them were to neglect this religious observance they would reckon us as godless and wild as the wolves of the desert. After the same manner the supposed holy waiters proceed from the highest to the lowest in their Synedrion [assembly or council] and when they have ended that awful solemnity they go round the whole square or quadrangular place and collect tobacco from the sanctified sinners according to ancient customs [quoted in Hale 1891:17].

Adair's observations are colored by his conviction that the Creek were descended from the Tribes of Israel, but his observations illustrate the ritual reverence with which ilex was drunk. Adair describes ilex, noting the drink contained other plants such as button snakeroot (*Eryngium cuneifolium*) and willow (*Salix* sp.; Hale 1891:18).

Mid-eighteenth century descriptions from Alabama and Florida note ilex was associated with calumet smoking (see Chapter 5). Bartram wrote in the 1770s:

> When the feast was over [the] chief with the rest of the white people in town took their seats according to order. Tobacco and pipes were brought. The calumet was lighted and smoked circulating according to the usual forms and ceremony and afterwards black drink concluded the feast. The king conversed, drank cassine and associated familiarly with his people and with us [Bartram 1928:200].

Bartram (1928:357) goes on to record one of the longest and most detailed observations of ilex:

> I was introduced to the ancient chiefs at the public square . . . and in the evening in company with the traders who are numerous in this town repaired to the great rotunda where were assembled the greatest number of ancient venerable chiefs and warriors that I had ever beheld. We spent the evening and greater part of the night together in drinking cassine and smoking tobacco. The great council house or rotunda is appropriated to much the same purpose as the public square but more private and seems particularly dedicated to political affairs. Women and youth are never admitted. . . . In the first place the governor or officer who has the management of this business with his servants attending orders the black drink to be brewed which is a decoction or infusion of the leaves and tender shoots of the cassine. This is done under an open shed or pavilion at 20 or 30 yards distance directly opposite the door of the council house.

Bartram goes on to describe the creation of an elaborate fire in the council house, then continues:

> Soon after this illumination takes place the aged chiefs and warriors are seated . . . in three classes or ranks rising a little one above or behind the other and the white people and red people of confederate towns in like order. The king's cabin or seat is in front, the next to the back of it the head warriors, and the third or last accommodates the young warriors etc. The great war chief's seat or place is in the same cabin with and immediately to the left hand of the king and next to the white people, and to the right hand of the king the most venerable headmen and warriors are seated. The assembly being now seated in order and the house illuminated, two middle aged men who perform the office of slaves or servants pro tempore come in together at the door each having very large conch shells full of black drink and advance with slow uniform and steady steps. Their eyes or countenance lifted up, singing very low but sweetly, they come within 6 or 8 paces of the king's and white people's cabin, when they stop together and each rests his shell on a tripod or little table but presently takes it up again and bowing very low advances obsequiously, crossing or intersecting each other about midway. He who rested his shell before the white people now stands before the king and the other who stopped before the king stands before the

> white people, when each presents his shell one to the king and the other to the chief of the white people and as soon as he raises it to his mouth the slave utters or sings two notes, each of which continues as long as he has breath and as long as these notes continue so long must the person drink or at least keep the shell to his mouth. These two long notes are very solemn and at once strike the imagination with a religious awe or homage to the Supreme, sounding somewhat like a "hoo ojah" and a "he yah." After this manner the whole assembly are treated as long as the drink or light continues to hold out and as soon as the drinking begins tobacco and pipes are brought [Bartram 1928:358].

Further associations between ilex and tobacco, and their relation to gender and social rank, are illustrated by Bossu, from Alabama:

> All the Allibamas drink the cassine. . . . They toast these leaves as we do coffee and drink the infusion of them with great ceremony. When this diuretic potion is prepared the young people go to present it in calabashes formed into cups to the chiefs and warriors, that is the honorable, and afterwards to the other warriors according to their rank and degree. The same order is preserved when they present the calumet to smoke out of. . . . The women never drink of this beverage which is only made for the warriors [quoted in Hale 1891:18].

Bossu describes the role of tobacco and ilex in social interaction when Natives and Europeans met in negotiations:

> The Chevalier de Emville held a speech to the assembly in his turn and made the nation a present which the governor had sent him. The Indians gave him the great calumet of peace to smoke all the soldiers and French inhabitants likewise smoked it in sign of a general amnesty. Afterwards they drank the cassine which is the potion of the white word i.e. the potion of oblivion and peace [quoted in Hale 1891:18].

Catesby writing in 1754 has a detailed description of ilex consumption:

> [Yaupon] is highly regarded by the Indians and used for many purposes, which gives it an even greater character. They say that the virtues of the shrub have been known since the earliest times and that for their use, it has always been prepared in the same manner as today. After drying or roasting the leaves in a pot over the fire, they are stored for use. From these they make their favorite beverage by preparing a potent decoction which they drink in great quantities, both for their health and also with great desire and good pleasure, without any kind of sugar or other additives. They drink great amounts of this, and time and again, and thus swallow many quarts. They have an annual custom in the spring in which the drinking takes place in a ceremony. The inhabitants of the village gather in the communal house after they have cleaned their own houses by burning all of their furniture and replacing this anew. The king is first served the drink in a great bowl or snail shell which has never been used before. After this, the other eminent personages receive the drink according to their rank. The women and the children are the last to receive the

> brew. They say it makes lost appetites return, that it strengthens the stomach, and that it gives them power and courage for war [quoted in Rätsch 2005:295].

This description is notable in including women and children, if in a subsidiary position to men.

Based on such sources, we can say ilex was prominent in Native lives in the Southeast during the eighteenth century, and likely throughout the contact period. While researchers have supposed ilex has a lengthy history (Hudson 1979; White and Weinstein 2008:255), this is based on little physical evidence. Three types of evidence are significant for the prehistoric distribution of ilex: botanical evidence, organic residues, and pottery and shell vessels.

Archaeobotanical evidence of ilex is rare, since processing the plant destroys much of the substance. Even in areas where its use was suspected, botanical evidence has been lacking: "University of Illinois archaeobotanical researchers have examined nearly 10,000 [liters] of Mississippian period soil samples, searching for carbonized Ilex remains, to no avail" (Crown et al. 2012:13948). Even in well-preserved, carefully excavated sites, where ritual feasting likely took place, botanical remains of ilex have proved elusive (Pluckhahn et al. 2006).

Some ilex seeds have been recovered in Southeastern and Midwestern Mississippian sites. Nine *I. vomitoria* seeds were recovered from the Grove's Creek site in Georgia (Keene 2004:676). Alabama's Moundville included a submound structure from which tobacco and ilex were recovered (Jackson and Scott 2003:559), while the Bottle Creek site, south of Moundville, produced ilex seeds from two mounds (Scarry 2003:110).

Pre-Mississippian evidence of ilex is scant. A site in Virginia produced ilex seeds dating between 1040 and 1220 CE, interpreted as evidence of gathering ilex (VanDerwarker and Stanyard 2009). A Late Woodland (590–780 CE) mound from Louisiana produced ilex seeds as well as seeds of morning glory (Sherwood et al. 2013:348). Researchers speculated about ilex among the Swift Creek culture (between 100 and 800 CE) in Alabama, Georgia, and Florida (Jones et al. 1998:239; Anderson 1998:278), but evidence is lacking. Ilex seeds associated with black bear (*Ursus americanus*) bones were recovered from a public structure at the contact period Cherokee site of Coweeta Creek in North Carolina (Rodning and VanDerwarker 2002:7).

Archaeologists have turned to other evidence. Ilex requires substantial processing; leaves must be roasted, or caffeine is not bioavailable and cannot be absorbed. Also, the infusion must be concentrated by decoction, or boiling off water. Researchers investigating pottery jars from Cahokia and nearby sites have identified interior sooting consistent with decoction (Miller 2015). This supports speculation (Emerson 1989:66) that such vessels were used in Mississippian-era ilex ceremonialism. Ilex teas are the only substances known to have been so prepared; and the vessels were recovered from ceremonial contexts, so the argument is plausible.

There have been some analyses of prehistoric artifacts for caffeine, theobromine, and theophylline residues of ilex. One study detected caffeine in buried experimental residues, indicating such residues can survive in archaeological contexts (Reber 2014; Reber and Kerr 2012). Similar results were presented by Tushingham et al. (2011). Swanton (1946) states ilex was prepared in large "cauldrons" (Hally 1986:270), so archaeologists can target specific vessels for analysis in the future. Thompson and Pluckhahn (2018:134) identify likely ilex-related shell vessels from Fort Center in Florida. This is a site of burial processing and intoxicant consumption, featuring pipes and shell vessels, many of which had been "killed" by breaking. Another study focused on "beakers" from Cahokia (Crown et al. 2012), likely drinking cups from renewal/cleansing rituals. Ilex compounds were detected using LC-MS/MS on pottery fragments dating from 1050 to 1250 CE.

Eight vessels from Cahokia were found to contain caffeine biomarkers. The project also identified compounds present in ilex but not in cacao (though researchers have contested this—see Washburn et al. 2014). The ratios of caffeine to theobromine in the samples indicate the most likely species was *I. vomitoria*, representing the earliest known chemical evidence of ilex use (Crown et al. 2012:13947; Emerson and Pauketat 2015). Washburn and colleagues (2014) conducted similar research, and found similar results, on vessels from two sites in Illinois (Washburn et al. 2014). The same researchers analyzed vessels from Arkansas, Florida, and Mississippi, which also contained caffeine residues.

The authors hypothesize ilex played a role in a spreading religious movement:

> It suggests that the beakers spread as part of a religious package including a suite of ritual accoutrements such as flint clay figures, Ramey Incised vessels, and accompanying icons and religious ceremonies. If their association with Black Drink is shown to be exclusive, then beakers add another distinctive artifact to those already associated with Cahokian religion during the Stirling phase (1100–1200 CE) [Crown et al. 2012:13948].

Washburn and colleagues (2014) argue chemical profiles of Mississippian vessels are consistent with cacao, not ilex. They propose Mississippians were trading with Mesoamerica for cacao. While cacao could not be cultivated outside the tropics, cacao beans could have been traded across the Gulf of Mexico or through Texas (White and Weinstein 2008:255). These assumptions are based on ratios of caffeine and related compounds, but many factors could change these ratios postdepositionally (Crown et al. 2015:11438). A follow-up investigation was conducted on 117 vessels from 18 sites ranging from 750 to 1400 CE (Crown et al. 2015). Forty samples tested positive for caffeine and related compounds. These vessels grouped by compound ratios fall into three groups: samples with high theobromine, indicative of cacao; samples with high caffeine, consistent with ilex; and samples with ambiguous ratios, possibly indicating a mixture. These results do support possible trade in cacao and ilex, pending additional research.

While botanical and chemical evidence is suggestive, most evidence of ilex is in the paraphernalia of its use: pottery vessels for processing, and pottery and shell artifacts for consumption. Shell artifacts are more pertinent as pottery vessels could have been multipurpose, while shell artifacts were likely only used for ilex. Shell cups similar to ones described in ethnohistoric accounts were used by Mississippian cultures throughout the Southeast and Midwest (Thompson and Pluckhahn 2018). The geographic distribution of cups indicates

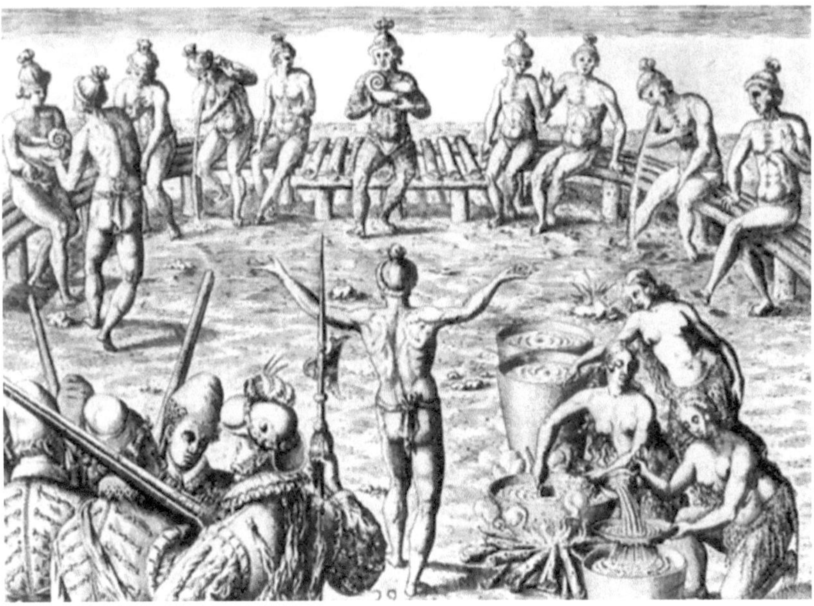

FIGURE 20 Black Drink Ceremony among the Timucua.

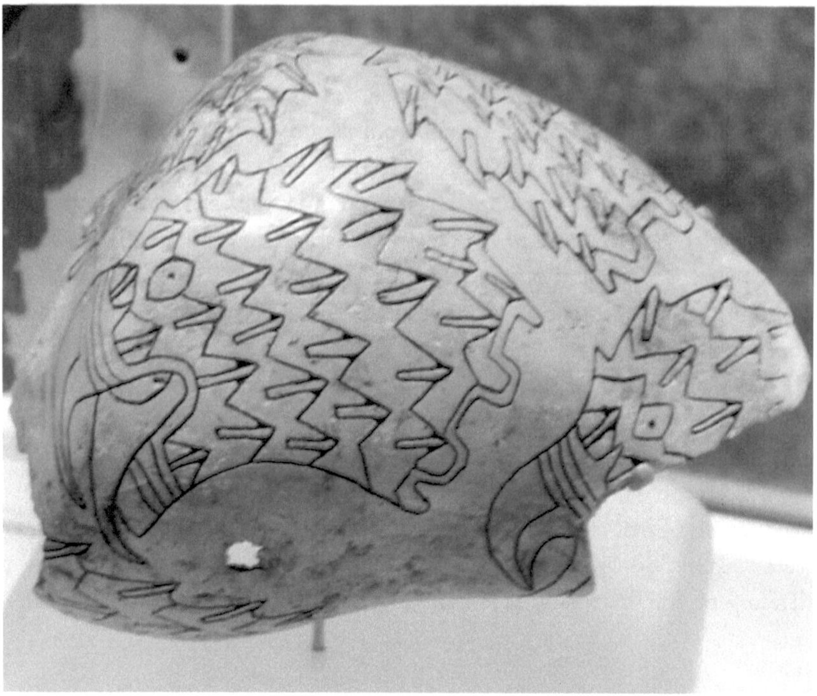

FIGURE 21 Shell cup with Raptorial Bird Engravings from Spiro Mounds.

a pre-Mississippian history (Milanich 1979:84). Accounts show their significance as ritual items and rank symbols. In the eighteenth century, Adair (1930 [1775]) noted shell cups in black drink ceremonies were made by older women but used by adult men. Le Moyne wrote of the sixteenth-century Timucua: "When a chief dies, he is buried with great solemnities, his [shell] drinking cup is placed upon the grave, and arrows are planted in the ground around it" (Le Moyne 1875:15). A woodcut by Le Moyne depicts Europeans observing a black drink ceremony; shell cups are prominent (Merrill 1979:47). Le Moyne depicts a nautilus shell likely not available to Natives of the area (Hann 1986:95), but this is unsurprising as he was not a direct observer. Swanton (1928) noted shell cups used in Creek busk or "Green Corn" ceremonies in the 1920s. The busk ceremony centered around renewal and purification; old fires are extinguished, new fires are lit, and copious spiritually cleansing ilex is consumed.

Some early examinations of Native earthen mounds noted the craftsmanship of shell cups. Holmes, during the late nineteenth century, described examples from Illinois, Arkansas, Georgia, Tennessee, Ohio, Iowa, and even New York (Holmes 1883). Archaeologists have long known the role marine shell played in Mississippian-era trade (Prentice 1987). Shell cups are associated with Mississippian elites (Cobb 2003:72), in mound burials and ritual contexts, but not in lower status burials. Cups were carved from shells of Gulf of Mexico lightning whelks (*Busycon contrarium*), emperor helmet (*Cassis madagascariensis*), or horse conch (*Triplofusus giganteus* or *Pleuroploca gigantea*) and traded throughout the Mississippian world (Milanich 1979:85).

The Spiro site in Oklahoma and Belcher Mound in Louisiana contain the most cups, though fragments have been recovered from most major Mississippian sites. A submound burial from Cahokia contained a shell cup (Trubit 2000:678). A cup was discovered from a single burial (out of more than 1,800) from the Upper Nodena site in Arkansas, dating between 1400 and 1600 CE (Fisher-Carroll and Mainfort 2000). A cup fragment was recovered from near Etowah Mounds in Georgia (Wauchope 1948:206). Numerous cups were recovered from high-status burials at Etowah (Larson 1971; King 2001) and from Moundville (Peebles 1971). Milanich (1979) reports specimens from Florida, and recent projects have identified similar specimens at other Floridian mound sites (White 2013:59). The distribution of shell cups ranges from the Mississippi River to the Atlantic, and from the Gulf of Mexico to the Great Lakes.

The "great mortuary" beneath Spiro's Craig Mound contained ritual items, including feathers, basketry, copper, lithics, and engraved shell cups. Phillips and Brown (1975, 1978) analyzed shell artifacts from Spiro, identifying 274 shell cups, plus 560 fragments (Wyckoff 1985). Many of these contained the residue of liquid contents. Five specimens had intentional holes, rendering them useless, "killing" a sacred object (Sievert 2003:191–193). Intentional disposal of artifacts for ritual intoxicant consumption represents a sacrifice of powerful religious paraphernalia. As mentioned previously, King and others (2017) have shown shell vessels from Spiro were also used to drink datura.

Eight shell cups were recovered from the Belcher site. Belcher is smaller than Spiro, with a single mound. While Belcher cups are fewer than for Spiro, all were recovered by excavation of submound burials (Webb 1959). One was interred with an adolescent, another with an adult female. Three cups were interred in a mass grave of children, and three were associated with a burial of an adult male, adult female, and a child. These are intriguing details, as the ethnographic record places shell cups and ilex in an adult male sphere. It is possible that cups and other artifacts were markers of high status as opposed to marking specific behaviors or possessions.

Dates for shell cups are rare due to the early excavation of so many specimens. AMS radiocarbon dates place some Spiro shell toward the Early to Middle Mississippian. One Spiro grave containing cups was dated 1038–1277 CE (Brown and Rogers 1999). Shell cup fragments from Mound 34 at Cahokia, a ritual location with ceremonial fires and a burned structure, are associated with a date from the late thirteenth to mid-fourteenth century CE (Kelly and Brown 2010:4).

The function of shell cups and spoons cannot be separated from their iconography. They were often engraved with images of humanoid figures and other motifs. Archaeologists have argued that these were depictions of deities (Phillips and Brown 1975, 1978:106; Prentice 1986:239). Religious motifs include decapitated humans, snakes or snake/human hybrids, and geometric symbols of cosmological significance such as the cross-in-circle (Knight et al. 2001).

Shell likely had cosmological significance, representing a watery underworld (Clark 2013). The spiral shells may have significance as well (Milanich 1979:86). Marquardt and Kozuch (2016) speculates that the whelk shell spiral is represented in the spiral patterns of ceremonial fires in which ilex was consumed and that the left-handed direction of the whelk shell spiral symbolized the path of the sun and the path of the dead (Marquardt and Kozuch 2016). This association of spirals with death is drawn from eighteenth-century observations of Natchez elite funerals observed by Le Page du Pratz (2006:365), who noted that the body was transported in a left-handed spiral path. Spirals have been repeatedly observed as symbols in shamanistic rituals.

Kozuch (2013a, 2013b) and Reed (2009) expand on the role of shell iconography, arguing the figures depicted represent souls following "the path of the dead." This interpretation differs from interpretations of Knight and others (2001) that figures depicted in Southeast Ceremonial Complex (SECC) art represent deities (Blitz 2009:22). One example from Spiro has been interpreted as representing the Green Corn ceremony or ilex harvesting, as well as vomiting humans experiencing its effects (Phillips and Brown 1975:115–116). Regardless of the meanings of the iconography, there is consensus that images depicted on shell cups are supernatural in reference, which in conjunction with their common ritual/ceremonial contexts and their primary use as a drug-delivery device, is further evidence of the religious role of ilex in Mississippian society.

There are two styles of art on Mississippian shell cups (Brown 1997). The

Braden style is centered in the north of the Mississippian world and likely developed during Cahokia's growth in the eleventh century. Braden style, in keeping with the SECC, includes warrior figures, birds or bird/man figures, bilobed arrows, and forked eye symbols. Since so many cups were recovered from Craig Mound, the form is dominated by the Craig style, which incorporates Caddoan symbolism west of the Mississippian heartland.

Shell cups have featured as motifs in artwork. A spiral whelk shell can be found on a flint clay figurine recovered from the East St. Louis mound group near Cahokia (Emerson and Boles 2010:478); the image depicts a noded spiral interpreted as a shell cup. The figure is an adult female, modeled as presenting a cup, which could relate to Adair's observations of females crafting the ceremonial vessels. Emerson (2003) makes a compelling argument that flint clay figures similar to the East St. Louis specimen represent shamans, further evidence that shell cups, and their intoxicating contents, were tools of religious expression.

There are ceramic representations of shells. Kozuch (2013a, b) has presented results of analysis of 31 Late Mississippian vessels from numerous sites in the American Bottom, including nine from Cahokia. These shell effigy vessels might have been involved in ilex preparation or consumption, as is the case for the vessels containing ilex alkaloids from Cahokia. Several vessels feature "spouts" opposite the spiral decoration, giving the shape of a shell cup (Holmes 1883; Kozuch 2013b:36–37). It is plausible that these vessels served the role of shell cups when shell was in short supply (Cobb 1991). Residue analysis could show whether they contained ilex. One attempt to identify residues on cups was unsuccessful, possibly due to the alkalinity of shell (Washburn et al. 2014:201). Complicating any study of residue on shell cups is the fact that so many of the known examples were recovered in uncontrolled excavations, most have been exposed to secondary residues, and many have been washed (Sievert 2003:190–191).

Marine shell's rarity and the religious content of the cups' engravings place them in the realm of sacred objects (Knight 1986). While historically ilex consumption was a means of purification and group building, researchers suggest additional implications. Emerson places cups, and their marine origin, in a symbolic context centered on fertility and renewal, associated with other under(water)world symbols such as the serpent (Emerson 1989). This is based on the marine origin of shell and possibly on the material's color (Claassen 1998).

Kozuch (2013b:41) argues the increase in shell cups and cup effigies between 1200 and 1400 CE represents an increased focus on renewal and purification in a time of increasing social unrest and warfare in Mississippian societies. The association of ilex consumption and Mississippian warfare has been previously demonstrated (Dye 2007). The purification associated with ilex consumption and the use of shell cups and other vessels is aptly summarized by Dye:

> The rituals that surrounded warfare emphasized purity in order that one might be in a pure state to solicit aid and power from the culture heroes. Purity was achieved in part through the consumption of sacred drinks brewed in and consumed from ceramic vessels [Dye 2020].

While the use of shell cups with ilex is a largely Mississippian phenomenon, dating after 1000 CE, there are earlier examples. Milanich (1979:87) and Marquardt and Watson (2005) note cups from Archaic sites in Kentucky, including Indian Knoll. A cup was recovered from the Middle Woodland (200–800 CE) Bowman Mound in Virginia (Carpenter 1950:308). Bowman likely dates at least 200 years prior to Mississippian sites. Shell cups seem to be absent in the Early Woodland (1000 BCE–200 CE). Milanich argues the earliest contexts where shell cups can be ascribed ritual use are Middle Woodland or later.

Based on ethnography, ethnohistory, and archaeology, we can make the following statements. Ilex was utilized throughout the Southeast at contact in circumstances requiring purification and intersocietal interaction. These rituals were formalized, with rank and gender divisions. Ritual ilex consumption has prehistoric roots at least as early as the Mississippian era around 800 CE. While it is possible ilex consumption has origins as early as the first millennium BCE, evidence for such claims is presently lacking. Systematic investigations of the prehistory of ilex are only just beginning, and hopefully recent developments in chemical analysis will produce additional data.

EPHEDRA

Ephedra has a global distribution. The number of species is a matter of contention, but there are dozens in temperate Eurasia. New World species are limited to the Andes and North American Southwest. Ephedra is the oldest known psychoactive. Ephedra pollen was identified at Shanidar Cave, dating over 50,000 years before present (Solecki 1975).

Ephedra contains ephedrine, as well as pseudoephedrine and norephedrine. These compounds are all similar to amphetamine. Until recently, ephedra was available for weight loss, but after cardiovascular side effects became apparent (Haller and Benowitz 2000), it was removed from US markets. Ephedra has desirable properties, including increased alertness and decreased fatigue, and

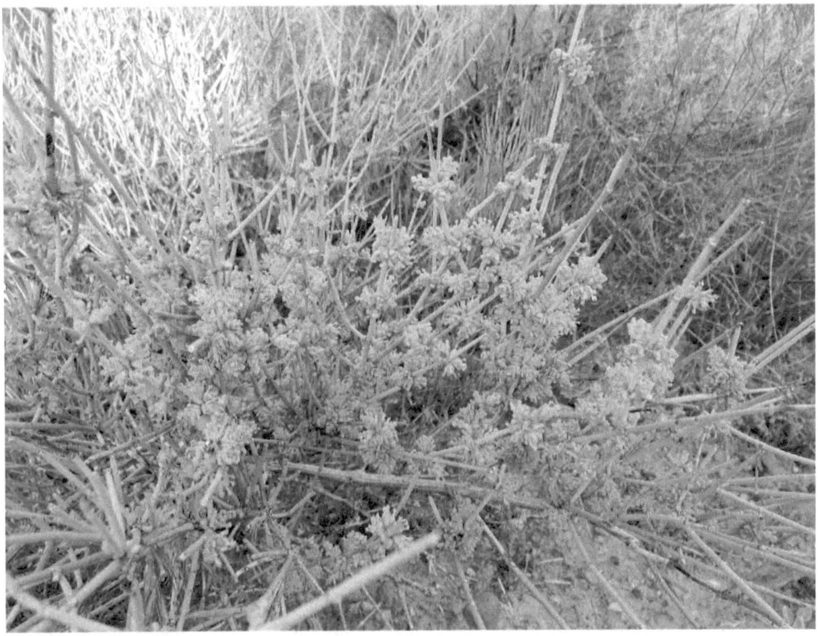

FIGURE 22 *Ephedra nevadensis.*

euphoria. Hyperactivity, irritability, hypertension, rapid heart rate, and nausea are all side effects, with increased danger of stroke or heart attack.

Southwest Natives have used two species of ephedra: *E. nevadensis* and *E. torreyana*. *E. nevadensis* has the common name "Mormon tea." *E. nevadensis* has been alleged to have aphrodisiac properties (hence, its other common name, "whorehouse tea") which may also contribute to its popularity (Morton 1977:36). Southern California Natives have used ephedra, for example, the Cahuilla brew *E. nevadensis* tea known as *tú-tut* (Barrows 1967:73). The Navajo use *E. torreyana*, "torrey joint fir" as an antidiuretic and analgesic (Rätsch 2005:233). Prehistoric evidence of ephedra has been recovered from Caldwell Cave in northern Texas, occupied from approximately 1200 to 1450 CE. Coprolites from Caldwell, as well as stomach contents of a natural mummy, indicate a high level of diarrhea, as well as ephedra pollen and pollen from mesquite or creosote (*Prosopis* spp. and *Larrea* spp.; Holloway 1983). Botanists have identified Native use of mesquite to combat gastrointestinal distress (Curtin 1984:94). A sample of 32 coprolites from Caldwell were analyzed for pollen from medicinal plants, three of which exhibited high levels of ephedra (Sobolik and Gerick 1992). All three were from individuals suffering from diarrhea, which ephedra has been used to treat (Burlage 1968). Similar results were found from coprolites from Baker Cave in Texas, where 15% of coprolites analyzed contained ephedra pollen.

Merlin (2018:80–84) cites several sites with evidence of ephedra. The earliest is from two caves in western Arizona dating as early as 600–900 CE. Ephedra charcoal has been recovered from a Pueblo II period (900–1150 CE) site in Colorado. There is also evidence of ephedra from California—from late prehistoric/historic caves used by the Chumash and from microscopic remains of ephedra on stone pounders. Merlin concludes based on the limited evidence for ephedra that a religious, psychotropic function is plausible.

SUMMARY

Some might question including stimulants in a volume on intoxicants. However, a broad and inclusive definition of "intoxication" is more in keeping with the scientific rather than the vernacular use of the term. Rather than focus on substances that cause "drunkenness" but instead on the intentional ingestion of toxins that create a range of ASCs, it is possible to see a more holistic picture of these ubiquitous social practices. Hyperstimulation is every bit as much an ASC as is a hallucinatory "trip," albeit an ASC of a very different character. Also, viewed globally, a huge proportion of intoxicants consumed across the world have a primarily stimulating effect. The evidence described for cacao, ilex, and ephedra, drawn from ethnography, ethnohistory, and archaeology, show that Native Americans were no different in their widespread use of stimulatory intoxicants.

Our discussion now turns to the idiosyncratic North American use of alcohol.

4 ALCOHOL

BASED ON EXAMPLES PRESENTED IN THE PREVIOUS CHAPTERS, WE CAN say with confidence that the Native use of intoxicants is extensive geographically and has a long history. Prehistoric North Americans were similar to all other prehistoric populations in that respect: they shared a desire for experiencing ASCs through consumption of intoxicants. Seemingly contradicting this trend, however, is a most intriguing pattern—the relative lack of evidence of the most common intoxicant in the rest of the world, alcohol.

There is literature on Native American alcohol use, but research largely evaluates the hypothesis that Native Americans are less able to metabolize ethanol than populations which colonized the Americas from the sixteenth century onwards. This is a matter of ongoing research, with some researchers arguing it is untenable (Saggers and Gray 1998). Alternatively, other researchers argue for a strong genetic component in alcoholism in general and among Native Americans specifically (see discussion in Earle 2014). Attempts have been made to explain modern Native alcohol use as due to contact period use of European beverages to achieve ASCs similar to those achieved through indigenous intoxicants (Smart and Ogborne 1986). There is no real evidence that Native populations ever used European beverages in such a fashion, however:

"There are no ethnographic records of Indigenous people drinking alcohol to achieve religious ends—as the Native American Church did with peyote—on a scale that would explain contemporary patterns of consumption (Saggers and Gray 1998:77). There is very little evidence of precontact use of alcohol at all, despite its Old World ubiquity.

Evidence of alcohol use in the Old World dates as early as the Neolithic in the Near East and Asia and is likely related to the development of farming. There is the question of whether the practice of brewing cereals into fermented beverages was a side effect of farming or a causative factor in the origins of agriculture. Either way, alcohol is one of the most pervasive modern intoxicants, alongside caffeine and nicotine. Some early researchers viewed past use of alcohol as a primitive marker in comparison with civilized society, which only drinks "for the taste and thirst-satisfying qualities of the beverage" (Lippert 1887, quoted in Loeb 1943). While alcohol has potential for abuse, there is reason to argue that the prehistory of alcohol was more culturally constructive.

Alcohol is among the most studied substances humans use to alter perceptions and cognition. Much research focuses on alcohol's role as food, dealing more with its role in consumption and social interaction and less with the specifics of its effects. Dietler (2011:179) observes: "alcohol, as a special form of food with psychoactive effects, has a particularly salient role in ritual because of its transformative properties." Alcohol is first and foremost an intoxicating drug with ritual associations.

Some researchers have posited a distinction between alcohol and other intoxicants, in that alcohol lacks reality-altering properties (Winkelman 1992:186). Rätsch (2005:15n) notes such arguments are ethnocentric, and that shamans have been known to use alcohol: "The effects of alcohol that we are familiar with (ranging from being slightly tipsy to delirium tremens) are thus at least partially conditioned by culture." Rätsch notes that ancient descriptions of ritualized alcohol consumption in the worship of Bacchus/Dionysus indicate a frenzied suspension of reality in the same vein as that experienced by shamans under the influence of hallucinogens. One might add the use of substances whose effect was stimulatory, such as ilex, discussed above. The shamanic and shamanistic practices of North America include a range of distinct ASCs, including those induced by alcohol.

The lack of evidence for intentional fermentation in North America is striking in comparison with the range of alcoholic beverages drunk in Mesoamerica and South America. La Barre (1938) lists numerous beverages made from fermented maize, cacti, succulents, and other plants. Even human urine can be fermented into an intoxicating brew (Greer and Greer 2003:115). Nearly all examples are Mesoamerican or Andean.

The lack of North American evidence has been summarized in a recent article: "The greatest mystery to an archaeologist is the absence of any prehistoric native alcoholic drink . . . north of Mexico (White and Weinstein 2008:254). Many researchers have remarked on the lack of alcoholic beverages in North America (e.g., Core 1967:202). One can go to nearly any part of the globe and find a long history of alcoholic beverages, but in North America, such a tradition is lacking. Alcohol in the New World, north of Mexico, is nearly entirely a postcolumbian phenomenon.

An exception is the use of fermented beverages in the Southwest. Several Southwest and Plains tribes fermented maize and other starchy plants into alcoholic beverages such as *tiswin* (also *tizwin* or *tulpi*). This was observed among the Apache and Pueblo native groups. The beverage is weak in alcohol content and was described by one source as "not much stronger than water" (Robinson 2016). Peyote could be added for a more potent brew (Stewart 1987:4).

The question remains of how early fermented maize can be documented in prehistoric contexts. A 2008 paper compared experimentally produced pottery used to brew maize beer with pottery used by the Tarahumara (Borek et al. 2008). Using dynamic headspace gas chromatography-mass spectrometry (DHGC-MS), they identified similar signatures from the two samples. The same methods were applied to sherds from New Mexico dating to the 1200s CE, identifying a similar chemical signature. While this is evidence of maize beer production in late prehistory, further research in this area is clearly warranted.

Another project focused on vessel use wear. NAN Ranch is a Mimbres site. The site has had other intoxicants ascribed to it, including acacia pollen, the ingestion of which may have had a sedating effect (Pendleton et al. 2003). One room contained metates and large pots, likely a storage and feast preparation area (Shafer 2003:76). Some pots had interior pitting due to maize beer brewing. These were similar to "fiesta pots" used by the Tarahumara (Shafer 2003:124). NAN Ranch dates from 750 to 1130 CE, and the vessels date to the latter half of that range, which makes this among the earliest evidence of brewing north of the Rio Grande.

Agave is another plant fermented in the Southwest, though its prehistoric ancestry is less well understood. Agave has been recovered from Mexico as early as 8000 BCE from caves in Tehuacán (Rätsch 2005:43). Cultivated agave (*Agavea murpheyi*) has been recovered from Hohokam sites in Arizona, and agave is known to have been gathered wild before that. Agave is drought tolerant, grows on marginal land, and produces starch and fibers. Agave sap can be fermented into a weak alcoholic beverage (Minnis 2004:126), which was drunk by Natives of Mexico, where it was known as pulque. Some observations of pulque come from sixteenth-century Spanish writings on the Aztecs. While pulque was used during ritual occasions, Sahagún writes that drunkenness was punishable by death, except for the elderly (Sahagún 1953:2:34). Drunkenness was less proscribed among Gulf Coast groups, where it was commonly featured in rituals (Rätsch 2005:46).

There is ethnographic evidence of fermented pulque in the Southwest where it went by numerous names, such as *tulapai* or *tulpi* among the Apache, who sometimes added datura (La Barre 1938:227, 231). There are observations of agave cultivation from 1613 among Piman Natives living in large pueblos (Dobyns 1988). These sources compare Piman agave fields to vineyards. Ethnographic accounts of pulque brewing exist for several Southwestern cultures, including the Pima, Apache, and Zuni (Castetter et al. 1938). Descriptions show agave being roasted, then pounded, and then buried for several days. The fermented juice would be squeezed out of the mash and allowed to ferment further (Castetter et al. 1938:60–61).

Rätsch (2005:45) notes the Apache used fermented agave in festivals. It is not known whether pulque has significant precontact history in the Southwest, and as with maize beer, agave fermentation north of the Rio Grande should be viewed as the northernmost extension of a Mesoamerican practice. Apache groups have stated that brewing was a recent import from Mesoamerica (Castetter and Opler 1936:51), though accounts indicate the practice goes back to the nineteenth century. Some fermented beverages were reported to be older than others, with agave and mesquite brews being oldest and maize-based beverages youngest.

Historic accounts name other fermented Southwestern plants. *Dasylirion*, or "sotol," a relative of asparagus, has been used to concoct alcoholic beverages in combination with, or independent of, agave (Driver 2011:109; Driver and Massey 1957:266). Sotol fibers have been recovered in Texas dating to approximately 500 CE, though it is unclear if this represents food or intoxicant use. Yucca shrubs (specifically *Yucca baccata*, *Y. macrocarpa*, and *Y. treculeana*) were fermented by the Chiricahua Apache into a drink called *aguardiente* (Spanish for "burning water"). Mesquite beans (*Prosopis juliflora*) were fermented along the Colorado and Gila Rivers (Havard 1896:37). The Yuma made a beverage termed *pissioina* from fermented wheat as a postcontact invention (Hrdlička 1908:28; La Barre 1938).

An early nineteenth-century observer in California described mesquite fermentation. After being accosted by an intoxicated Native woman, Hardy (1829:337) observed the cause of her drunkenness:

> I afterwards examined this mixture, and found it to be the pod of the Mesquite-tree steeped in water. It is naturally very saccharine, and from its sour smell, must have undergone fermentation. The inhabitants of the island of Tiburow [Tiburón] have the same dirty practice. The pods in this state last for months, with the addition, occasionally, of a few fresh ones; and each goes to it in his turn, with as much pleasure as sailors to their quid of tobacco!

Other related plants have ethnohistoric references to being fermented, for example, screwbean, also known as screwbean mesquite or *Prosopis pubescens*. This particular species was fermented by Natives along the Colorado River (Bell and Castetter 1937:33).

While these anecdotes are interesting, they do not indicate that the practice of mesquite fermentation had much antiquity, as Natives had been in contact with Europeans by that point and could have learned of fermentation recently. Alternatively, Natives of Baja and Tiburón could have been adapting Mexican practices to local starchy plants.

Several groups in Arizona and northern Mexico, including the Akimel O'odham, Maricopa, and Tohono O'odham, made beverages from fermented saguaro cactus (*Cereus giganteus*) of the Sonoran Desert. This species contains several compounds similar to those found in peyote. Gigantine has hallucinogenic properties, and dopamine has been detected in saguaroas well (Furst 1976:111n).

A member of the 1540–1542 Coronado expedition notes saguaro fermentation as follows: "They drink wine made of the pitahaya which is the fruit of a thistle which opens like the pomegranate. The wine makes them stupid" (Winship 1896:516). Few details beyond this are offered, but this provides plausibility for precontact saguaro fermentation. Over two centuries later, a Spanish priest observed saguaro intoxication on the occasion of Akimel O'odham in California welcoming his arrival (Coues 1900:438–440):

> This extravagant shouting, a thing foreign to the seriousness of the Pimas, I knew came from drinking, which produced various effects. Some came and took me by the hand, saluting me.... Others made the sign of the cross, so that though I felt very angry at such

> general drunkenness, there did not fail me some gusto to hear the good expressions into which they burst, even when deprived of reason.

Upon complaining of what seemed an ungodly display, he was chastised by the local leader:

> [He] told me that it only happened a few times and in the season of saguaro, and adding that it made his people vomit yellow and kept them in good health.

His last observation provides a gendered view on the practice:

> What most pleased me was to see that no woman got drunk; instead of which I saw many of them leading by the bridle the horse upon which her husband was mounted, gathering up at the same time the clothes and beads that the men scattered about, in order that none should be lost.

Much remaining evidence is more recent. Fermented saguaro among the Tohono O'odham played a role in rain magic. Castetter and Bell (1937:12) put this in a seasonal context:

> These Indians returned from the [winter camp] in late June or early July to pick the ripe sahuaro fruit which they carried to their summer villages for their great yearly ceremony. This was held just before the rainy season and at this time the fruit was fermented and drunk, accompanied by dancing, singing, and oratory. Although the Papago year contained numerous ceremonies, the most important was, and is, this great drinking ceremony which brought the rain and initiated the Papago calendar year.

Driver (2011:110) cites the underlying rationale for the ritual, stating: "Everyone drank, believing that as men saturated themselves with liquor so the earth would be saturated with rain." Castetter and Bell (1937:24–25) provide several late nineteenth- and early twentieth-century observations of saguaro intoxication among Tohono O'odham, Akimel O'odham, and Apache. In most cases, it is described as a seasonal activity. One observation of the Akimel O'odham notes "drinking of [saguaro] made their New Year's season one of debauchery."

Underhill (1936, quoted in La Barre 1938:232) quotes a Tohono O'odham informant:

> "Much, much liquor we made," said a Papago woman, "and we drank it to pull down the clouds." In its preparation the men dance in a great circle around a fire, following a leader with a rattle, and later the women join them so that men and women alternate in the circle. Thus they dance and sing for two nights, while the medicine men make magic with strings of eagle feathers and sprinkle the dancers with eagle down, which symbolizes clouds. Next the liquor is strained through baskets and a gourd is passed around until all the liquor in

> the council house is consumed. Then they visit from house to house and drink the liquor which each woman has brewed and buried in the ground with the injunction, "Do you ferment and let us get beautifully drunk." No family may drink its own liquor lest the house burn down, but they drink at other houses, vomit, and go on to visit others and sing songs.

Saguaro wine plays a significant role for the Akimel O'odham, Maricopa, and Yuma:

> It is upon [saguaro] liquor that the Pimos, Maricopas, and Yumas get drunk once a year, the revelry continuing for a week or two at a time; but it is also a custom with them to take regular turns so that only one-third of the party is supposed to indulge at a time, the remainder being required to take care of their stimulated comrades and protect them from injuring each other or being injured by other tribes [Havard 1896:36, citing one Col. Cremony].

Other cacti were also fermented by the Southwest Natives. *Stenocereus thurberi*, the organ pipe cactus, was fermented and drunk by many of the same Native groups that fermented saguaro. It was used alongside or in place of saguaro in the southern part of Tohono O'odham territory, as well as by Native groups in Sonora.

La Barre (1938:233) and Havard (1896:35) state that there is little historic evidence of fermentation, of any plant, among the pueblo-dwelling tribes, despite their long history of settled agriculture. While residue and pottery analysis cited previously points to the fermentation of maize beverages, it is possible that this practice was attenuated in late prehistory or during the contact period. Havard (1896:37) attributes this to a geographic and historical accident:

> It appears that the only United States Indians preparing these liquors were those of our southwestern border. The most obvious reason for this geographical peculiarity is that these Indians have always had relations with the Mexican natives and were visited at a very early date by white men; thus Arizona and New Mexico were pretty thoroughly explored by Spaniards before Hudson entered the Bay of New York or the May Flower landed at Plymouth Rock.

La Barre attributes the lack of evidence for alcohol to the structure of Puebloan religion:

> The heavily institutionalized and ritualized religions of the pueblos evidently found little place in them for such orgiastic experiences as the California datura-intoxication, the Yuman alcoholic or dreamed vision, or the individualistic Plains peyote-vision (La Barre 1938:234).

The evidence from NAN Ranch and other Southwestern sites of Ancestral Puebloan peoples would seem to contradict this narrative. Spanish suppression of Native religious practices is a more likely cause of the absence of contact-period drinking. As sedentary people, Pueblo groups such as the Navajo or Hopi were far easier to regulate than their more mobile neighbors.

When considering evidence for alcohol in the Southwest, it is important not to let one's biases color interpretations. Alcohol is the dominant intoxicant in modern, Western society, and it is tempting to view Native use as having similar meanings. It is equally possible that alcohol's intoxicating properties were secondary. Much of the alcohol produced today is not consumed but used as fuel or as solvent. This characteristic was surely of value to Natives. Alcohol is an effective solvent, and many intoxicant compounds dissolve in it. Previous chapters mentioned how red bean, peyote, or datura could be added to corn beer or pulque. Natives intentionally used the solvent properties of alcoholic beverages to extract and ingest these more powerful intoxicants.

This would have several benefits. Alcohol would suppress harmful microbes. Also, only compounds soluble in alcohol and water would be extracted, which could remove less desirable substances, reducing side effects. Most significantly, this would allow for more precise dose control. Active compounds in many intoxicants are unevenly distributed in the tissues in which they are found and can vary between specimens. Making a tea or infusion averages out these differences and reduces the likelihood of an overdose. While that is less important with peyote or hallucinogenic mushrooms, with red bean or datura, dose control is a matter of life and death.

While research on Southwest maize beer is the best prehistoric and historic evidence of Native alcohol use, there are accounts of the use of fermented beverages in other regions. McGovern (2009:227) mentions berry wines along the Northwest Coast. John Smith allegedly recorded fermented persimmons and hickory nuts in Virginia (Core 1967:202; Driver and Massey 1957:268), though references to Smith's observations are brief and unsourced. Smith's 1624 volume does not mention fermenting persimmons or hickory, though it does refer to Native grapes and of their utility for wine making. These passages refer to English settlers making wine from Native grapes, not Native wine making. Persimmons do grow in Europe, so it is plausible but unproven that Smith had observed their use there.

Some seventeenth-century observations of fermented beverages are recorded by Smith (Smith 1630). For example:

> For their Feasts, they have all sorts of Beasts, Birds, Fish, Fruits, and Herbs they can get, but the more variety of wild ones is the best; to which they have excellent Drink made of Rice, Millet, and Honey, like Wine.

This sounds more like a beer or a mead than a fruit-based wine. Smith (1630) also notes:

> Though the Ground be fertile, they sow little Corn, yet the Gentlemen have Bread and Hony-wine; Grapes they have plenty and Wine privately.

There are no details on the fruit the wine was made from, no discussion of fermentation practices, no reference to the social contexts in which it was drunk (tobacco was referenced nearly 20 times in the same volume). Other references relate to European beverages.

Beverley's 1705 volume, which references Smith's work, in addition to not including references to fermentation, includes the following passage:

> Among all this variety of Food, Nature hath not taught them the use of any other Drink than Water; which tho they have in cool and pleasant Springs every where, yet they will not drink that, if they can get Pond Water, or such as has been warm'd by the Sun and Weather. Baron Lahontan tells of a sweet juice of Maple, which the Indians to the Northward gave him, mingl'd with Water; but our Indians use no such Drink. For their Strong drink, they are altogether beholding to us, and are so greedy of it, that most of them will be drunk as often as they find an opportunity; notwithstanding which, it is a prevailing humour among them, not to taste any Strong drink at all, unless they can get enough to make them quite drunk, and then they go as solemnly about it, as if it were part of their Religion (Beverley 1855:140).

This contradicts any tradition of fermentation, though it does not rule out the possibility of small-scale fermentation. It would be odd, if fermentation was a common practice, that there was no attempt to ferment maize, which would have been available in far greater quantities and could have provided greater volumes of alcohol.

In the Southeast, there are anecdotes regarding the ilex black drink (see Chapter 3). These suggest the beverage was occasionally allowed to ferment and then drunk for intoxicating effect. This is plausible, for if the beverage was stored, natural fermentation would be expected, though probably not to the degree for sugar-rich fruit or starchy plants. That said, there is no ethnohistoric support, nor has the issue been explored archaeologically.

Evidence of precontact fermentation seems to be similarly absent in the Northeast. Sagard, echoing Beverley's writing, wrote in 1636:

> Our savages, in their feasts, are, thank God, free from such misfortune, for they use neither wine, beer nor cider; if any one among them asks for a drink, which very rarely happens, he is offered fresh water, not in a glass, but in a dipper or off the kettle itself from which he freely drinks and is thus saved from drunkenness, a great blessing to the body and

> soul, for it is likely that if they had wine they would become as intemperate as ourselves [quoted in Havard 1896:33].

Carr (1947) cites eighteenth-century accounts of persimmon wine, but these are of English wine making. Carr cites accounts of Southwest mesquite and corn beer, for which there is ethnohistoric support, as if these support his arguments regarding fermentation in the East, for which he marshals only anecdotes. He cites Native informants from the Catawba, Cherokee, and Rappahannock, attesting to persimmon fermentation, but the earliest is from the 1920s. This is not to say these observations are untrue, only that they are not evidence of a long-standing, precolumbian tradition of fermented beverages in the Eastern Woodlands. The more plausible interpretation is that Natives adopted the practice during or after the contact period.

Available explanations for the absence of fermentation in North America lack plausibility. Suggestions that tobacco replaced earlier alcohol in the Americas is speculative and archaeologically unsupported. It is unlikely that environmental yeast sufficient for fermentation would be absent across the entire continent. The dominance of tobacco as the primary intoxicant is a likely factor (McGovern 2009:228), yet we see alcohol in Mesoamerica and South America alongside tobacco. It is possible the late adoption of maize in North America played a role, leaving centuries for tobacco to dominate. However, evidence from Mesoamerica points to fermentation being one of the first practices associated with maize domestication, if not the cause of domestication in the first place (Smalley and Blake 2003). McGovern (2009:229) noted Northwest Asia is lacking in fermentable substances, so ancestral Native populations may have lost the tradition, resorting to hallucinogenic mushrooms and rediscovering the practice in Mexico and South America millennia later.

Another possible reason for the lack of indigenous fermentation has to do with the cultural context in which fermentation typically develops. Fermentation is closely tied to food production. While hunter-gatherers take advantage of natural fermentation in fruits or other sugar-rich resources, there is little ethnographic evidence of hunter-gatherers engaging in large-scale fermentation. The fermentation of large amounts of cereals historically co-occurs with domestication of those plants and the adoption of agriculture. This is not to say that "only farmers drink," but there is a correlation between farming and fermentation.

The only region in North America with significant evidence of fermentation is the Southwest, which is also the area that has been farming maize for the longest. For most of North America, maize farming has a history of less than two and a half thousand years, and even following the development of sedentary farming villages, foraging for wild plants was never fully abandoned. Perhaps, given time, the practice would have taken root beyond the Southwest. But the late onset of farming, as well as the presence of a reliable alternative in tobacco, prevented this from happening. It is to this dominating intoxicant, tobacco, we now turn.

5 TOBACCO

> Smoked tobacco . . . mediates domains of existence and facilitates relations with others, traversing borders and acting as a broker, in the same way in which the shaman does [Rahman 2015:348].

TOBACCO IN NATIVE NORTH AMERICA

This quote summarizes tobacco's significance in Native America, historically and prehistorically. At contact, tobacco was the most widespread Native American intoxicant (Moerman 1998), with a wider distribution than maize. Paper (1992:163) writes: "the ritual use of tobacco is unique to aboriginal America as well as pervasive." Tobacco was commonly remarked upon by early explorers and was a focus of early ethnographers (e.g., Linton 1924b).

Only the extreme northern and southern latitudes do not have evidence of tobacco. Tobacco in the arctic was acquired from southern neighbors or European or West Asian sources. Tobacco did not play a major role in arctic shamanism, another indicator that tobacco was recent, in that it had not integrated into religious practices. Tobacco was more significant among subarctic Athabascans and Algonquians in Canada and Alaska but was only available by trade.

Tobacco was hugely significant in the Eastern Woodlands. Winter (2000b:16) notes that Iroquoian cultures "depend on [tobacco] for their very spiritual and cultural survival." The Khionontateron, named "Petun" by the French, after the Brazilian term for tobacco, were major suppliers to surrounding tribes. While

Iroquoian and Algonquian speakers are distinct cultures, both share reverence for tobacco. When the Huron speak of desire for tobacco, they use the same verb for the desire for food, water, urination, or other physical needs; different verbs are used for things that are "optional" while tobacco is fundamental (Steckley 1985:15). Hamell (1987:77) places tobacco in a category of sacred substances in Iroquoian culture which: "gave assurance of physical, spiritual, and social well-being, of long life through spiritual resuscitation and success, especially in the conceptually related activities of courtship, hunting, and warfare."

Few Great Plains tribes cultivated tobacco as most of the region is too arid. Winter (2000b:20) writes:

> Most plains tribes had to obtain tobacco indirectly, through trading expeditions, raids, and other means, from the Crow and other tobacco-growing Plains Indians or from Mexican settlers and pueblo Indians in the Southwest, who grow and gather several tobacco species.

Groups such as the Crow, Hidatsa, Mandan, and Arikara were exceptions, growing so much they supplied neighboring groups. *N. quadrivalvis* (see below for details on species) was a valued trade good, as its cultivation was limited to the upper Missouri River. Setchel (1923) shows the Great Plains divided between west/central Plains, where wild *N. attenuata* was gathered, with the Natives of the eastern Plains growing *N. rustica*. Adair (2000:172) argues most of the Plains are unfavorable to *N. attenuata* and Setchel's map should be used with caution.

Tobacco is central to Plains religious rituals, be they long-standing traditional practices or newly introduced, such as peyote rituals. Plains Natives so venerate tobacco that smoking pipes became one of their most potent symbolic items: the calumet. The significance and implications of calumet pipes are discussed later in this chapter.

Tobacco was absent in southern British Columbia until the 1200s and absent in Alaska and coastal British Columbia until the historic period (Keddie 2016:157). In other Northwest Coast cultures, such as the Haida or Tlingit, tobacco was cultivated and chewed with lime. There was speculation that a different plant was chewed, but historic documentation indicates tobacco (Heizer 1940). Winter (2000b:26) notes it is remarkable that Northwest Coast Natives cultivated tobacco, given their diet was dominated by marine resources, with little cultivation. Lime is alkaline and may help release nicotine and aid nicotine absorption. Thompson and Pluckhahn (2018:134) argue that lime was used in smoking pipes as well. Tobacco may have been given to Drake by Northwest Coast Natives in 1574 (McGuire 1899:423).

Tobacco use in California is complex due to a diverse cultural landscape. Winter (2000b:28–37) breaks the region into seven subregions. Native tobacco species are significant throughout, featuring in Native religion, ritual, and myth. These are mostly foraging peoples who would still grow or trade tobacco, which they would ingest using a range of means (smoking, snuffing, chewing, drinking, etc.). Complicating the role of tobacco in Californian religious practices is the role of datura, especially among southern populations discussed in Chapter 1.

A similar situation held in the Great Basin, though tobacco was more significant than datura. Natives pruned or weeded wild species, dispersed seeds, and set fires to encourage new growth (Adams and Toll 2000:144–145). Winter (2000b:41) indicates the medicinal importance of tobacco was emphasized in the region:

> Tobacco in all of its forms was used for numerous medicinal purposes and was recognized as an extremely potent magical force—so much so that the supernatural beings were afraid of it.... It was also employed for many other reasons, including infanticide and suicide (by overdosing) and killing rattlesnakes with the plant's spiritual power.

The Southwest has a tobacco tradition similar to the Eastern Woodlands:

> Indeed, it is possible that the diverse species utilized, with their long archaeological record, represent one of the oldest tobacco-growing and tobacco-gathering complexes on the continent, with roots that reach back to well before the arrival of cultivated food plants in the region [Winter 2000b:41].

Nearly all Southwest cultures cultivated tobacco, and many gathered wild species. Tobacco shamanism, in some cases incorporating datura, is characteristic of less settled groups in the northern Southwest, tobacco farming key among Pueblo cultures. Tobacco features in Pueblo religious rituals, such as the Navajo "blessing way."

Tobacco still plays a role in Native American religious life. Hultkranz (1997:10) states: "It is ... obvious that indulging in tobacco (*Nicotiana rustica*) afforded such subjective experiences that they could be interpreted within a religious framework." Furst (1976:23) summarizes the role that tobacco plays in Native spirituality:

> In much of the traditional Indian world tobacco was and still is considered to be the special gift of the gods to humanity, given to assist mankind in bridging the gulf between "this" world and "the other"—the world of the gods themselves. In many cases this view involved employing tobacco to attain precisely the kinds of mystical states, or the characteristically shamanistic ecstatic trance, that we commonly associate only with the better recognized vegetal hallucinogens.

TOBACCO SPECIES

Tobacco belongs to the genus *Nicotiana*, comprising 95 species—in the Americas (74 species), Africa (one species), and Australia (20 species; Winter 2000c:90). Most are native to South America, likely the genus origin. Several grow in Western North America. Some early twentieth-century authors suggested, based on linguistic evidence, that tobacco was introduced by enslaved Africans, but data show there are numerous native species (Setchel 1923). The original range of North American tobacco is difficult to ascertain due to human range extension (Tushingham and Eerkens 2016:218). Relations between native species are difficult to assess due to artificial selection. What follows is a summary of indigenous species, their ranges, and their cultural associations with Native peoples.

Nicotiana attenuata, "coyote tobacco," is native to Western North America and was used medicinally and ceremonially in several tribes, including the Hopi (Fewkes 1896:19), Navajo (Elmore 1944:75), Zuni (Setchel 1923), Apache (Reagan 1929:158), Akimel O'odham, Paiute, Shoshone (Train et al. 1941), and Blackfoot (Johnston 1970:319). Winter (2000c:114) notes it is the most widely used wild tobacco. Among the Hopi it was rarely inhaled but used to create smoke to bring rain or carry prayers. Hopi folklore contains stories of ordeals where characters inhale smoke in contest with a spirit (Malotki and Gary 2001:xxxviii).

An early sample of *N. attenuata* was recovered from a site near Tucson. Adams and Toll (2000:152) cite a date range of between 398 and 169 BCE, which until recently was the oldest botanical North American tobacco date. This species becomes widespread in the Southwest in the third century CE and was ubiquitous by the Basketmaker and Pueblo periods. Adams and Toll (2000:154–155) list 30 sites prior to 750 CE that contain *N. attenuata* remains.

N. attenuata's range extends as far as British Columbia and Montana. It was typically smoked in corn-husk cigarettes. Brandt (2000) notes Natives at Zuni pueblo distinguish between coyote and commercial tobaccos. Coyote tobacco was gathered and smoked by men for ritual occasions. As mentioned in Chapter 1, a ninth-century CE Arizona village yielded coyote tobacco in association with pipes and datura seeds (Sebastian 1985:172). This is currently the earliest association of the two plants, predating Mississippian examples by several centuries.

Nicotiana clevelandii, "Cleveland's tobacco" grows in the Sonoran and Coloradan Deserts, and was used by the Cahuilla (Bean and Saubel 1972:90). In

Cahuilla mythology, a man transformed into the first tobacco; he then serves as go-between for people and gods (Godlaski 2013:2–3). Cleveland's tobacco was used in Baja California, Southern California, and southwestern Arizona, but is not used anymore north of Mexico. Hammett (2000:132) notes *N. clevelandii* has been identified at coastal Californian shell middens.

Another wild tobacco is *N. glauca*, known as "tree tobacco," due to the height (10 m) to which it can grow. Of recent South American origin, it lacks nicotine, containing only the similar but less intoxicating compound anabasine (Winter 2000a:8). It has been used among the Chumash, and Winter (2000c:122) claims it was recovered from late prehistoric sites on the Channel Islands. Goodspeed (1954), however, considered it of recent, Mexican origin.

Nicotiana obtusifolia, also termed *N. trigonophylla* or "desert tobacco," grows in deserts throughout the Southwest and was used by the Cahuilla (Bean and Saubel 1972:90), Havasupai (Weber and Seaman 1985:240), Hopi (Whiting 1939:90), Tohono O'odham and Akimel O'odham (Castetter and Bell 1942; Castetter and Underhill 1935), Navajo (Elmore 1944:75), and Yuma (Castetter and Bell 1951). The Navajo are reported to smoke and use as incense *N. palmeri*, "sleeping tobacco," but few references are available (Rätsch 2005:390). Winter (2000a:7) refers to it as "coyote's tobacco" though that term is applied to *N. attenuata*. Winter (2000c:125) cites evidence from sites dating between 950 and 1200 CE in southern Arizona. Winter also notes that while *N. obtusifolia*/*N. trigonophylla* overlaps range with *N. attenuata*, Natives preferred *N. attenuata* due to a more palatable taste and higher nicotine content.

Nicotiana quadrivalvis is native to the West Coast where it is known as "Indian tobacco," a term more often applied to *N. rustica*. This designation replaces older nomenclature, including formerly distinct species (including the often-cited *N. bigelovii* and *N. multivalvis*) in one taxon, though one can still find references to the older designations (Winter 2000c:115). Variation within the species has contributed to this confusion. There are four major varieties (Hammett 2000:128) that diverge from the original variety as one moves north and east within its modern range.

N. quadrivalvis is found throughout California, Oregon, and Washington State, and southern British Columbia. Winter (2000c:119) depicts this species along major rivers of the Great Basin and Great Plains as far east as the Middle Missouri River. Two varieties (*N. quadrivalvis* var. *quadrivalvis* and var. *multivalvis*) no longer self-seed and are functionally domesticated (Hammett 2000:129).

N. quadrivalvis was used by several California tribes including the Costanoan (Bocek 1984), Chumash (Timbrook 1990), Karok (Schenck and Gifford 1952), Kawaiisu (Zigmond 1980, 1981), Miwok and Midoo (Setchel 1923), Kashaya (Goodrich and Lawson 1980), and Tolowa (Baker 1981). This species was traded and cultivated beyond its native range and was used as far as southern Alaska (Keddie 2016:170); it is unable to propagate naturally in these regions which are far colder than its origin. *N. quadrivalvis* has been described as the most potent native North American species, capable of rendering a smoker unconscious (Rätsch 2005:390), though it likely falls below *N. rustica* in intoxicating potential. Zigmond (1981:43) notes it was seen as stronger than *N. attenuata* in the region. Male and female Kawaiisu chewed *N. quadrivalvis*, but only men smoked it. The plant is the only one the Kawaiisu tended, and in Kawaiisu origin myths, it was one of the First Medicines. A Spanish priest traveling in California in 1776 recorded the effect of ingesting lime and *N. quadrivalvis*:

> My companions the [Mohave] having tried it were attacked at once with vomitings so violent that I thought one of them would die, which those of the Rancheria greeted with great laughter. . . . I have been abel to ascertain that they drink this sort of gruel to cure fatigue and consequently it is customary to offer it to all their guest [Zigmond 1981:45].

Zigmond (1980:1999) describes hallucinations associated with *N. quadrivalvis*; they were described as akin to the buzzing of bees. Adair (2000:183) notes the nicotine concentration of *N. quadrivalvis* was low; this may be due to geographic variation in a heterogenous species.

Drake observed Natives smoking *N. quadrivalvis* in 1579, and it was observed by Lewis and Clark, who remarked on the distinctiveness of Plains tobacco in comparison with that in the East (Adair 2000:175). The Crow consider it so sacred they do not smoke it, but simply grow it, as consumption is too profane for food for spirits (Winter 2000c:120). Winter (2000e:326) proposes wild tobaccos (*N. attenuata, N. quadrivalvis*, etc.) are derived from species that date to the Pliocene, and these species were encountered by Natives during the late Pleistocene. Domesticated tobaccos (*N. rustica, N. tabacum*) are later developments associated with food production in the mid-to-late Holocene.

All varieties of tobacco have been propagated through population movements and exchange. This propensity to trade tobacco has led to questionable interpretations. One of the most implausible assertions involved residue analysis of Egyptian mummies (Balabanova 1993; Balabanova et al. 1992). This analysis supposedly identified nicotine and cocaine dating prior to precolumbian Egyptian contexts. This was criticized as due to contamination (Bjorn 1993;

Schafer 1993). The researchers have maintained that their results are accurate (Balabanova et al. 1995, 1997) with little support.

Early researchers (e.g., Dixon 1933; White 1942) concluded tobacco in Western North America was recent, within the past six hundred years. Tobacco was thought to postdate 1000 CE in the East and have been adopted during the historic period in the West (e.g., Ford 1981, 1985). Researchers (e.g., de Rios 1984) have shown indigenous tobacco species have a long history, predating food crops. Wilbert (1994:47) writes:

> A . . . good argument can be made that the discovery of hallucinogenic potential of different species, including various Solanaceae other than the nicotianas, owes nothing to agriculture, and that the shamans of archaic hunter-gatherer peoples—who as we know, relied as heavily, if not more heavily, on the vegetable kingdom for sustenance as they did on game—could have consciously searched the environment for the plant allies used to this day.

Winter (2000b) argued tobacco not only predates maize and beans but also preadapted Native North Americans to farming. Early tobacco horticulture could have provided a foundation for later farming. Furst (1976:27) noted tobacco's "spectacular aboriginal distribution" as well as the "striking similarity of tobacco ideology" suggested a deep history for tobacco, and that there was evidence of tobacco preceding domesticated crops: "There is no reason of course why the first cultigens should not have been intended to feed the spirit rather than the stomach." Early migrants may have brought with them a propensity for intoxicants and adapted to local plants, primarily tobacco. Questions remain about the timing by which tobacco species spread. Conventional wisdom was that *N. rustica* spread north from South America, into Mexico, and then north and east (Wagner 2000:185). Western indigenous species were ultimately overshadowed by *N. rustica*, though some indigenous species were traded as far as the Mississippi River valley.

Smoking pipes in the Eastern Woodlands predate maize, and some of the earliest pipes were used to smoke tobacco. While some have assumed early pipes were used to smoke *N. rustica* (Rafferty 2002, 2006), pending botanical evidence, this cannot be assumed. Pauketat and colleagues (2002) identified *N. quadrivalvis* (not *N. rustica*) at Cahokia between 1040 and 1100 CE, and Haberman (1984) identified *N. quadrivalvis* in the Middle Missouri at 1000 CE. Previous discoveries of tobacco at contemporary sites have been published, perhaps erroneously, as *N. rustica* (see for example, Johannessen 1984; Parker 1992).

This indicates that western tobaccos were traded east, where they were exotic in comparison with *N. rustica*. We see several centers of tobacco use, both foreign and native, interacting across the continent (Winter 2000e:306). We know Natives in other regions with access to indigenous tobacco would trade for exotic species, as was observed in California (Davis 1961). Tushingham and Eerkens (2016:213) propose western tobacco in the Eastern Woodlands was replaced by *N. rustica*.

Modern commercial tobacco is *N. tabacum*, distinct from *N. rustica* (Goodspeed 1954; Winter 2000c:88). This is a hybrid of South American species, cultivated for a lower nicotine level than *N. rustica*, likely itself an older South American hybrid (Winter 2000c:103). *N. tabacum* is adapted to a tropical environment, while *N. rustica* is adapted to a cooler, dryer environment (Heister 1992:55). *N. tabacum* flourished in the Caribbean and Southeast, while *N. rustica* dominated the Northeast and eastern Plains.

Wilbert (1995:97) notes: "The principal species of tobacco utilized in the Indian Americas, *Nicotiana rustica* and *N. tabacum*, are cultivated hybrids and thus represent the end products of long processes of experimentation." There is one identification of *N. tabacum* from North America, north of Mexico and outside of the Caribbean, from Double Butte Cave, where Haury identified cane cigarettes as *N. tabacum*. Winter (2000c:96) argues this was "questionable and probably unfounded."

Selective breeding of *N. tabacum* created a milder, less intoxicating drug than *N. rustica*. *N. tabacum* diffused to the Caribbean via the Amazon and was observed by Columbus and later explorers of the region. Europeans found it more palatable than N. rustica, found to be "poore and weake and of a byting taste" by comparison (Winter 2000c:96). *N. tabacum* was introduced into Eastern North America by the early seventeenth century (Winter 2000c:93). *N. tabacum*, "Virginia tobacco," was exported to the Old World (Goodman 1995). French contact with Natives in the northeastern Great Plains during the 1700s may have introduced *N. tabacum* (Adair 2000:174), but this has not been demonstrated. *N. tabacum* was identified historically among the Omaha; their oral history suggests they previously cultivated *N. quadrivalvis* (Gilmore 1913).

Winter (2000e:326) writes:

> The domestication of tobacco and its widespread use by Native Americans has had profound effects upon the rest of the world. Previously used by Indians primarily as an offering and a way to communicate with the spirit world, tobacco is now ingested as a recreational, addictive drug all around the planet, with enormous economic and medical consequences.

N. rustica is sometimes referred to as "Indian tobacco" and is observed in too many North American tribes to cite. Native selection created numerous

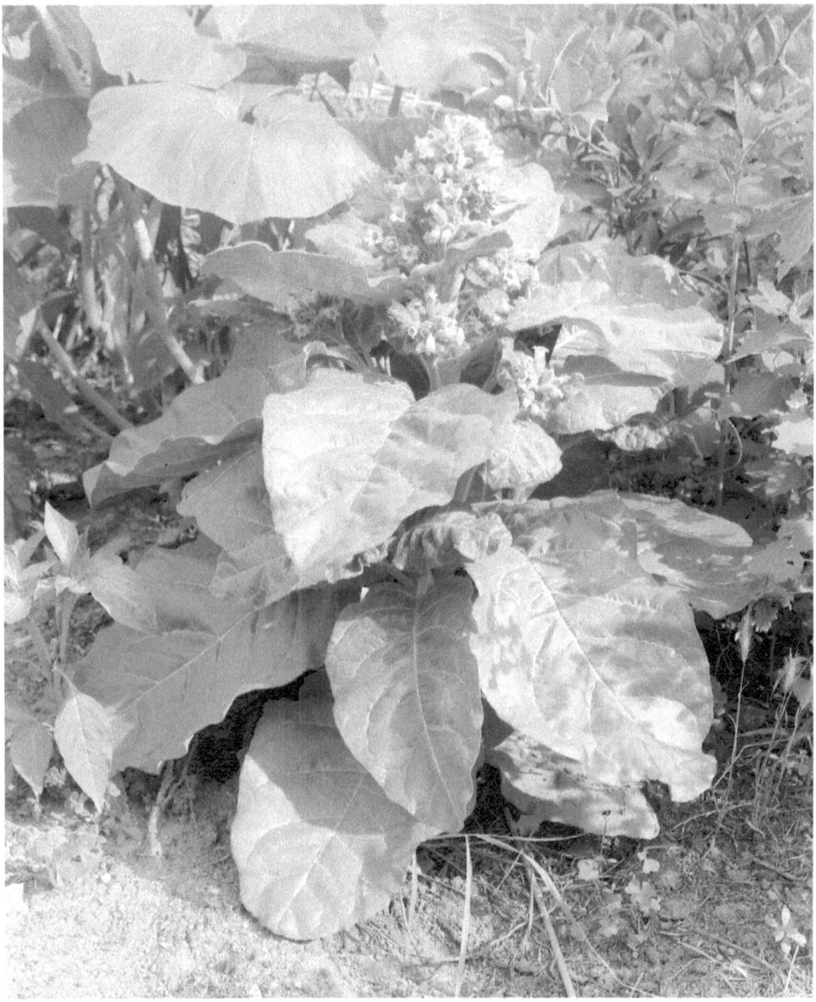

FIGURE 23 *Nicotiana rustica* Tobacco.

subspecies. Winter (2000c:103) notes three varieties in the Rio Grande Valley alone. *N. rustica* has one of the highest nicotine contents, up to 18.5% (the average ranges from 1.8% to 4%), compared with *N. tabacum*, which is generally 1.5% nicotine (Winter 2000e:307). Adams and Toll (2000:143) state:

> Nicotiana is composed largely of pioneer species that occupy coarse soils in disturbed sites. ... Tobacco plants are highly adapted to move into recently opened habitats through their enormous production of minute seeds that are dispersed by wind, water, and animals.

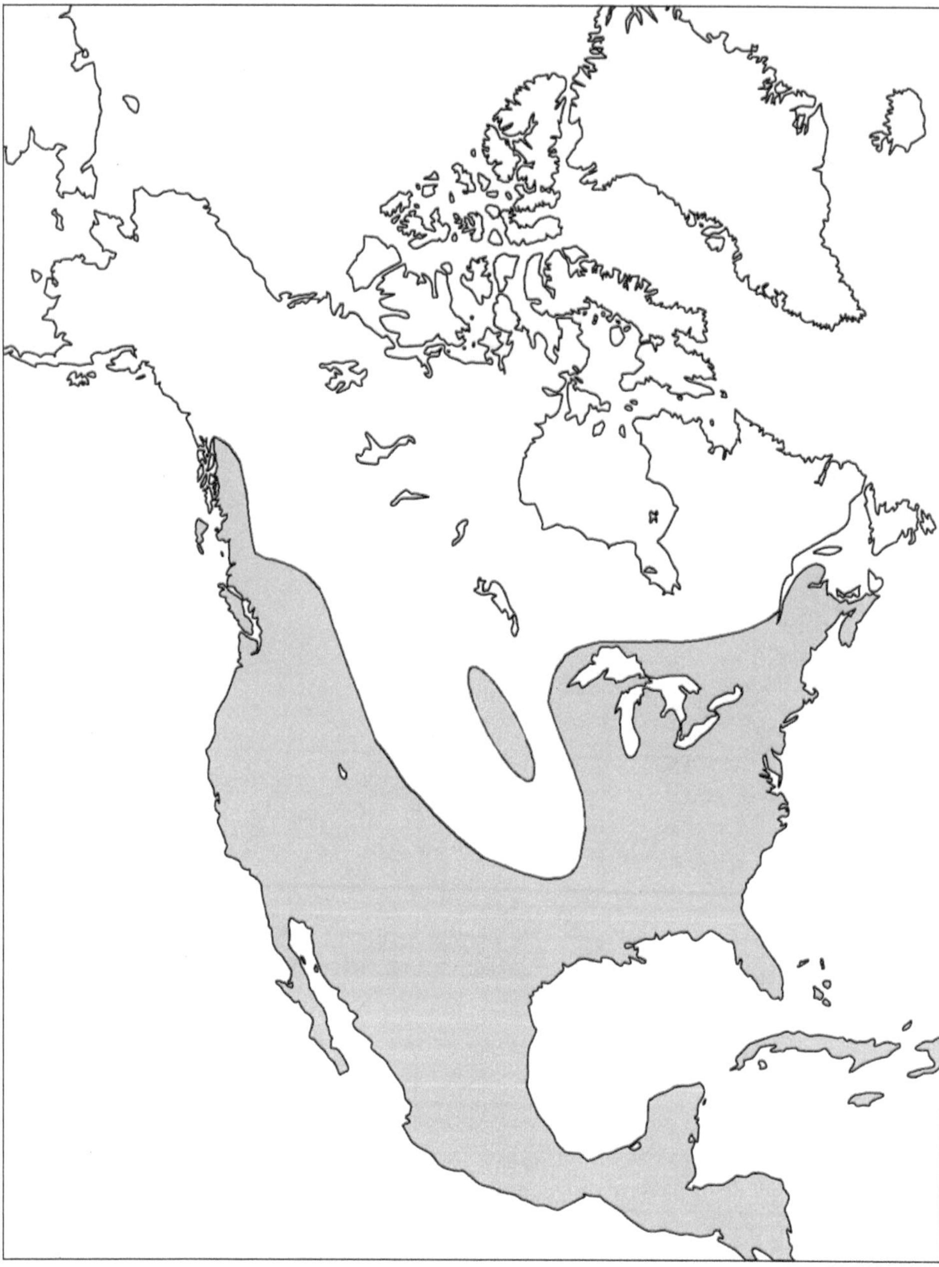

FIGURE 24 Range of Native and Foreign Tobacco Species. (Author's map.)

This means humans and tobacco were inevitably going to come into proximity since the plants were preadapted to human sites, and humans were preadapted for intoxicants.

ARCHAEOLOGICAL EVIDENCE OF TOBACCO

In 2016, reports were circulated of a Paleoindian campsite 12,300 years in age in Utah (Duke et al. 2018). The Wishbone site contained what was reported as tobacco seeds, comprising not only the oldest evidence of tobacco, but some of the oldest evidence of prehistoric intoxicants anywhere. Communication with one of the researchers indicate that the seeds were burned, found in a well-defined and intact cultural soil feature, with well-associated radiocarbon dates (personal communication, D. Duke, March 31, 2019). This argues for the accuracy of the finding, which has significant implications for North American tobacco use.

Paleoindian populations migrated from Siberia through Alaska and Canada. *N. obtusifolia* grows wild in Utah but is adapted to a desert climate; and Utah would have been wetter during the Pleistocene, so species such as *N. quadrivalvis* are more likely. It is unlikely any *Nicotiana* species were available in Siberia or northern Canada. Even though migrating populations likely possessed a shamanistic world view, they would have moved away from traditional intoxicants. This evidence implies these populations adopted local intoxicants in the more temperate Great Basin. This corresponds with Von Gernet (1992) and Winter (2000d:265) who proposed a migration by Siberians leaving behind traditional intoxicants and adopting tobacco.

Winter (2000e:314–315) writes:

> When the earliest hunters and gatherers arrived in the New World from Asia, they already possessed a set of magical and medicinal practices that used plants by drinking, smoking and otherwise ingesting their chemical powers. As the paleo-Indians slowly moved south . . . they encountered other psychotropic plants, including the various wild species of tobacco. . . . As they came increasingly to depend on tobacco . . . they developed tobacco shamanism and other religious rites organized around large-scale ingestion of nicotine.

This contradicts research (e.g., Ford 1985:343–344; Wilbert 1987:149–150; Yarnell 1964:85) that tobacco developed with agriculture and that other plants were smoked earlier (Winter 2000e:312).

Tobacco is an ideal intoxicant for a shamanistic society. Nicotine causes increased heart rate, blood vessel constriction, and increased alertness.

Overdose can cause convulsions and death; some South American shamans have died (Wilbert 1987), but the toxic dose is quite high. Neurological research shows nicotine is addictive (Pontieri et al. 1996), which surely played a role in its widespread consumption (Winter 2000e:308):

> Humans, plants, and spirits are linked together in a complex chemical and ideological relationship. At the heart of it is a pharmacological explanation—a chemical dependency—but it is shrouded in sacred smoke and explained by religious belief.

Nicotine can have hallucinogenic effects in high doses (Joniger and Dobkin de Rios 1973, 1976; Parrott 1998; Winter 2000d:267). Some species may include hallucinogenic compounds (Schultes 1979:152). Nicotine can interfere with color perception, rendering one able to perceive only yellow, black, or white. Casas Grandes pottery depictions of tobacco smoking do not use red, despite its prominence in other Casas Grandes pottery (VanPool 2009:184). Hallucinatory tobacco shamanism is primarily a South American phenomenon (Wilbert 1987), though Von Gernet (1995, 2000) hypothesizes North American tobacco shamanism existed in the past.

Botanical evidence for early *N. rustica* in South America is limited; the oldest known dates are from Peru, between 2500 and 1800 BCE (Pearsall 1992:178). Tobacco alkaloids were detected in materials from a Bolivian cave dating to approximately 375 CE, in addition to ilex, in what was interpreted as a shaman's tomb (Bruhn et al. 1978). Conservatively, the South American origin for *N. rustica* smoking is between 3,500 and 4,000 years ago. The timing of *N. rustica*'s entry into North America is complicated by morphological overlap with other species, making identification difficult (Asch and Asch 1985; Ford 1985; Winter 2000c:105).

Prior to the possible recovery of Paleoindian tobacco, seeds from the Southwest had been recovered from 1000 BCE (Bohrer 2004; Winter 2004). This contradicts speculations of ethnographers such as White (1942) who argued tobacco was of postcolumbian origin, echoing arguments posed by late nineteenth-century ethnographer Bandelier (1890:37). However, Bandelier is an unreliable source (Castetter 1943:321), and there is significant evidence of precontact tobacco use in North America.

The earliest tobacco from Eastern North America is in the Mississippi Valley between 100 and 200 CE (Asch 1991, 1994:45; Haberman 1984:271; Wagner 2000; Winter 2000a), and most dates fall between 200 and 800 CE. Wagner (2000:191–194) provides a list of radiocarbon dates. The oldest is the Naples-

Abbot site in the Illinois River Valley between 100 BCE and 250 CE (Asch 1991; Asch and Asch 1985). Another is the Hopewell Strait site in Ohio, dated between 220 and 260 CE (Burks 2001; Dancey and Burks 2006). A potentially later date (70 BCE–320 CE) for early *N. rustica* in the Eastern Woodlands is the Smiling Dan site in Illinois (Asch 1994:45; Asch and Asch 1985:196; Haberman 1984:272–273; Wagner 1987:840). Wagner (2000:190) notes unpublished data of tobacco from the Meriden Hills site at 100–200 CE.

These are the earliest botanical tobacco remains in Eastern North America. These dates agree with *N. rustica* from caves in Northeast Mexico, on the path into North America (Blanton 2015:17). There is little evidence for *N. rustica* in the Caribbean (Godlaski 2013:2; Heister 1992; Wagner 2000:185). *N. rustica* was reported from Newt Kash rockshelter in Kentucky, from contexts as early as 3400 years BP, but it was never directly dated (Asch 1994:45; Winter 2000c:105). Newt Kash has occupations that would predate current evidence. *N. rustica* was reported from Salts Cave in Kentucky, which may date to 3500 BP (Winter 2000c:105).

Winter (2000c:108) notes *N. rustica* in southern Illinois by 300 CE and in Ontario by 700 CE, though chemical evidence from the Northeast argues for tobacco as early as 300 BCE (see below). *N. rustica* appears in Arizona by 950 CE, augmenting or replacing native species. Tobacco seeds have been recovered from along the Missouri River, with the earliest dating to 450–600 CE from northwest Iowa (Adair 2000:178).

These data leave a gap between evidence for tobacco and evidence of smoking pipes. The earliest pipes in Eastern North America are over a thousand years before the earliest botanical evidence. A stone pipe from the Robeson Hills site in Illinois dated to 3490 ± 100 years BP (Winters 1969:69), among the oldest pipes from Eastern North America and contemporaneous with tobacco from Newt Kash. A similar specimen was recovered from the Middle Archaic Eva site in Tennessee. Several researchers have tried to address this discrepancy using chemical analysis.

TOBACCO AND RESIDUE ANALYSIS

Dixon and Stetson published an analysis of Basketmaker pipe residue in 1922. Two pipes had no provenance, while a third came from Arizona. There are few specifics, only: "The material was given to a well-known firm of analysts, who made a very careful chemical and microchemical investigation" (Dixon and

Stetson 1922:245). Gas chromatography was available; GC-MS was not until 1959, so available techniques were limited. This report claims negative results but states "preliminary tests gave what appeared to be a faint indication of nicotine"; however this was not confirmed. The researchers declared this negative, though I suspect confirmation bias, as Dixon believed tobacco was a late introduction. It is impossible to say more than results were equivocal.

Later attempts to identify nicotine in precolumbian pipes were successful but unpublished beyond a 1959 conference paper and a reference by Switzer (1969:13). Wagner (2000:195) notes unpublished identification of nicotine in a pipe from North Carolina between 900 and 1000 CE, conducted by tobacco company scientists. These attempts demonstrated nicotine can be extracted from residues and detected.

In 1995 this author began study of smoking pipe residues. Data were collected on the earliest pipes in the Eastern Woodlands—their shape, decoration, context, associations, and for pipes from burials, who they were buried with. Results have been published (Rafferty 2004, 2007, 2008), but to summarize, the earliest pipes in Eastern North America were tubular, incorporated in burials in mounds or cemeteries, buried primarily with adult males, and associated with a range of other objects of religious significance.

The initial research design for the project called for collecting residue from numerous pipes. Over one hundred pipes were investigated; regrettably only two yielded residue samples. The exceptions were a pipe from the Adena Cresap Mound site in West Virginia (Dragoo 1963) and a pipe from the Boucher site, a site in Vermont occupied through the first millennium BCE (Heckenberger et al. 1990). Nicotine and nicotine metabolites were detected in the Cresap pipe (Rafferty 2002) and the Boucher site pipe (Rafferty 2006). The Cresap pipe may date as early as 500 BCE; the Boucher site pipe was dated to ca. 300 BCE. A third pipe dated to ca. 300 BCE from Pennsylvania was later analyzed using GC-MS and the results again identified nicotine (Rafferty et al. 2012).

This author was involved in another recent residue analysis of a smoking pipe from Eastern North America conducted on a blocked-end tube pipe from the Niles-Wilford site in Ohio. Scientists from the University of Washington analyzed residue from this pipe using ultra-performance liquid chromatography (UPLC). Results indicated the presence of compounds consistent with tobacco, such as nicotine, cotinine, or anabasine, any of which would comprise strong evidence for tobacco (Marley et al. 2018).

In total, four pipes, including specimens from Ohio, Pennsylvania, Vermont, and West Virginia, dating to between 500 and 300 BCE, have tested positive for nicotine. Results from two pipes from Pennsylvania and one from Ohio were suggestive but not conclusive. These are some of the oldest pipes in Eastern North America (though they postdate Late Archaic pipes). These results extended the tobacco chronology to the mid-first millennium BCE.

Researchers have investigated pipes from the West Coast (Eerkins et al. 2012; Tushingham et al. 2010; Tushingham et al. 2013). Two pipes from the CA-ALA-554 site in California, from approximately 1000 to 1500 CE, contained residue, which was subjected to GC-MS analysis. Both tested positive for nicotine. The researchers note they cannot identify a species of tobacco (a pertinent issue in California where there are numerous species).

Two sites in Northern California contained pipes that were subjected to GC-MS. One pipe and 15 fragments were tested. Six tested positive for nicotine. Four were from a nineteenth-century plank sweat lodge. Two were older, with median radiocarbon dates of AD 863 and AD 1225 (Tushingham et al. 2013:1402). The authors associate tobacco along the Northwest Coast with the arrival of Athabascan populations after 700 CE and the establishment of villages.

Residue analysis was conducted on Late Woodland and Mississippian pipes from Tennessee (Carmody 2015; Carmody, Caffrey et al. 2017). Fourteen pipes were analyzed using pollen analysis and GC-MS. Three contained *Nicotiana* pollen. Tobacco pollen is rarely recovered, and there is a problem with contamination (Cummings 2000). *Nicotiana* pollen overlaps in shape the genus *Lycium* (boxthorn), which occurs throughout the Southwest (Gish 2000:256). This creates potential for misidentification, though this is not an issue for this study of Eastern specimens. One Mississippian pipe tested positive for nicotine, which is not surprising. Pollen results are of greater interest. Five pipes contained pollen of plants known to have been smoked, including the Asteraceae family, Poaceae family, Ericaceae family (which includes *Arctostaphylos uva-ursi*, bearberry, or kinnikinnick), and Solanaceae family (which includes tobacco and datura). This research has been expanded to samples from Alabama, Georgia, Mississippi, and North Carolina (Carmody et al. 2016). In total, 55 pipes were analyzed. Twenty-six from Moundville tested positive for nicotine, as well as seven late prehistoric and historic pipes. Two pipes push dates back for Southeast tobacco, including one Hopewellian pipe from North Carolina and a Copena pipe from Alabama, dating ca. 200–500 CE.

Carmody and colleagues (2018:905) have recently published results from a Late Archaic site in northern Alabama that comprise the earliest residue-based evidence for North American tobacco. A limestone tube from the Flint River site was recovered from a soil stratum with an associated radiocarbon date of

1685–1530 BCE. Residue from the tube was examined using both GC-MS and liquid chromatography-high resolution mass spectrometry (LC-HRMS), and results were consistent with nicotine in both cases. These results are notable in that they are corroborated by two different analytical techniques and are from a recently excavated and extensively radiocarbon-dated context. At the time of this publication, this is among the earliest tobacco in Eastern North America, dating to the pre-horticultural Archaic, with only Paleoindian seed evidence from Utah (referred to earlier) being of greater age. These results further indicate that tobacco was a widespread intoxicant from an earlier date than has previously been supposed and strengthens the argument that the smoking pipes of the Late Archaic period were used primarily to smoke tobacco.

Another analysis of ancient tobacco has been conducted by Eerkens and others (2018) that will likely have far-reaching implications in terms of the methodology of smoking pipe analysis. The material analyzed was dental calculus from eight individuals from prehistoric California. Dental calculus contains microdata on diet and environment, such as phytoliths, starch grains, proteins, or DNA. Eerkens and colleagues hypothesized that dental calculus might preserve molecular residues of intoxicants as well. Using UPLC-MS, they found calculus from two specimens tested positive for nicotine. Both were adults, one male, one female. These specimens are fairly recent, at most 600 years old, so the identification of tobacco is not surprising, but the direct analysis of human remains is groundbreaking. This approach has the advantage of identifying individuals who used intoxicants, providing evidence on the social context of intoxicant use. We may be able to tell whether tobacco was used by specific individuals (adults only, one sex only, etc.) or whether it was ubiquitous. The mode of use might affect this method; tobacco was smoked and chewed in the region, and chewing is more likely to leave dental residue.

Residue analysis is a promising methodology. However, tobacco was likely more widely distributed than smoking pipes. Pipes leave clear evidence, but this may bias interpretations away from other data. When tobacco was observed by Europeans in the late fifteenth century, it was chewed. Much tobacco use in South America does not involve pipes, but large cigars (Wilbert 1987). Spanish observations of tobacco chewing in South America date as early as 1502, and even in the mid-eighteenth century there was no recorded tradition of pipes in South America. There is a reference to "poor awkward tools" used to smoke by Native and enslaved African populations (McGuire 1899:404), so it is unclear whether pipes might have been used. Regardless, chewing still was the primary means of ingestion. A recent discovery from Arizona (Adams et al. 2015) indicates chewing has historical depth in North America as well.

Evidence from an Arizona cave indicates chewing tobacco is as old as pipe smoking. Numerous masses of plant material, termed "quids," have been recovered in the Southwest, the Great Basin, northern Mexico, and Texas. These were chewed and discarded. Material from Antelope Cave in Arizona includes "thousands of artifacts, including arrows, sandals, basketry, nets, twine and rope, feather ornaments, gourd and ceramic vessels and quids" (Adams et al. 2015:312). The site dates to approximately 1–1000 CE; dates on two quids are 680–890 CE and 710–960 CE, contemporary with West Coast residue results. In total, 345 quids were analyzed from Antelope Cave, all of which consisted of Yucca fiber, with seeds and plant material of wild tobacco mixed in. This shows chewing occurred as early as the seventh century CE. Quids are fragile and even in the Southwest are only found at sheltered sites. Stone or ceramic pipe fragments preserve more easily. Tobacco chewing may have a hidden history, and the seeming dominance of smoking pipes in the Southwest may be due to preservation bias.

It is also possible tobacco chewing was a short-lived phenomenon. The authors note quids from Antelope Cave date as early as the early first millennium CE. However, there is little historic evidence of tobacco chewing overall. There is some evidence from the Pacific Northwest (Dixon 1933), and the Natchez of Louisiana may have chewed tobacco at the time of contact (McLeod 1930). On the whole, there is little evidence in North America, so evidence from the Southwest may represent a local practice.

The Southwest has produced evidence of smoking using cane "cigarettes." Cane grows in wetlands and along rivers throughout the continent, so it is possible that cane was used outside of the Southwest and that favorable preservation again creates a recovery bias. Mid-nineteenth-century researchers identified cane smoking in California (Steen 1943). An 1849 observer showed their place among the Akimel O'odham in healing rituals:

> One Indian was smoking tobacco through a piece of reed, blowing the smoke with all possible force through his nostrils upon the bare back of the sick Indian, at the same time pressing it with a cloth as if to smother the smoke upon his back to prevent its escape. He continued this process for about fifteen minutes, when another Indian took his place, going through the same process. During this time all, except the one engaged in smoking, were singing at the top of their voices a song to the tune I had heard at Santa Rosa. The performance was kept up all night [Steen 1943:641].

Cane tubes observed in the Southwest were often wrapped in insulating cordage (Ariss 1939). Cane tubes containing tobacco were recovered from Double Butte Cave (Haury 1945:194). Cane tubes of *N. attenuata* were recovered from Arizona caves dated to approximately 650 BCE (Raffauf 1960). Jones (1935) reported cane cigarettes from Casa Grande in Arizona. Botanical analysis of the site (Fewkes 1912) identified *N. attenuata*. One room contained a bowl of *N. attenuata*, though Jones (1944) questioned this, and the samples were lost (Adams and Toll 2000:152). The species in Casa Grande reed pipes was not identifiable, but Jones (1935) concluded *N. attenuata* most likely. None of the cigarettes had been smoked, though similar cigarettes in the region were smoked. This suggests the Casa Grande cigarettes were for a symbolic or sacrificial purpose.

Casa Grande was associated with the Hohokam culture and was occupied from the early thirteenth century CE to approximately 1450. Cane cigarettes were common in Hohokam sites near Casa Grande. These cane tubes occur with tubular clay and stone pipes, raising the question of whether cane was a precursor to the tubular pipe that is typically the earliest style throughout North America. Given earlier dates for cane cigarettes from cave sites in the region, and for tube pipes throughout North America, it is likely the two modes of smoking coexisted.

HISTORICAL ACCOUNTS OF TOBACCO

Tobacco's significance is demonstrated in ethnographic and ethnohistoric observations. Some have supposed that tobacco was smoked less frequently by prehistoric Natives than in recent times (Goodman 1993; Linton 1924a; McGuire 1899) and was unknown to some groups in precontact times (Robert 1949; Goodman 1993; McGuire 1899). This seems dubious given the range of historic, ethnographic, and archaeological records on the practice. To see how historic tobacco use relates to archaeological patterns, we need to go back to the earliest direct observations. We are fortunate in that the use of tobacco was such an alien practice to Europeans that it was generally recorded.

The earliest European observations of tobacco use cover a wide area from the late fifteenth to early seventeenth centuries. Primary sources can be drawn from explorations of the Caribbean, Central and South America, and Gulf Coast between 1492 and 1555. Other accounts come from the French in Canada, between 1535 and 1640. Accounts from Jamestown between 1606 and 1609 also contain references. These are the earliest sources to specifically address tobacco (Brooks 1937). Later observations are colored by European adoption of the practice.

Tobacco was first observed by sailors with Columbus. One of their observations reads:

> Under date of October 15 [1492] the admiral found a man in a canoe, between the island of Santa Maria de la Conception and the island of Fernandina, who bore dry leaves of great estimation among the natives and samples of which the admiral says were offered to him as a present while he was at San Salvador or Guanahani [Thatcher 1912, quoted in Brooks 1937:17].

This is the earliest observation of tobacco, although it was not published until 1571. This points to tobacco's value and social function as a gift to newcomers. Additional observations came from Columbus's men:

> These two Christians met on the road (says he) many people who were proceeding to their villages, women and men, always the men with a firebrand in their hands and certain herbs to take in their incense burners, which are dry herbs wrapped in a certain leaf, also dry, after the manner of a musket made of paper which the boys make at the feast of Pascua del Espiritu Santo; and having lighted one end of it, at the other they suck or inhale, or receive within with the breath, that smoke, with which the body is soothed and which almost intoxicates, so that they do not feel fatigue. These muskets, or whatever we shall call them, they call tabacos. I knew Spaniards on this Island of Hispaniola who were accustomed to taking them, and, being reproached for so doing because it was a vice, they replied that they could not stop the habit. I know not what savor or benefit they found in them. Here may be seen the origin of our cigars. (Navarrete, quoted in Safford 1917:389)

Las Casas (in Brooks 1937:243; West 1970:30) related observations made in 1492 on San Salvador. These include the earliest observation of cigars. They mention Native smoking of cigars "dulls their flesh" and "intoxicates them and so they say that they do not feel weariness." This shows tobacco was widespread on the island, and they mention men always carried a cigar. Men and women smoked, one of the few early examples of female smoking (West 1970:30). The mention that smoking "dulls the flesh" may be a reference to a condition documented among South American shamans, where smoking large amounts of tobacco leads to changes in skin tone, eyesight, and body odor (Wilbert 1987).

In 1507, describing islanders off Venezuela, Vespucci describes tobacco chewing: "In looks and behavior they are repulsive, and each had his cheeks bulging with a certain green herb which they chewed like cattle, so that they could scarcely speak" (Waldseemüller 1507, quoted in Brooks 1937:189). While pejorative, this contains useful information. It generalizes tobacco chewing to males, all of whom carried tobacco; women did not partake. In another incident Vespucci's party requests water but was offered tobacco. This indicates tobacco was given the same esteem as life-sustaining resources and had the properties of staving off thirst.

Another account is from Oviedo in 1535. Oviedo was a historian who resided Haiti, Central America, Peru, and Patagonia between 1513 and 1514 (Milanich and Milbrath 1989). He described Haitian smoking as follows (quoted in Brooks 1937:202):

> The Indians of this island, among others had a very wicked vice, to wit: they took smoke which they called *Tabaco*, in order to go out of their senses. They did this with the smoke of a certain herb, which, as I have been able to ascertain, is of the quality of henbane.... They take it in this manner: the caciques, or principle men, had some hollow sticks about a span long, and as thick as the small finger on one hand. These pipes had two hollow tubes, merging into one ... and the whole forms one piece. And these two [ends] they put in their nostrils and the other [end] in the smoke of the burning herb. This instrument was smooth and well-polished. They burned the leaves of this herb ... and they inhaled the smoke once, twice, thrice, or as often as they could endure it, until they lost their senses and for a large space of time they lay stretched out on the ground, drunk and in a deep and profound sleep.... The Indians considered this herb very precious ... they let it be understood that taking this herb and its smoke was not only a healthy, but also a very holy thing to do.

Oviedo's account has been criticized (Brooks 1937:202). He ascribes the word "tabaco" to the act of smoking as well as to a v-shaped pipe, rather than to the plant: "It is to this instrument with which they take the smoke the Indians give the name *tabaco* and not to the herb or the profound stupor in which they fall, as some have believed." This may not be damning for the account, given the term was derived from Arawak for "cigar" (Driver 2011:105). However, the pipe may not have been for tobacco, but for snuffing cohoba, hallucinogenic *Anadenanthera peregrina* (Emboden 1979a). Tobacco is occasionally confused with other hallucinogens, and smoking was sufficiently new to Europeans that they may have missed such distinctions. Oviedo's account raises several issues. He mentions high-rank males smoked, but implies the practice was widespread. If accurate, this would be the earliest description of a pipe. He deduces tobacco's botanical affiliation, placing it among solanaceous plants—it is unclear whether he means the plant's appearance, its effects, or both (Heister 1992:55). His observations support psychoactive properties of tobacco. Finally, Oviedo is the first to unequivocally note that tobacco smoking was sacred to Natives.

Oviedo's account is more intriguing when considered with observations of Ramon Pane who accompanied Columbus in 1499. Pane observed "priests" snuffing *A. peregrina*: "They drink the powder of a certain herb, by whose quality they are driven into a fury. At which time (as they say) they learn many things by revelation of the Zemes" (Martyr ca. 1500, quoted in Brooks 1937:193–195). "Zemes" is a term for spirits. The writings of Pane and Oviedo indicate Natives of Haiti used psychoactive compounds, including peregrina and tobacco, to contact spirits.

While Oviedo probably never observed tobacco, an early seventeenth-century observation by Purchas in Brazil describes taking tobacco through a forked tube:

> [The Natives] had tobacco in religious estimation, not only for a sanity, but for sanctity also, as Oviedo writeth, the smoke whereof they took into the nose with a forked pipe fitted to both nostrils, holding the single end in the smoke of that herb burning in the fire until they became senseless. Their priests most used this, who, coming to themselves after this sleepy fume, delivered the oracles of their zemes or devils, which some times spake by them [Purchas 1626, quoted in McGuire 1899:402].

De Soto's 1539 entrada is notable in that tobacco is not mentioned, despite his encountering numerous Native groups. McGuire (1899:411) used this absence to argue for the absence of smoking. Adair (2000:173–174) noted that Spanish expeditions through the Great Plains, including Coronado in 1541 and Oñate in 1601, made no mention of tobacco, and argued that, as pagan ceremonies, tobacco rituals may have been ignored by Christian observers. Smoking was a convivial practice to establish positive social relations, and de Soto's interactions were often antagonistic, so it is not surprising he did not observe the practice. Archaeology shows smoking was widespread in the Southeast for at least 3,000 years. McGuire (1899:412) noted sixteenth-century observations that do not mention smoking, such as Verrazano's 1524 exploration of the Atlantic coast, Frobisher's 1577 descriptions of Hudson Bay, or sixteenth-century observations in Florida. However, he argues smoking was present but restricted to ritual circumstances, becoming widespread following interaction with Europeans.

Another account is from Thevet (1558, quoted in Brooks 1937:217) who traveled Brazil in 1555. He wrote:

> There is another peculiar herb, called *petun* by the Indians in their language. They most commonly carry this herb about them, for it is marvelously useful for many things. . . . The Indians pick this herb very carefully and let it dry in the shade within their small huts. They use it in this manner: when dried they wrap a quantity of this herb in a very large leaf of a palm tree, and thus they make rolls the length of a candle; they set fire to one end and receive the smoke thereof by their nose and by their mouth. . . . They commonly use it if they have to discuss some matters among themselves; they draw in the smoke and then

> speak. . . . It is true that if too much of the smoke or perfume is taken, it rises to their heads and harms them in the same manner as strong flavored wine does.

Thevet describes physiological effects in the humoral medical theory of the day and compares it with drunkenness. The effects are described as potentially dangerous; Europeans smoking for the first time experienced sweats and drunkenness, or even unconsciousness. Thevet was among the first to point to tobacco's role in decision making, noting that smoking was integral in councils. Thevet also stated tobacco smoking was a male behavior (Thevet 1558, quoted in Brooks 1937:217). Thevet would later describe tobacco in Canada (see below).

Another source is Benzoni, a traveler in Central America and the West Indies from 1541 to 1555. He described making and smoking cigars (Benzoni 1565, quoted in Brooks 1937):

> When these . . . leaves are in season, they pick them, tie them up in bundles and suspend them near their fireplace, till they are very dry; and when they wish to use them, they take a leaf of their grain [maize] . . . and putting one of the others into it, they roll them round tight together; they set fire to one end, and putting the other end into the mouth, they draw their breath up through it, wherefore the smoke goes into the mouth, the throat, the head, and they retain it as long as they can, for they find a pleasure in it, and so much do they fill themselves with this cruel smoke, that they lose their reason.

Benzoni links tobacco smoking and intoxication with medicine men or shamans:

> In La Española and other islands, when their doctors wanted to cure a sick man, they went to the place where they were to administer the smoke, and when he was thoroughly intoxicated by it, the cure was mostly effected.

Benzoni noted tobacco used as medicine in the West Indies for a wide range of ailments (West 1970:47). Benzoni mentioned the power of tobacco, noting:

> And there are some who take so much of it, that they fall down as if they were dead, and remain the greater part of the day or night stupefied. Some men are found who are content with imbibing only enough to make them giddy.

Benzoni noted that tobacco intoxication could lead to hallucinations. In describing a man undergoing a curing ritual, he stated:

> On returning to his senses, he told a thousand stories of having been at the council of the gods, and other high visions.

Benzoni's aversion is apparent in his description of tobacco as "truly diabolical and stinking" and "a pestiferous and wicked poison from the devil." He only mentioned men smoking, never women. Benzoni may have confused the meaning of the term "tobacco" as referring to the plant, when it indicated the cigar or tube by which it was consumed. This became incorporated in the European lexicon as referring to all Nicotiana species (West 1970:30–31).

There are observations of tobacco in Mexico among the Aztec. Tobacco was widespread in Aztec society, where it was known as *piciétl*. As with Caribbean and South American cases, Mexican accounts accentuate tobacco's intoxicating power, again comparing it to henbane (Elferink 1988:430).

There is the sixteenth-century account of Monardes (1925:75–90, quoted in Schleiffer 1973:142–143). Monardes was not a direct observer and confuses details. He described throwing tobacco into a fire and sucking the smoke, probably conflating smoking and tobacco sacrifice. His account described tobacco used for appetite suppression and endurance. While he attributed tobacco to the devil, he provides an account of a shaman using an intoxicant to enter an ASC to commune with spirits.

> One of the merveilles of this Hearbe . . . is the maner how the priests of the Indas did use of it, whiche they did in this maner: when there was amongst the Indians any maner of businesse, of greate importaunce . . . then thei wente and propounded their matter to their chief Prieste, forthewith in their presence, he toke certain leaves of the Tabaco, and caste theim into the fire, and did receive the smoke of them at his mouthe, and at his nose with a Cane, and in taking of it, he fell doune upon the grounde, as a dedde manne, and remainyng so, according to the quantitie of the smoke that he had taken, and when the hearbe had doen his woorke, he did revive and awake, and gave theim their aunsweres, accordying to the visions.

Monardes also described secular tobacco:

> In like sorte the reste of the Indians for their pastyme, doe take the smoke of the Tabaco, for to make theim selves drunke withal, and to see the visions, and thinges that doe represent to them, wherein thei dooe delight: and other tymes thei tooke it to knoe their businesse, and successe, because conformatble to that, whiche thei had seen beeying drunke themrewith, even so thei might judge of their businesse.

Monardes attributes such knowledge as deriving from the devil, "who had virtue of the knowedlge of herbes."

An eighteenth-century account shows smoking endured over centuries of Spanish rule:

> The Aztecs gave to tobacco the name "pycietl," which they were not satisfied to smoke in the shape of cigarettes wrapped in corn leaves, but also inserted it in fine powder in their noses. The powder thus employed served to clear the head, and its virtue was so highly appreciated in Spain that it was called the "sacred herb" [Clavigero 1787, quoted in McGuire 1899:403].

The sixteenth-century record of tobacco in North America is less detailed than that of the Caribbean, and South and Central America. Von Gernet (2000:59) describes early accounts as "awkward, circumlocutory," attributing this to unfamiliarity with an "unprecedented" practice, though it was no less so in regions already discussed. He notes increased detail with European adoption of the practice.

D'Anghiera makes a reference to tobacco in South Carolina in 1525 (quoted in MacNutt 1912:265):

> When the priest has finished his speech, he inhales the smoke of certain herbs, puffing it in and out, pretending to thus purge and absolve the people from their sins. After this ceremony the natives return home, convinced that the inventions of this impostor not only soothe their spirits, but contribute to the health of their bodies.

While based on secondhand information, this reference is evidence that, while pipes and tobacco were common by late prehistory, they still played a role in the actions of the social elite.

Verrazano wrote in 1524, noting of North Carolina Natives: "if they are wounded, they cure themselves with fire," (quoted in Tarrow 1970:139–140) potentially referring to tobacco healing. Cabeza de Vaca (1983 [1542]:99), in the same passage where he described black drink, states: "Everywhere they produce stupefaction with a smoke, and for that they will give whatever they possess." This 1528 statement is among the earliest descriptions of tobacco. It is difficult to draw conclusions from a brief statement, and it is not clear whether pipes were being used or whether tobacco was the source of the smoke. Later observations support this assumption. Cabeza de Vaca's reference indicates tobacco's commonplace status, in comparison with his detailed account of ilex.

A reference to the Tejas or Asinai (along Cabeza de Vaca's route) from the early 1700s describes their shamans (Hatcher 1927:167):

> They offer drinks to the prospective medicine men. The latter consume great quantities of tobacco. This, with their drinks, causes them to lose their senses, to make faces, and to fall upon the ground like drunken men. Here they remain either really senseless or pretending to be, for twenty-four hours, as if dead, until they decide to come to and begin to breathe. They then relate what they have dreamed or whatever their imagination suggests to them. They say that their souls were far from them.

Von Gernet (1992:176) included this passage as evidence for the power of Native tobacco. However, he edits the quote to elide the reference to a drink, which may be datura. There is a reference in the document of using tobacco in interactions with strangers (Hatcher 1927:151):

> Each captain took a handful of the powdered tobacco they use and placed it upon a curious and beautifully crafted deerskin. They all stirred it around to show their union of wills. They then put some of the tobacco in a pipe adorned with many white feathers as a sign of peace among them. One of the principal Indians lighted it and, after taking a whiff, he passed it to the priests and other Spaniard, for this is their most usual ceremony when receiving friends.

Cartier did not mention tobacco during his first voyage, which is intriguing as he took part in trading with Natives. However, his course circumnavigated St. Lawrence Bay and Newfoundland, mostly encountering hunting and foraging Micmac and Beothuk (Cook 1993:25). It is plausible that tobacco did not play a role in these groups, but Cartier's concern was geographic; his interest in Natives was confined to how they could aid his explorations. He may have seen smoking as irrelevant. Also, Natives shared tobacco with those with whom they wished to forge relationships, but Verrazano and Cartier's first actions were to kidnap Native informants.

Cartier did describe smoking during his 1535 voyage down the St. Lawrence, where he interacted with Iroquoian groups. He wrote of the Saint Lawrence Iroquois (quoted in Cook 1993:69–70):

> They have a plant, of which a large supply is collected in summer for the winter's consumption. They hold it in high esteem, though the men alone make use of it in the following manner. After drying it in the sun, they carry it about their necks in a small skin pouch in lieu of a bag, together with a hollow horn of stone or wood. Then at frequent intervals they crumble this plant into powder, which they place in one of the openings of the hollow instrument, and, laying a live coal on top, suck at the other end to such an extent that they fill their bodies so full of smoke that it streams out of their mouths and nostrils as from a chimney. They say it keeps them warm and in good health, and never go about without these things. We made trial of this smoke. When it is in one's mouth, one would think one had taken powdered pepper it is so hot.

Cartier made the first description of pipes, as a "horn" of stone or wood. The term "pipe" would not come into use until the 1590s. Pipes were more popular in North America than Central America, South America, and the Caribbean, and were unfamiliar to sixteenth-century observers. The earliest depiction of a pipe from those regions is from 1565 of the Timucua. Observations in Spanish territories were of cigars or chewing, which do not feature in North America. Thevet contrasted pipes and cigars, likely in reaction to Cartier descriptions (Schlesinger and Stabler 1986:10, 47). Cartier again describes smoking as a male practice; all males used it and always had pipes. He points to health benefits as a panacea, but Cartier found it unpleasant.

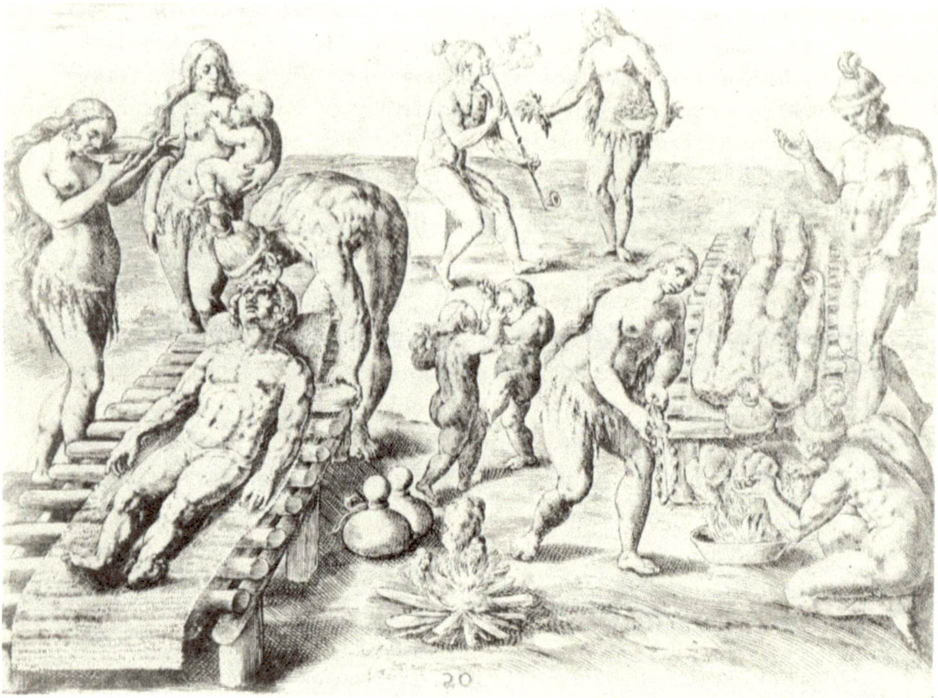

FIGURE 25 Pipe Smoking in Florida, 1564–65.

Thevet, in addition to describing smoking in Brazil, collated mid-seventeenth-century descriptions of Canadian geography, wildlife, and Natives. In France in 1557, he published a volume with a passage describing pipes (quoted in Schlesinger and Stabler 1986:10–11):

> There is besides a very fine little seed resembling seed of marjoram, which produces quite a large plant. This plant is highly prized and they dry it in the sun after collecting heaps of it. They wear it around their neck in little pouches of the skin of some animals in a kind of cylinder with a hole in the end in which they stick a piece of this dried plant which, having rolled it between their hands, they set fire to it and take the smoke of it into the mouth by the other end of the cylinder. And they take it in such quantities that it comes out of their eyes and nose. Thus they perfume themselves at all hours of the day.

Thevet's description was likely based on Cartier's. A 1575 work includes a similar passage, naming tobacco (*theniot*) and comparing Canadian pipes (*coronet* or "horn") and Brazilian *petun* cigars (Schlesinger and Stabler 1986:47–48).

Pipe smoking was referenced in Southeastern accounts. McGuire (1899:411) quotes John Hawkins, who described the Timucua of Florida in 1565:

> The Floridians in 1564 were said . . . to have used in traveling a dried herb, which, with a cane and an earthen cup in the end, they "with fire and the dry herbs put together do suck through the cane the smoke thereof, which smoke satisfieth their hunger and there with they live four or five days without meat or drink, and these all the Frenchmen used for this purpose."

The reference to French tobacco use shows how European use had grown. When Champlain arrived in 1604, he ordered tobacco given to Natives to establish cordial relations (Grant 1907:46). Champlain's references duplicate observations made by Cartier, but with greater comprehension. He took advantage of smoking and exchange in establishing alliances.

The rapidity with which tobacco spread in Europe is remarkable. The first to Spain was in 1518, the first written description in 1524; by the seventeenth century tobacco use was established in Europe and developing into a cash crop in North America. Observations of Native smoking from then on carry European biases about smoking, which, while common, was seen as a vice. The potential dangers of nicotine were published in 1597 (Emboden 1979a:36). King James I sought to curb tobacco, and his moral judgement affected European views of Native smoking. Some Natives cast aspersions on white smoking, criticizing their addiction (McGuire 1899:421).

Anti-tobacco opinions ultimately held little sway. By 1640, over one million tons was imported into England and sold in over 1,700 shops (Emboden 1979a:37). Both domesticated species, *N. rustica* and *N. tabacum*, were introduced into Europe in the mid-sixteenth century, *N. rustica* into Portugal and *N. tabacum* into France (Wagner 2000:186). *N. tabacum* would win out, in part due to Thevet's efforts to popularize it at the French court. Raleigh introduced *N. tabacum* in Virginia, contributing to its domination of seventeenth-century trade.

Most seventeenth-century observations of Northeast Native tobacco are from Canada, from two sources: Lescarbot (1907–1914 [1609]), and the Jesuit Relations (Thwaites 1959). Lescarbot came to New France in 1606 where he observed Micmac Natives. These observations contain one of the earliest descriptions of tobacco (Lescarbot 1914 [1609]:3:252–253):

> Our savages also plant great store of tobacco, a thing most precious with them, and universally among all those nations . . . the smoke of which they suck up with a pipe. . . . After they have gathered this herb, they dry it in the shade, and have certain small leather bags,

> hanging about their necks, or at their girdles, wherein they always have some, with a calumet or tobacco-pipe, which is a little horn with a hole at one side, and within the hole they fit a long quill or pipe, out of which they suck the smoke of the tobacco, which is within the said horn, after lighting it with a coal which they lay upon it. They will sometimes endure hunger for five or six days with the aid of that smoke. And our Frenchmen who have frequented them are for the most part so bewitched with this drunkenness of tobacco, that they can no more be without it than without meat or drink, and upon it they spend good money.

This description closely follows that of Cartier cited previously and was likely based on it as much if not more so than Lescarbot's own observations, as it was the practice at the time to essentially plagiarize the content of earlier accounts.

He also provides one of the earliest detailed descriptions of pipe smoking (Lescarbot 1914 [1609]:253):

> This tobacco smoke taken in at the mouth by sucking, as does a child at the breast, they send out through the nose, and by its passage through the breathing conduits the brain is warmed and its humidities dried up. It also in some sort makes one giddy, and as it were drunk, it opens the bowels, calms the passions, induces sleep, and the leaf of this herb, or the ashes that remain in the pan, heal wounds. I shall add that this nectar is so sweet to them that the children sometimes suck in the smoke that their fathers send out of their nostrils, to the end that nothing be lost.

Lescarbot also describes tobacco intoxication. Comparing tobacco to alcohol (177):

> Our savages . . . are far from these delights [alcohol], and have only the tobacco of which we have spoken to warm their stomachs and to give some smatch to the mouth, having in common with many other nations a love for what is biting, as is the said tobacco, which like wine or strong beer, when taken in smoke, numbs the senses and tends to bring on sleep; so that the word drunkard is used among them.

Lescarbot (1914 [1609]:33) includes a secondhand description of tobacco sacrifice:

> After carrying their canoes to the foot of the fall, one of the company takes up a collection, plate in hand, into which each man puts a piece of tobacco. The collection finished, all dance about the plate, singing after their fashion, and after the dance one of the chiefs makes an oration, pointing out to the young men that from the time of their ancestors they make in this place an offering which insures them against their enemies, and that if they omitted to perform this, evil would befall them. Then the orator throws the tobacco into the basin, and all together raise a great shout, and they think that without this offering their journey could not be a success.

John Smith observed in 1607: "Tobacco, they offer the water in passing in fowle weather" (quoted in Gardner 1907:51). Paper (1992:163) describes this as "ubiquitous throughout North America."

Lescarbot includes numerous references on tobacco. He notes Natives were excellent at carving figurines, but that this was done only for "personal tools" such as pipes (Lescarbot 1914:99), indicating that he didn't understand tobacco's sacred associations. He acknowledges the potency of tobacco (164) while misattributing its role in Native mores. He attributes what seemed paradoxical Native propriety ("One might think that the nakedness of this people would make them more lecherous, but the contrary is the case") to "their frequent use of tobacco, the smoke of which dulls the senses, and mounting up to the brain hinders the functions of Venus." Throughout his account is a mix of superstition; tobacco can "warm the stomach" offsetting a fish-based diet, which would "extinguish their natural heat." In the same passage he compares sharing tobacco with social drinking (176) and notes how not sharing a pipe would be an insult.

Du Creux (1969:I:108) also published an early description of pipes in 1664:

> The Indians are passionately fond of smoking the dried leaves of a plant which was first introduced into France in the last century. At the time it was called *nicotiane* from the name of the man who introduced it [Jean Nicot]. Today it is generaly called *tabac* or *petun*, and form the latter comes the French name of a tribe known in Canada as the Tobacco or Petun Indians. This tobacco has a wonderful effect in drying up the brain, as European explorers were the first to learn; today both Europeans and Canadians use it to produce intoxication. The Indians will not go anywhere without the longish pipe through which they inhale the smoke, generally to inebriation; for the smoke affects the brain and finally produces an intoxication like wine. Certainly they spend a great part of their time in this perilous business, and will buy the noxious dust at any price.

Du Creux's account was based on the Jesuit Relations. He supports previous observations of tobacco's potency, as well as Native dependence. Also, his description of the "longish" pipe is interesting. Iroquoian pottery pipes are seldom beyond 10 cm. It is possible he is conflating personal pipes with calumet pipes, with a long detachable stem. An accompanying figure (Du Creux 1969:I:117) of a Huron smoking a pipe does show a pipe with a long stem.

The Jesuit Relations are reports from New France to France between 1632 and 1673. They provide descriptions of lifeways in over sixty volumes. Two individuals dominate. The first is the 1616 relation of Biard from Port Royal, Acadia. This predates documents considered "The Jesuit Relations" but was collected and translated (Thwaites 1959) with later documents. By this point many Natives were dependent on the French for tobacco; Sagard (1939:85) laments in 1636 of constant requests by the Huron.

Biard writes of the Micmac (Thwaites 1959:3:117):

> They also use tobacco, and inhale the smoke as is done in France.... It is the sole delight of these people when they have some of it, and also certain Frenchmen are so bewitched with it that, to inhale its fumes, they would sell their shirts. All their talks, treaties, welcomes, and endearments are made under the fumes of this tobacco. They gather around the fire, chatting and passing the pipe from hand to hand, enjoying themselves in this way for several hours. Such is their inclination and custom.

Biard stated smoking was necessary to stave off hunger and noted excessive use was injurious. He gave the impression smoking was universal. The degree to which European tobacco use had grown by the seventeenth century is interesting. Cartier was impressed by the behavior's novelty, but 71 years later Biard used French smoking to describe Native practices.

Most observations come from Le Jeune, Jesuit Superior of New France from 1633 to 1640. Le Jeune made over 30 references to tobacco, including entries relating to its value to Natives and the privation of going without. Of the Montagnais he wrote:

> The fondness they have for this herb is beyond all belief. They go to sleep with their reed pipes in their mouths, they sometimes get up in the night to smoke; and it is the first thing they do when they reenter their cabins.... I have often seen them gnaw the stems of their pipes when they had no more tobacco, I have seen them scrape and pulverize a wooden pipe to smoke it. Let us say with compassion that they pass their lives in smoke, and at death, fall into the fire (Thwaites 1959:7:137)

Montagnais were a hunting culture who did not grow tobacco (Winter 2000e:306). This description of Native dependence is echoed by many accounts. Sagard (1939:88) relates Huron astonishment at his declining tobacco, to them a physical necessity.

Le Jeune noted tobacco trade. His concern seems practical, as Jesuits seized upon tobacco exchange as a means of influence and bribery. Le Jeune's accounts are one of few attempts to look at tobacco from the Native perspective (Thwaites 1959:10:219):

> They believe that there is nothing so suitable as Tobacco to appease the passions; that is why they never attend a council without a pipe or calumet in their mouths. The smoke, they say, gives them intelligence, and enables them to see clearly through the most intricate matters.

According to Le Jeune, tobacco fulfilled many functions and was used by nearly all Natives. Women used it, based on an observation of Montagnais women giving tobacco to a man they had insulted (Thwaites 1959:7:175), though he did not mention women smoking. Shamans would demand tobacco be burned during rituals (Thwaites 1959:13:259). Tobacco was sacrificed into fires, water, onto people's bodies, or simply onto the ground. Jean de Brébeuf observed Huron tobacco sacrifice in 1636 (Thwaites 1959:10:159):

> They address themselves to the Earth, to Rivers, to Lakes, to dangerous Rocks, but above all, to the Sky; and believe that all these things are animate, and that some powerful Demon resides there. They are not contented with making simple vows, they often accompany them with a sort of sacrifice. . . . They throw some Tobacco into the fire; and if it is, for example, to the Sky that they address themselves, they say, "O Sky, here is what I offer thee in sacrifice; have pity on me, assist me." If it is to implore health, "Heal me."

He referenced Huron sacrificing tobacco to a river spirit (255–257): "Spirit, you who live here, here is some tobacco. It is a present I give you to make you like a field prepared for planting [i.e., peaceful]."

Sagard in 1636 (1939:171) made similar observations of the Huron; spirits had dominion of natural features, and tobacco was the price for safe passage. Tobacco was burned during sweat lodges "by way of sacrifice and offering" (Sagard 1939:198). Iroquois false face societies "fed" tobacco and maize to false face masks (Winter 2000d:283). Rogers (1966:3) describes: "Certain Iroquois were instructed in their sleep to carve masks in the likenesses of the Faces. These they put on at festivals, and invoked the help of the spirits by burning tobacco and chanting curing songs." Sagard's 1632 account of the Huron referred to tobacco in special feasts (1939:112): "Sometimes they hold festivals at which nothing is consumed except tobacco in their pipe or calumet, which they call *Anondahoin* . . . and usually these are festivals prompted by dreams, or held at command of the medicine man." This shows the Huron engaged in marathon smoking at the instigation of spirits.

A last Jesuit reference is from 1666 among the Illinois (Thwaites 1959:61:47–49):

> They practice a kind of dance, quite peculiar to themselves, which they call "the dance of the tobacco-pipe." It is executed thus: they prepare a great pipe, which they deck with plumes, and put in the middle of the room, with a sort of veneration. One of the company rises, begins to dance, and then yields his place to another, and this one to a third; and thus they dance in succession, one after another, and not together. . . . After they have all danced, one after the other, around the pipe, it is taken and offered to the chief man in the whole assembly, for him to smoke; then to another, and so in succession to all. This ceremony resembles in its significance the French custom of drinking, several out of the same glass;

> but, in addition, the pipe is left in the keeping of the most honored man, as a sacred trust, and a sure pledge of the peace and union that will ever subsist among them as long as it shall remain in that person's hands.

This account includes many aspects of Native American tobacco including the association with male identity; the ritual reflects and reinforces the social hierarchy, while binding participants in a collective, aided through intoxication. The pipe is a symbolically charged element.

Late sixteenth- and seventeenth-century references are found in English accounts from the mid-Atlantic, such as Hariot's 1588 report on Virginia (Hariot 1972:16):

> There is an herbe which is sowed a part by it selfe & is called by the inhabitants vppówoc: In the West Indies it hath diuers names, according to the seuerall places & countries where it groweth and is vsed: The Spaniardes generally call it Tobacco. The leaues thereof being dried and brought into powder: they vse to take the fume or smoke thereof by sucking it through pipes made of claie into their stomacke and heade; from whence it purgeth superfluous fleame & other grosse humors, openeth all the pores & passages of the body: by which meanes the vse thereof, not only preserueth the body from obstructions; but also if any be, so that they haue not beene of too long continuance, in short time breaketh them: wherby their bodies are notably preserued in health, & know not many greeuous diseases wherewithall wee in England are oftentimes afflicted. This Vppówoc is of so precious estimation amongst them, that they thinke their gods are maruelously delighted therwith: Wherupon sometime they make hallowed fires & cast some of the pouder therein for a sacrifice: being in a storme vppon the waters, to pacifie their gods, they cast some vp into the aire and into the water: so a weare for fish being newly set vp, they cast some therein and into the aire: also after an escape of danger, they cast some into the aire likewise: but all done with strange gestures, stamping, somtime dauncing, clapping of hands, holding vp of hands, & staring vp into the heauens, vttering therewithal and chattering strange words & noises.

Accounts were made at Jamestown. Archer traveled the James River in 1607, and observed tobacco cultivation (e.g., Barbour 1969:1:85). Several passages highlight its role in gift exchange (e.g., Barbour 1969:1:94). One passage relates to tobacco's power: "They sacrifice Tobacco to the Sun, fair picture or a harmful thing, as a sword . . . they sprinkle some into the water in the morning before they wash" (quoted in Barbour 1969:1:104).

Percy made a similar observation in 1607:

> These people have a great reverence to the Sun above all other things. At the rising and setting of the same, they sit down lifting up their hands and eyes to the Sun making a round Circle on the ground with dried Tobacco, then they began to pray making many Devilish gestures with a Hellish noise foaming at the mouth, staring with their eyes, wagging their

> heads and hands in such a fashion and deformity as it was monstrous to behold [quoted in Barbour 1969:1:143].

Percy later describes tobacco offerings, related to him by William White.

Percy was no friend to the Natives and would lead forces against them; but by then tobacco was a constant in English life, and it is unlikely he misrepresented Native use. One description is of a leader brandishing weapons and a pipe (quoted in Gardner 1907:14):

> At our landing, there came many stout and able Savages to resist us with their Bowes and Arrowes, in a most warlike manner. . . . Amongst the rest one of the chiefest, standing before them cross-legged, with his Arrow readie in his Bow in one hand, and taking a Pipe of Tobacco in the other, with a bold uttering of his speech, demanded of us our being there, willing us to bee gone.

The implications of the weapons are obvious—of the pipe, less so. Given the role of pipes in social relations, this is saying, "This can go one of two ways; which is it going to be?" Violence was avoided, though there is no mention of tobacco sharing, indicating Native ambivalence.

John Smith made several observations. Smith published a volume anonymously in 1608 and another under his name in 1624. His observations are more positive than those of Percy. Smith, as mentioned, noted tobacco sacrifice. While held captive among the Powhattan, he describes a shaman (quoted in Gardner 1907:51):

> One disguised with a great Skinne, his head hung round with little Skinnes of Weasels and other vermine, with a Crownet of feathers on his head, painted as ugly as the divell, at the end of each song will make many signes and demonstrations, with strange and vehement actions, great cakes of Deere suet, Deare, and Tobacco he casteth in the fire.

In 1612, he includes blood among the materials burned and describes an altar. Du Creux (1969:1:117) notes similar use of bear fat in New France in 1624. A century later the Spanish would make similar observations in Texas, suggesting sacrifice of rare and/or fundamental substances (fat, tobacco) was widespread in late prehistory and the contact period. In a Cherokee medicinal, Mooney (1932) notes burning tobacco wards off witches, a major cause of illness.

Smith's references to a costume and mask, singing, and burning food and tobacco show shamanic practice. Smith provides little context, so it is impossible to determine its purpose; Smith equated it to the *pater noster*. The passage describes other practices, such as rattles and sucking out "blood and flegme," though no mention is made of an ASC. Other observations of Smith's relate to social distinctions. Tobacco was a requirement for an afterlife, attainable only by chiefs and priests (Barbour 1969:2:368). It appears that the social significance of tobacco was differentially expressed depending on status.

Smith also made an early description of a pipe (quoted in Gardner 1907:80): "One had the head of a Woolfe hanging in a chaine for a Jewell; his Tobacco pipe 3 quarters of a yard long, prettily carved with a Bird, a Beare, a Deare, or some such devise at the great end, sufficient to beat out the braines of a man." This was a trading party, and likely represents an item for interacting with strangers. The pipe is typical of effigies from as early as 500 BCE. Offering a pipe was a first step in peaceful interaction, particularly trading (e.g., Gardner 1907:314). Percy made a similar observation of a "pipe made artifically of earth as ours are, but far bigger, with the bowle fashioned together with a piece of fine copper" (quoted in Gardner 1907:12).

Eighteenth-century observations in Florida are relevant. Bartram (1792:351) described tobacco smoking by rank prior to drinking black drink among the Cherokee:

> After partaking of this simple but healthy and liberal collation and the dishes cleared off, Tobacco and pipes were brought, and the chief filling one of them, whose stem, about four feet long, was sheathed in a beautiful speckled snake skin, and adorned with feathers and strings of wampum, lights it and smoaks a few whiffs, puffing the smoak first towards the sun, then to the four cardinal points and lastly over my breast, hands it towards me, which I cheerfully received from him and smoaked, when we fell into conversation.

There is also this excerpt from a lengthy description of a black drink ceremony:

> As soon as the drinking begins, Tobacco and pipes are brought. The skin of a wild cat or young tyger stuffed with Tobacco is brought, and laid at the king's feet, with the great or royal pipe beautifully adorned. . . . A skin of Tobacco is like-wise brought and cast at the feet of the white chief of the town, and from him it passes on from one to another to fill their pipes from, though each person has besides his own peculiar skin of Tobacco. The king or chief smokes first in the great pipe a few whiffs, blowing it off ceremoniously, first towards the sun, or as it is generally supposed to the Great Spirit, for it is puffed upwards, next towards the four cardinal points, then towards the white people in the house, then the great pipe is taken from the hand of the king by a slave, and presented to the chief white man, and then to the great war chief, whence it circulates through the rank of head men and warriors, then returns to the king. After this each one fills his pipe from his own or his neighbours skin [453].

Bartram published observations that showed smoking fundamental to social interactions:

> A man goes forth on his business or avocations, he calls in at another town, if he wants victuals, rest orsocial conversation, he confidently approaches the door of the first house he chooses, saying "I am come"; the good man or woman replies, "You are; its well." Immediately victuals and drink are ready; he eats and drinks a little, then smokes Tobacco, and converses either of private matters, public talks or the news of the town [Bartram 1791:491].

A critical view must be maintained. Some observers did get aspects wrong, such as Oviedo's confusion of tobacco and peregrina. While most of these were exploratory voyages, or specifically tasked to observe, the possibility of bias remains. Regarding the gender of smokers, observers were men from patriarchal societies. It is possible females were using tobacco but that this was not observed because women were not observed. An observer's presence may have affected what they were observing; high levels of tobacco use were a reaction to culture shock of contact, and Native Americans were likely using it for comfort and explanation.

Several aspects of these observations are useful for the hypothesis that smoking served spiritual functions. These accounts show tobacco was widespread, not an artifact of contact. The earliest Europeans to reach the New World observed tobacco in widely separated areas. The distances between these regions supports the assertion that tobacco was integrated in Native culture on a vast scale. Several accounts indicate tobacco had effects in excess of what we would be familiar with, including trance and hallucinations (Goodman 1993:7; Joniger and Dobkin de Rios 1973, 1976; Ripinsky-Naxon 1993:141; Wilbert 1987:135). These effects are sought in societies with beliefs in a spirit world, which would explain the sacred associations of tobacco (Bourguignon 1973). Von Gernet (2000:70) argues that tobacco cultivation was a male-dominated ritual practice, different in character than any other plant . . . it was a "symbolically distinct product." Blanton (2015:24) notes: "The inclusion of tobacco smoking in any event . . . almost certainly had the objective of sanctifying the subsequent proceedings."

These observations agree with accounts of tobacco ingestion by shamans (Dobkin de Rios 1984; Wilbert 1987). Writing on the Warao of Venezuela, Furst (1976:31) observes:

> Their astonishingly complex metaphysical universe is quite literally held together and sustained by tobacco smoke, through the agency of their shamans, who smoke incessantly to fulfill the primordial promise to the gods that there be abundant tobacco smoke as their proper and only food and as the shaman's means of communication with the Otherworld. . . . In the course of shamanizing, shamans may smoke ten, twenty, thirty and even more . . . giant cigars, never exhaling but "eating" the smoke until it suffuses their entire system.

> So "lightened" by tobacco, the shaman's ascend in their ecstatic trances to the zenith and travel to their respective master spirits on celestial bridges constructed of tobacco smoke, as are the houses to which they retire after death.

The account of Warao shamans and their copious tobacco consumption agrees with the ethnohistoric record and points to the hallucinogenic potential of nicotine.

Finally, these accounts relate to sacred and secular contexts for tobacco. Several accounts describe tobacco as restricted to ritual specialists or individuals of status as a means of contacting spirits or healing. This does not mean that tobacco was entirely religious in nature. But tobacco did have a sacred mode, alongside everyday use. Intoxicants need not be limited to specialists or elites to be sacred; there are numerous examples where drug use is widespread in society as "personal vision quests" (Dobkin de Rios 1984; Harner 1972). There are observations of tobacco serving secular and sacred functions, notably for the Cherokee, with the sacred associations depending on tobacco being ritually "remade" (Hudson 1976:353). These examples provide analogues for prehistoric ritual smoking, while showing differences in the scale of social regulation of such behavior.

TOBACCO ETHNOGRAPHY

Several early ethnologists were aware of tobacco's significance to Native Americans (e.g., Lowie 1919; Morgan 1972). Lowie, for example, studied Crow tobacco societies. The Crow engaged in vision quests using self-torture and smoking to induce visions (Winter 2000d:287). The visions were central to success in "war, hunting, working and life in general" (Winter 2000d:288), and tobacco was a facilitator in acquiring those visions.

Tobacco plays an important role in many Native American rituals. The Oglala Lakota holy man Black Elk recorded this chant from the Sun Dance (Brown 1953:88–89):

> I am making sacred smoke; In this manner I make the smoke; May all the people behold it! I am making sacred smoke; May all be attentive and behold! May the wingeds and four-leggeds be attentive and behold it! In this manner I make the smoke; All over the universe there will be rejoicing!

This shows the power of tobacco, not just for the user, or for society, but for the natural world. Black Elk describes how a pipe is filled by a ritual leader and then passed about a circle of participants, each paying homage to their ancestors and gesturing to sacred directions (Brown 1953; Bucko 1998:54). The pipe was a medium of prayer and purification. Bird symbolism features in the account, with each direction having an associated bird, foremost of which was Wanbli Gleska, the spotted eagle, messenger from Wakan Tanka, the Great Spirit: "According to Black Elk, the birds make sure that all the people of the world are symbolically included in the pipe. The pipe, like the lodge itself, is an inclusion symbol" (Bucko 1998:57).

Ethnologists recorded how tobacco plays a role in daily interaction with the spirit world. McElwain (1992:267) points to tobacco use in personal ritual among the Seneca: "Burning tobacco with its rising smoke is typical of sky-spirit petitions. Tobacco offered to another type of being is generally not burnt in Seneca narrative. The choice of sky beings to whom tobacco invocations may be made is quite broad." Every hunting expedition began with an invocation to spirits (McElwain 1992:261–262; Curtin and Hewitt 1918). Similar invocations were made in preparation for war (McElwain 1992:267). Such petitions often involved tobacco, held to be desired by the spirits.

Tobacco plays a role in Native myths, especially myths of origins or cosmology. Many myths show tobacco as a gift from the gods. A Fox myth tells how Great Manitou gave humans tobacco, keeping "not even one pipe" (Furst 1973:24[no Furst 1973 in bib]). The Menomini have a myth where a hero steals tobacco from giants (Godlaski 2013:3). The idea of tobacco as a gift from spirits, who are then dependent on obligatory human smoking, is common (Winter 2000e:308–309). Whenever Natives smoked, there was always an invisible partner in the exchange (Hamell 1987).

White Buffalo Calf Woman first gave Plains people tobacco. Iroquoian groups believe tobacco grew from the grave of the first woman (Winter 2000d:281–283). Some Eastern groups include tobacco in "earth diver" myths, where an animal creates land from a primordial sea. Blanton (2015:21) summarizes Southeastern origin myths. These groups relate "cult bringer legends" of migration from the land of spirits and the dead. Prior to migration, people are given sacred plants, including tobacco, yaupon holly, red button snake root, and red root. Blanton speculates these stories derive from a prehistoric migration from the Midwest (Pauketat 2010). Similar legends are common for the origins of other intoxicants. Myths relating to peyote mirror myths of tobacco, with a supernatural origin (Vecsey 1988). Some myths center on material culture. Sagard (1939:168) related a myth where a pipe was given by God, and so long as Natives possessed it, no harm came to them. The pipe was lost, and misfortune entered the world.

Native gods are said to crave tobacco but are dependent on human offerings. Tobacco smoke rises to spirits, and as discussed previously, tobacco is sometimes burned or thrown into water. Humans are dependent on spirits, so the relationship is reciprocal. This relationship between tobacco, intoxication, and spirits can be embedded in language. Steckley (1985) notes the Huron term for a tobacco-induced ASC ("to make dizzy") includes "-oki-," a term for spirit. To say one is intoxicated by tobacco in Huron is to say one is interacting with spirits. Steinmetz recognized the importance of the pipe in Oglala myths (Kaiser 1984:19). "Mythology is the primary source of the Sacred Pipe's sacramental nature" (Steinmetz 1984:30). He notes pipes and tobacco are featured at the creation of the world. Among Pacific Northwest groups such as the Karok and Yurok, spirits used tobacco to create the world, and humans repay that debt in tobacco (Winter 2000d:295).

As mentioned, the Lakota associate tobacco with White Buffalo Calf Woman (Furst and Furst 1983:12–13; Steinmetz 1984:34–36) as well as such cultural fundamentals as corn, beans, and squash; horse riding; and buffalo hunting (Furst and Furst 1983:13; Kaiser 1984:2–3). Black Elk states the Sacred Pipe played a role in most Lakota rituals (Brown 1953; Steinmetz 1984:33–34). He recounts the White Buffalo Calf Woman's giving of the pipe:

> Behold this and always love it! It is *lela wakan* (very sacred), and you must treat it as such. No impure man should ever be allowed to see it; for within this bundle is a sacred pipe. With this you will, through the winters to come, send your voice to Waken-Tanka, your Father and Grandfather.

Part of the importance of smoking is due to smoke itself; smoke is a sacred substance. Smoke is a means of communication with the spirit world, as smoke rises to the sky and passes between different realms. Among the Pawnee, the smoke hole in the roof is said to "carry messages to the celestial gods" (Chamberlain 1992:227). Tribes in southern Arizona believe that burning releases the spirit of tobacco (Russell 1908). Von Gernet (2000:72–73) writes:

> Transforming a leaf into smoke had unparalleled symbolic importance; not only could both interior and exterior parts of a body be exposed to an empowering substance, but the smoke could also reach the lofty and normally inaccessible realms where many of the spirit beings resided. It is, perhaps, for these reasons that smoking became the most popular form of tobacco consumption.

Williamson (1992:65) writes in reference to the Alabama busk ceremony: "The smoke participated in unifying the Earth and Sky, just as the entire Busk ceremony was thought of as unifying the various discordant elements that had developed within the tribe throughout the year." The busk is a renewal ritual intended to restore harmony. Blanton (2015:24) summarizes:

> In view of tobacco's unique status and sacred connotations, the significance of the timing and associations in its use in the Green Corn ceremony becomes clearer. It was routinely displayed and consumed at the outset and at the conclusions of the ceremony, presumably to signal the sanctity of the collective proceedings, or in other terms, as respective statements of both consecration and consummation.

Smoking began and ended the ritual, purified participants, and appeased spirits. The ritual is likely a holdover from Mississippian cultures (Blanton 2015:25).

Smoke is an analogue for breath in the busk ceremony: "Smoke, as a kind of visible breath, served as a communication medium between the realms" (Farrer and Williamson 1992:286). This communication could be two-way: among the Navajo smoke transmitted the natural and social order to infants (Pinxton and Van Dooren 1992:106–107). Von Gernet (1992:179) states:

> Certain properties of tobacco allowed the free soul to cross thresholds into mythical realities, and the plant therefore became a vehicle of communication. If tobacco could convey diaphanous souls from the center of the world to other cosmic realms, it could also relay the tiny invisible voices of men to the abode of the spirits. Hence, speeches were accompanied to tobacco invocations, during which the powdered leaf was sprinkled on fires, so that the words could "ride" the smoke to the upper world.

Observations from California show the importance of Native tobacco. The Chumash ate wild tobacco as a drug and panacea. Spanish accounts describe tobacco chewing with lime or drinking a blend of tobacco and water and/or urine. Such mixtures were served at social gatherings and caused vomiting, seen as "healthful" (Timbrook 1987:175) as in black drink ceremonies. The Chumash smoked tobacco, usually to blow smoke as a blessing (Priestley 1937). Pipes were sacred for the Chumash and were cared for by individuals who would charge for their services.

Rituals involving the sacred pipe, such as peyote rituals of the Native American Church (Anderson 1996; Pego et al. 1995; La Barre 1972) or the Plains Sun Dance (Walker 1991), model cosmology. Sacred pipe rituals feature presentations of the pipe to cardinal directions, to the sky, and to the earth. This represents a spherical cosmos as opposed to the Western perception of spirituality oriented upwards. The pipe holder is situated at the universal center. The circular offering represents relations with human (family, clan, and nation), animals (terrestrial, avian, and aquatic), and spirits (Paper 1987:301).

Pipes were used in Winnebago funerals (Paper 1988:30); a pipe was interred "so that it may offer them to the spirits it meets on the road and make requests of them." These gifts are called "spiritual" tobacco and food (Steinmetz 1984:50). Nipistingue warriors were interred with their pipes in their mouths, their weapons in hand (Thwaites 1959:70:149–151). De Smet reported a custom where several days after death, relatives would smoke at the grave, hanging presents including tobacco. These were gifts to the individual's spirit (Thwaites 1959:27:166). A similar observation was made for the mid-nineteenth-century Ojibwa (Jones 1861). Other tribes threw tobacco into a grave (West 1970:79). The Plains pipe was held during a Keeping of the Soul ceremony for the dead (Steinmetz 1984:50).

Strachey writes of the burial of a chief in the early 1600s; the man was buried with "all his ritches in severall basketts his Apooke [tobacco] and Pipe, and any one toy which in his life, he held most deere in his fancy" (Strachey 1967:94–95). Wilbert (1995:97) draws a connection between tobacco growth and human burials:

> Certain species of Nicotiana, tend to grow spontaneously in disturbed soil—that is, at the edges of paths, trails, and roadways, on fields, and especially on the turned-over and enriched soil of burial sites. It is likely because of this latter characteristic that tobacco became widely identified with the ancestors, whom many Amerindian peoples credit with causing it to sprout from their graves as a special gift from the spirit world to their surviving kin. This, in combination with its utility as a vehicle for ecstasy, made tobacco a sacred plant.

No other pipe has received as much attention as the calumet (Hart 1980). The calumet was a Plains and Eastern practice where pipes facilitated interactions (Brown 1989:311). This led to the term "peace pipe," but not all interactions were peaceful. Sagard (1939:150) describes Huron councils smoking while debating whether to go to war. The calumet was part of meeting rituals involving processions, speech-making, gifts, and feasting (Brown 1989:314). Rodning notes the pipe's color, white stone used for peace, red or black for war.

The term "calumet," from French for reed (Brown 1989:312) refers to a detachable stem, used with a stone elbow or disk pipe (Steinmetz 1984:60). The stem was important by itself (Furst and Furst 1983:15; Pego et al. 1995:154; Steinmetz 1984:60). Some pipes had multiple stems (Stone 1955), and some cultures would use undrilled stems. Despite the stem's significance, the power of the pipe was not manifested unless bowl and stem were joined (Furst and Furst 1983:16), a union of male and female elements (Paper 1987:302; 1988:40).

A range of practices is included under the term "calumet." Blanton (2015:27) notes:

> It is important to add that the true form of the calumet ceremony, as practiced by native groups of the Plains, upper Mississippi, and the Great Lakes Regions . . . was not a feature of southeastern Indian ceremony outside its limited adoption in the lower Mississippi River valley, such as among the Choctaw.

Outside of those boundaries, the term refers to a range of tobacco rituals for interacting with strangers. Blanton argues this should not be equated with the calumet. The expansion of the term is a product of Europeans seizing upon the practice to facilitate their interactions with Natives. The distinctions that make the calumet unique include a stone pipe of particular materials and a detachable, decorated stem, both kept and maintained by particular specific individuals.

The earliest observation of a calumet ritual was by Spanish among the Apache in 1634 (Blakeslee 1981). The power of the calumet was described by Marquette in the 1670s (Thwaites 1902; Hamilton 1970). Marquette was among the earliest Europeans to contact tribes in the lower Mississippi. He described the calumet in his journal:

> There remains no more, except to speak of the Calumet. There is nothing more mysterious or more respected among them. Less honor is paid to the crowns and scepters of Kings than the Savages bestow upon this. It seems to be the God of peace and of war, the Arbiter of life and of death. It has but to be carried upon one's person, and displayed, to enable one to walk safely through the midst of Enemies—who, in the hottest of the Fight, lay down their arms when it is shown. For that reason, the Illinois gave me one, to serve as a safeguard among all the Nations through which I had to pass during my voyage [quoted in Thwaites 1959:59:129–131].

He was not speaking hypothetically. While travelling, Marquette's party was attacked; Marquette displayed a calumet given to him by the Illinois, at which point their attackers apologized and withdrew (Thwaites 1959:59:15). A similar event occurred among the Illinois, in 1679, when members of La Salle's party were saved from Native aggression by the presentation of a calumet (Cox 1905:1:78–79). Le Page du Pratz (2006) described seventeenth-century Louisiana Natives presenting a calumet to the French governor.

There has been debate about the calumet's origins. Turnbaugh (1979) depicted the practice as a response to European entry of the Mississippi based on a supposed lack of accounts prior to the late 1690s. Blakeslee (1981) referred to documents that described calumet rituals during the 1660s and 1670s. He (1981:760) attributed Turnbaugh's error to misunderstandings of seventeenth-century documents by Fenton (1953) and Swanton (1946). He also noted that, since seventeenth-century Apache pipes were distinct from the calumets they

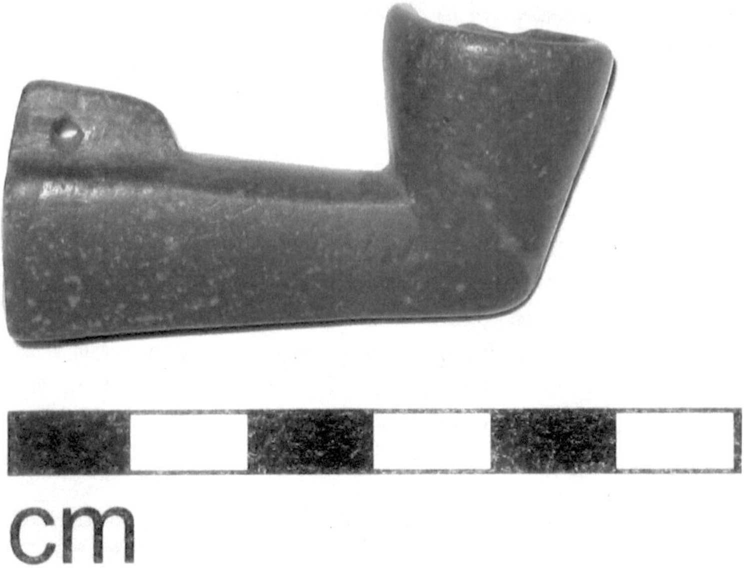

FIGURE 26 Redstone Pipe, Wamampito Site, 17th-century Iowa.

also used, the calumet was not an Apache innovation and must have had a prehistoric origin. Pipes similar to calumets appeared in the Plains around 1200 CE. Blakeslee (1981:763) notes a shift from obtuse-angled clay pipes to right-angled stone pipes during the mid-thirteenth century, arguing for the calumet's origin at that time.

Pipestone is found in the Midwest and Great Plains, particularly Minnesota, where "catlinite" originates. Catlinite is often used to refer to any red pipestone, but without clear origin, the general term "redstone" should be used. This material was traded in late prehistory; examples are found hundreds of miles from sources (Thomas and Ray 2002). Calumets are typically elbow- or disc-shaped, and need not be redstone, but redstone specimens dating to the second millennium CE were probably calumets. When such pipes are found outside the Midwest, they are rarely found with redstone debris, indicating they were traded as finished items (Rodning 2014:432).

Calumet rituals likely originated from mourning/adoption ceremonies (Brown 1989:313–314), and their ability to maintain peace was responsible for their spread (Brown 1989:314; Hall 1987:30). Late seventeenth-century explorers note the calumet as far south as Mississippi (Springer 1981:222–223). Brown (1989) observed it was unknown in the Northeast, where its role was fulfilled by wampum exchange (Springer 1981). There is uncertainty regarding the calumet in the Southeast. While sixteenth-century Spanish sources note meeting rituals, no smoking was recorded. Springer (1981:226) feels this was due to Spanish hostility, but Brown (1989:315) maintains the calumetwas absent in the Southeast and that the calumet in the Eastern Woodlands was due to seventeenth-century French promotion. The French, he argued, seized upon the ritual to ensure a "measure of predictability" in Native interactions (Brown 1989:315–316). Contrary to Brown, Hall (1977, 1987, 1997) argues the calumet in the Eastern Woodlands was the product of development starting in the Middle Woodland. To Hall, Middle Woodland platform pipes were associated with atlatl spear-throwers. Over time, pipes and weapons became conflated into the calumet. The pipe/weapon association was illustrated to Marquette who observed a mock battle among Illinois where one person bore a weapon, the other a calumet (Thwaites 1959:59:134–137). There are also contact period examples of tomahawks that incorporate a pipe bowl in the ax-head.

The calumet was found through much of the Eastern Woodlands at contact, and it is doubtful the French could have widely disseminated the behavior in the absence of existing pipe rituals. French traders did play a role in introducing the practice to the Cherokee, though Native migration from the Gulf Coast also played a role. The distribution and associated trade relations of the practice were extensive. Pawnee hako ceremonies, and Iroquois eagle dances exhibited aspects of the calumet. The eagle dance features elements of tobacco symbolism and pipe smoking (Fenton 1941; Winter 2000d:285). At least one Upper Midwest redstone pipe was recovered from a historic Cherokee site in North Carolina (Rodning 2014).

Timberlake relates eighteenth-century observations of Cherokee calumet use:

> As in this speech several allusions are made to the customs of the Indians, it may not be impertinent to acquaint the reader, that their way of declaring war, is by smoaking a pipe as a bond amongst themselves, and lifting up a hatchet stained in blood, as a menace to their enemies; at declaring peace this hatchet is buried, and a pipe smoaked by both parties, in token of friendship and reconciliation [King 2007:113–114].

These observations agree with Marquette's, though it is probable the practice was introduced with European encouragement. Reaction to European encroachment could have encouraged the spread of the practice. Calumet rituals encouraged harmony and may have been selected for during the tribulations of contact. By whatever means the practice spread, ritually smoking tobacco in a sacred pipe was key and based on centuries of exchange since the Archaic period.

KINNIKINNICK

Other plants were smoked besides tobacco (Brown 1989; Hall 1977; Springer 1981; Knight 1975; Yarnell 1964). Ethnobotanists have recorded 55 genera smoked by Natives (Moerman 1998). These plants are often included under the name "kinnikinnick," Algonquian for "mixture" (Chamberlain 1902:246; Rätsch 2005:762), and were usually used instead of tobacco, but could occasionally contain tobacco. Brown (1989:313) and Knight (1975:129) argue kinnikinnick was used to dilute *N. rustica*; Knight argues it was added to stretch tobacco supplies. Some use the term without specifying whether they mean tobacco, tobacco with additives, or materials besides tobacco (e.g., Hilger 1944:565).

Common ingredients include dogwood (*Cornus* sp.), juniper (*Juniperus* sp.), sumac (*Rhus glabra*), and bearberry (*Arctostaphylos uva-ursi*; Springer 1981:220). West Coast Natives smoked a wider range of plants, including California black oak (*Quercus kelloggii*), common mistletoe (*Phoradendron villosum*), creeping sage (*Salvia sonomensis*), jimsonweed (*Datura* sp.), madrone (*Arbutus menziesii*), sagewort (*Artemisia douglasiana*), salal (*Gaultheria shallon*), and yew (*Taxus brevifolia*; Tushingham et al. 2013:1399). Natives in western Canada, in addition to bearberry and red osier dogwood, would add canby's lovage (*Ligusticum canbyi*), said to act as a relaxant (Keddie 2016:159). Dwarf wild rose (*Rosa virginiana*) and mountain valerian (*Valeriana uliginosa*) were used as tobacco flavoring in British Columbia. Yew (*Taxus brevifolia*) needles were smoked in Washington State (Keddie 2016:174). Species of bearberry, such as manzanita (*Arctostaphylos pungens*) were smoked among Puebloan peoples (Castetter 1943:320), in addition to fir and pine needles, mint, mullein (*Verbascum*), and borage (*Onosmodium*), and even feathers (Adams and Toll 2000:151).

Some sources apply kinnikinnick to specific plants, a linguistic misunderstanding. Kinnikinnick was used to refer to bearberry used by the Assiniboin by Prince Maximilian in 1843 (VanStone 1996:9). Northwestern Natives traded bearberries as well as tobacco (Turner and Loewen 1998:55). Hall (1997:158) and Knight (1975:130) argued smoking bearberry predates tobacco, plausible as bearberries grow throughout North America while *Nicotiana* are native only in the West. Steckley (1985:14) argues since Huron has a word for tobacco mixed with dogwood, bearberry, sumac, or red willow, the practice predates tobacco.

Bearberry was documented as food for Northwestern groups in 1866 (Wilson 1866:282). The Blackfoot added them to pemmican (Zarrillo and Kooyman 2006:477), and natives of California ate them raw (Gifford 1939:307). Bearberry (also called hog cranberry, mountain cranberry, Indian whort, or hardberry) is reputed to have intoxicating properties (Moerman 1998:87–89). Some Great Plains tribes used it as an analgesic, blowing smoke into the ears of someone with an earache (Hart 1979:281). The Cheyenne would drink bearberry tea as a diuretic (Grinnell 1905:41). Overindulgence could be hazardous:

> A few years ago, an Indian from the Quileute tribe smoked *Arctostaphylos uva-ursi* and became so inebriated that he danced barefoot in the fire until his soles were burned to a crisp and his feet were crippled forever. Several years before that, another old Indian became drunk from the inhaled narcotic after smoking the leaves of the plant. He was so drunk that he fell into the fire, burned his hands, burned his nose completely off, and also parts of his lips. He lived like this for many years [Rätsch 2005:764].

There are references to "narcotic" effects of bearberries among Northwest Coast Natives (Turner and Bell 1971:82, 1973:282). Chemical analysis has isolated numerous compounds (Pegg at al. 2008), none of which are known intoxicants. The only known effects are astringent, diuretic, disinfectant and possibly antibacterial (Hussey 1974). If the intoxicating effects are real, other substances were probably involved. Bearberry was clearly a valued substance, with some marking "real" tobacco by the inclusion of bearberry (Gatschet 1899:157).

One benefit for studying kinnikinnick is that it is easier to recover than tobacco. Bearberry seeds are much larger. While early evidence of tobacco is limited, there are numerous examples of bearberry seeds. Hearths dating back 2,000 years in British Columbia contain bearberry seeds (Pokotylo and Froese 1983:141). Charred seeds have been recovered from an Alaskan rockshelter from 50 CE (Lepofsky et al. 2001:54). These seeds could be evidence of food, however. When evidence is recovered from nonutilitarian contexts, the likelihood is that the plant was exploited for ritual reasons. A dog burial from Michigan from between 1250 and 1400 CE contained bearberry seeds (Clark 1990:267). There were no other plant remains in the feature, and the dog was not butchered or cooked. Researchers interpreted this as evidence of household ritual, and the bearberry implies a nonutilitarian association.

Tushingham and colleagues (2013, 2016) identified a biomarker compound for bearberry in experimental samples. This compound should be added to future pipe residue analyses. Even in known tobacco pipes, there is the possibility of identifying mixtures of smoked plants.

Another ingredient is dogwood (*Cornus stolonifera*). An observation of the Blackfoot describes extracting the material:

> A few branches about three-quarters of an inch thick and four or five feet long are procured, and the outer bark, scraped off after having been warmed over a fire. A knife is then pressed against the inner bark and drawn upwards for six or eight inches, until the whole of the inner bark is gathered in curly clusters around the stick. The stick is then thrust into the ground over hot coals and roasted until dry when, mixed with equal portions of tobacco, it forms the favorite kinnickinnik of the North West Indians [Hind 1860:vol.1:315

Dogwood has alleged "narcotic" properties, and there is an example of dogwood in a Utah coprolite (Ellis 2000:444).

A list of ingredients for smoking mixtures (Rätsch 2005:764–765) includes intoxicants, such as tobacco or datura, but also plants which include potentially mind-altering compounds, the effects of which are unstudied. As discussed, one Mississippian pipe has tested positive for atropine, indicating datura. While tobacco was the primary plant smoked by Native Americans, there is substantial work to do on other smoked plants.

We should address the fact that tobacco use has significant health effects. Numerous studies have shown correlation between tobacco and a range of illnesses. It is reasonable to ask what the health effect of ritual tobacco use was and how that compares with modern effects. This is difficult to address archaeologically as most tobacco-related deaths would not leave any skeletal signature. Samet (2000:338) cites data from modern Native populations that deaths due to tobacco are fewer than among other populations. Samet speculates that where tobacco use was ritualistic, addiction rates would be low. Winter and colleagues (2000:354) argue:

> Addiction was probably an important factor in the domestication and spread of tobacco. . . . Nevertheless, most Native Americans probably used tobacco infrequently and in small amounts, mainly because of religious proscriptions concerning its dangerous spiritual power.

Addiction rates would climb where smoking was intense and secular. However, since most tobacco-related deaths occur after long-term use, younger age at death for prehistoric populations might conceal negative effects.

SMOKING PIPES IN NORTH AMERICA

The earliest pipes in Eastern North America are from ca. 4000 to 1000 BCE (Concannon 1993:74; Custer 1987:42; Dragoo 1963:241; Walthall 1980:77). Webb and Baby (1957:22) reference tubular pipes from shell mounds in Alabama and Kentucky. The Eva site, occupied from 5000 to 1000 BCE (Lewis and Lewis 1961), is particularly significant due to two ground stone conical pipes. These are among the first pipes in Eastern North America. The Eva pipes were used in funeral practices from 1000 BCE to as early as 2500 BCE.

Turnbaugh (1980:16) observed the following:

> The durability of smoking pipes through the centuries as a major element of Native American culture lies in their symbolism and mystical associations. Even apart from the importance of tobacco, the pipes themselves are linked with life forces and other elemental beliefs in many New World societies. Every aspect of pipemaking and smoking—from the choice of raw materials, their shapes and ornamentation, to the rules governing use, and the substances tamped into their bowls was a matter of considerable importance in many native societies.

While pipes appear during the Late Archaic, they are rare, so it is difficult to draw conclusions. Given their rarity and careful construction, they were not for everyday use and there was little rank to mark in egalitarian cultures. It is most likely that these early pipes were ritual objects. From their common funeral contexts, we can conclude they were tools used to dispose of the dead and for renewing relationships among the living.

VanPool (2009:182) lists pipes among objects central to shamanic practices:

> Shamanic rituals also involve a variety of tools such as pipes or other paraphernalia to ingest drugs, "curing sticks" or tubes that are used to find and remove illnesses, shrines or altars that serve as entry points into the spirit world, and sand paintings or rock art that summons the spirits for the shamans. . . These "tool kits" should be observable in the archaeological record. Further, this sacra will provide direct evidence about the content of shamanic ritual and provide insights into the culture's cosmology, especially in regards to the composition of the spirit world.

More early pipes come from the Williams site in Ohio. Williams corresponds to the Glacial Kame culture (ca. 1200–900 BCE), which consists largely of cemeteries on natural promontories. Nine stone pipes were recovered from a mass cremation at Williams. They all had a narrow mouthpiece and a rounded opening, with an average length of 15 cm. In addition to pipes, burials at

Williams contained ritualistic bone specimens, particularly bear skulls. Bears are common in Native folklore and mythology (Rafferty 2009), evidence of the shamanic character of the burials.

Perhaps the most remarkable early site is Poverty Point in Louisiana. This massive array of earthen mounds is one of the most elaborate sites in Eastern North America, predating agriculture. It was the hub of an exchange network with raw materials that originated from as far away as the Great Lakes. Stone and clay tube pipes have been found on Poverty Point sites dating to 2000–850 BCE (Webb 1982:44). Some contained soot showing their use as pipes. Other Poverty Point tubes showed no evidence of use (Gibson 2001:153). Gibson (2001) suggests these were shamanic instruments. Webb and Snow (1974:86) argued subsequent Early Woodland tubes were not all intended for smoking but were sucking tubes for removing objects from a body, a common shamanistic explanation for illness. Others may have been used for applying pigment (Frison and Van Norman 1993; Howes 1942). While some early tubes likely had functions aside from smoking, many specimens have burned residue (Jordan 1959).

While originating prior to 1000 BCE, most tubular pipes in Eastern North America date from 1000 BCE to 200 CE (Gehlbach 1982; Meuser 1952; Rafferty 2004, 2006, 2016; Rafferty et al. 2012; Salkin 1986; Stephens 1957). These are made from several materials, including a type of Ohio Valley limestone (Stewart 1989; Thomas 1971:77). These are again recovered from burials, sometimes intentionally broken. Tube pipes are often interpreted as evidence of Ohio Valley Adena Mound Builders (Ritchie and Dragoo 1960; Webb and Baby 1957; Webb and Snow 1974). Dragoo noted pipes were prominent in Late Archaic and Early Woodland cultures in the Eastern Woodlands, suggesting they were used in a "cult of the dead" (Dragoo 1963:245).

While tube pipes are associated with Ohio Valley sites (Bense 1994:129), they were more widely distributed. Similar pipes have been recovered from New York, Pennsylvania, New England, southeastern Canada, and the mid-Atlantic (Carpenter 1950; Concannon 1993; Dent 1995:231–235; Haviland and Power 1994; Heckenberger et al.; Kraft 1976; Loring 1985; Ritchie and Dragoo 1960; Spence and Fox 1986:32; Thomas 1971). The presence of Ohio Valley–style artifacts so far away demonstrates trade of prestige artifacts (Stewart 1989), and their mortuary contexts suggest smoking was associated with burial ritual across Eastern North America. Contemporary pipes are found as far as the Gulf Coast, Tennessee (Faulkner 1971:102), and southern Mississippi Valley (Ford and Quimby 1945:29–32). While these southern pipes are different in style, they are also most often recovered from ritual sites.

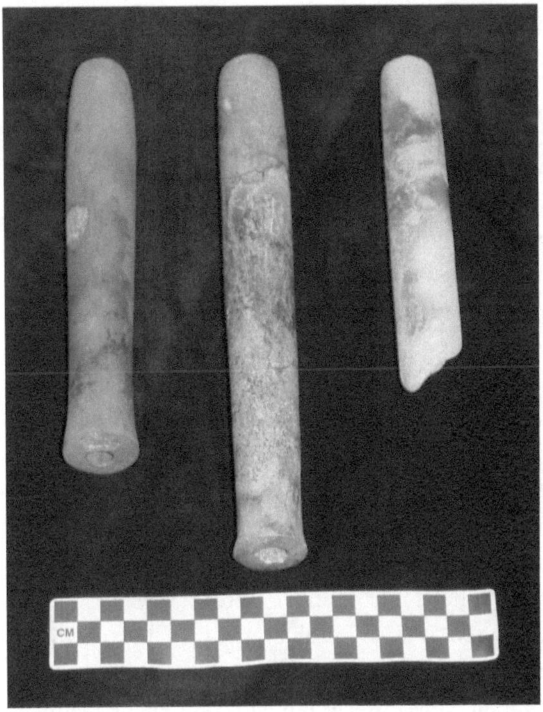

FIGURE 27 Early Woodland Pipes from Eastern North America. (Author's photo.)

The period from 200 to 1000 CE (Middle Woodland) saw the introduction of platform pipes (Gehlbach 1982). These have a flat base with a bowl at the center or far end. There are many animal effigy forms, often birds, but plain pipes were most common. Researchers have questioned whether the association of tobacco, pipes, and birds might have a physiological explanation (Von Gernet 1992:137, 2000:80; Von Gernet and Timmons 1987; Wilbert 1987:184): "Tobacco shamanism is always associated with bird imagery, perhaps because the physiological and biochemical reaction from nicotine intoxication causes people to 'see' flashes of movement that are commonly interpreted as birds" (VanPool 2009:182). Given these facts, the association of birds and pipes should come as no surprise.

Platform pipes are most associated with Ohio Valley Hopewell (King 1977:11), though some predate 200 CE, and they persisted after 900 CE (Seeman 1981). Tremper Mound and Mound City in Ohio contain caches of platform pipes (Brose 1985:62–63; Otto 1992; Weets et al. 2005:537–539) interpreted as disposal of profaned sacred artifacts (Otto 1992:11). Some were made from exotic catlinite though the site is near a local pipestone source (Emerson et al. 2005). Material analyses of Tremper and Mound City pipes provide a picture of their exchange role (Emerson et al. 2013). In the early Hopewell, raw materials were acquired from as far away as Minnesota and Illinois. Lack of manufacture debris at Ohio sites indicates pipes were made near distant sources and then traded. Only later are pipes made locally. Animal effigy platform pipes are mostly non-prey and likely totemic (Otto 1992:7). Totemic figures are common in shamanism (Winkelman 2002:75), which is consistent with the role of intoxicants. This would also explain human effigies, as mythic figures. This assumes shared symbolism among Hopewellian cultures, which is plausible as effigy forms are similar across Hopewell sites (Brose 1985:67).

Platform pipes were not limited to the Ohio Valley. Sites in New York, Ontario, and the Midwest include platform pipes as well as other "Hopewellian" artifacts (Brose 1985:62–67; O'Connor 1995:17; Ritchie 1980). Some are made of traded Ohio Valley stone (Penney 1985). Platform pipes are also found on mid-Atlantic sites (Bollwerk 2012:201–203; Dunham 1994:Table 15; Irwin et al. 1999), but their association with Hopewell is unclear.

Gulf Coast Middle Woodland sites also contained locally made platform pipes (Toth 1979; Brose 1985:62). Copena burials in Alabama feature pipes that differ from contemporaneous examples and include early elbow pipes, as well as large effigy tubes and platforms (O'Connor 1995:17; Walthall 1979, 1980). While Copena effigy pipes include similar forms, Copena effigies face away from the smoker, while Hopewell effigies face inward. Self-facing effigies are personally oriented symbols, while outward-facing pipes imply group orientation (Brasser 1980).

Late prehistory extends from roughly 1000 CE to contact. During this period the Northeast is dominated by elbow pipes. Early in this period, pipes had wide-angled bowls (Bradley 1987:17–19). Elbow pipes became more highly angled, and by 1300–1400 CE, most had bowls at a right angle (Bradley 1987:30; Noble 1992:42–43). A variety of animal and human effigy pipes were used (Kuhn 1986; Mathews 1980; Noble 1992; Wonderley 2005), and a range of geometric designs are also found. Miniature pipes were manufactured, presumably as exchange items (Kapches 1992). Pipe bowl shape varied over time, including barrel, square, flaring, and "trumpet" (Bollwerk 2012:Table 7.2; Noble 1992:41).

Effigy pipes played a role among the Mississippian chiefdoms in the Mid-

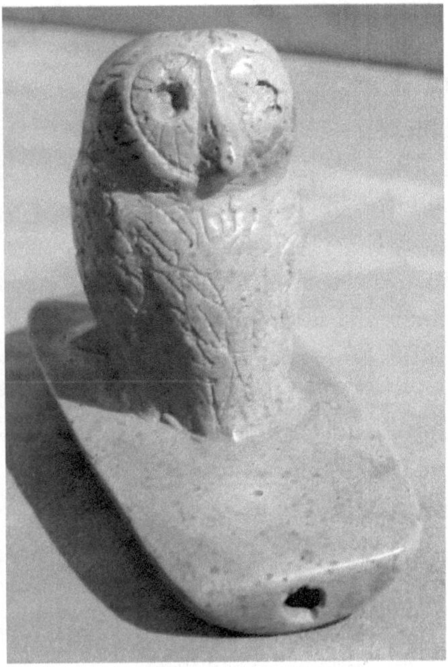

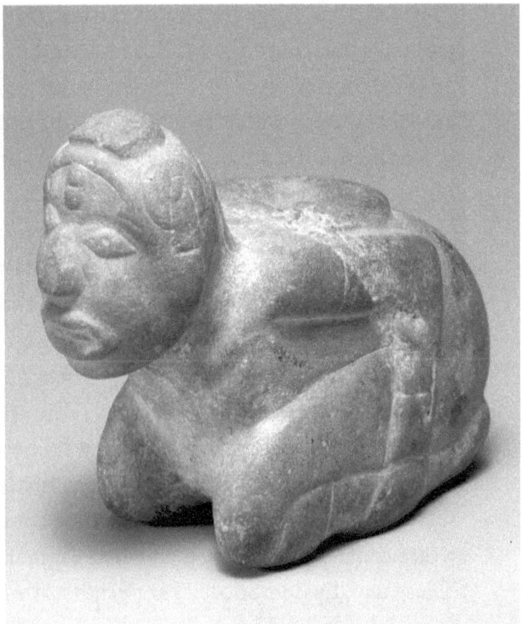

FIGURE 28 Left, Hopewell Owl Effigy Pipe.
Right, Mississippian Kneeling Prisoner Effigy Pipe.

west and Southeast. A famous pipe of the late period is the "Big Boy" from Spiro in Oklahoma (Brown 1985:102). This bauxite pipe depicts a kneeling elite male (Hall 1989:240). The pipe was a figurine refashioned into a pipe (Emerson 1982). Mississippian effigy pipes often include SECC artistic motifs, including horned serpents (Brown 1985:127) or other snake symbols. Snakes are powerful symbols in Native cultures. Examples include the Piasa Creek pipe, which depicts a kneeling shaman with a snake over his back, as well as the Schild Pipe, which shows a female kneeling on a coiled serpent (Emerson 1989:56). Other SECC pipes include war motifs such as kneeling prisoners. A pipe from Piasa Creek Mound depicts a kneeling figure (Brown 1985:156–157; O'Connor 1995:41). These effigy pipes tend to be found in mound burials or other ceremonial contexts. A ceremonial structure from the BBB Motor site included burials containing effigy pipes (Emerson 1989:48–49).

Other effigies give insight into additional associations of smoking (Blanton 2015, 2016). These include frog effigies found near Cahokia (O'Connor

1995:40). One effigy frog holds rattles, thus termed "Rattler Frog." Similar effigies have been found at Nodena Mound in Arkansas and from sites in Louisiana (O'Connor 1995:40). The frog is an underworld symbol in the Southeast, associated with water, fertility, rebirth, and life. Emerson (2003) interpreted this as communicating shamanistic concepts. The biological ambiguity of amphibians (not quite lizard, not quite fish), and their ability to move between land and water, makes them ideal spirit animals. Several pipes show frogs or humans holding frogs and/or rattles. Rhythm instruments feature in shamanistic traditions, with drums common in the arctic and subarctic (Van Deysen 2004) but rattles more common in the rest of the Americas (Vitebsky 2001).

Other Mississippian effigy pipes may not exhibit the same degree of craftsmanship. A sandstone pipe from the Humphrey site, ca. 1000–1250 CE, in Missouri has been interpreted as a feline predator (Johnson 1994), though others have interpreted it as a bison, turtle, rabbit, badger, beaver, or owl. It was discarded in a refuse pit. The pipe contained tobacco (Benn 1981). This is a rare artifact for the western Mississippian margins, with few similar effigies. These usually do not occur at peripheral villages, indicating emulation of elite material culture. This was a multifunction object, with one face showing wear indicative of hematite grinding and the base used to sharpen awls. This may indicate the pipe was associated with tattooing. A contemporary human effigy pipe with facial tattoos and hematite staining was recovered from a trash pit in Kansas (O'Brien 2003).

Hedden (2016) describes Mississippian pipes from Iowa, mostly clay elbows typical of the period. A small number are stone, including one red pipestone specimen similar to later calumets. The assemblage includes several effigies, including birds and faces. Another is a mace effigy, an elite symbol. Further symbolism is expressed on a clay pipe featuring an eye-in-hand symbol. Hedden ties these symbols to rituals allowing a soul's passage to the land of the dead.

While Mississippian effigy pipes are impressive, most late prehistoric pipes are less elaborate (Shriver 1983). Thomas's nineteenth-century mound survey illustrated examples , mostly elbows (Thomas 1985:233–234), including specimens from the Hollywood Mounds in Georgia (De Baillou 1965). At least five stone elbow pipes were recovered from the Nelson Triangle site from North Carolina, one from a mass grave (Thomas 1985:339–341). One elbow was found at Tennessee's Big Toco Mound (Thomas 1985:383), while the Lenoir Mounds contained elbow pipes in burials, generally near the head or hands (Thomas 1985:402–403).

Blanton (2015, 2016) observes Mississippian pipe decoration change in relation to cultural changes. Focusing on Etowah, he notes pipes early in the site's expansion are plain pottery pipes. As Etowah coopted surrounding sites after 1100 CE, pipes became elaborately decorated and standardized, incorporating foreign styles, often with detachable stems. Blanton argues smoking shifted from a less formalized mode to a dogmatic, elite-dominated mode. Elaboration in material culture has adaptive value as visible expressions of status. Those accruing status overextend themselves in consumption (such as pipe manufacture) and use those symbols to exhibit status.

While pipes had a role in maintaining power structures, this was not inevitable. Mass production of pottery pipes, as well tobacco replacing datura, allowed for a "democratization" of smoking (Von Gernet 1992:178; 1995). However, such a democratization of a ritual practice should not be seen as a secularization of that practice. Knight (1975:125) notes:

> By the end of the Middle Woodland Period, a definite dichotomy in pipe forms begins to become established. The simple, unembellished clay elbow pipe occurs quite commonly, while the beautifully made carved stone forms also occur. One might interpret this as an increasing secularization of smoking. With the introduction of pottery, the labor formerly involved in the manufacture of pipes must have been significantly reduced, making pipes available to individuals of lower status in the by now well-developed ranked societal structure. If smoking was formerly a prestige activity linked with ritual, as the pipe evidence indicates, then it was now less so, though not necessarily implying a divorce with ritual in smoking.

We see similar trends in Western North America. In California, some groups viewed tobacco as sacred, while others used it for pleasure (Underwood 2002). While pottery made pipe construction easier, ethnographies show ease of manufacture did decrease significance.

Looking to Western North America, we see many trends similar to the East. The earliest pipes are typically tubular or conical, while elbow pipes were used in late prehistory and after contact. Tube pipes are used as index artifacts for early cultures in the Southwest and northern Mexico (Jennings et al. 1956). While elbow pipes come to dominate eastern assemblages, tube pipes are common in the West into the contact period (Driver and Massey 1957:264): "The tubular pipe remained popular in the Southwest longer than it did to the east with the possible exception of the Northern Plains area" (Jennings et al. 1956:102).

Elbow pipes do not appear until Pueblo periods in the Southwest and were "rare and exotic" (Jennings et al. 1956:83). Sacred associations continued into the late prehistoric, with elbow pipes in burials and in kivas, in addition to domestic contexts (e.g., Martin et al. 1936:62). In the interior Pacific Northwest, California, southern Southwest, and southwestern Texas/northwestern Mexico, elbow pipes do not appear until the protohistoric. Elbow pipes probably developed in the East as a derivation of platform pipes. There are first-millennium CE platform pipes with the bowl at the end, essentially an elbow pipe with a platform stem, a transitional form. Since platform pipes are not found in the West, it is not surprising that elbow pipes are not found in large numbers either. It is reasonable to conclude that elbow forms were developed east of the Mississippi, then spread west in late prehistory.

Some early Southwest pipes were quite large; one sandstone example from northern Mexico is over 26 cm long (Di Peso 1957). This and similar examples could have been "cloud blowers" where smoke is blown out the pipe's end. Similar tubes are found from southern Arizona, including Ventana Cave. The cave featured in Tohono O'odham (Papago) mythology as the home of the whirlwind, and the cave's significance is enhanced by a permanent spring (Murray 1988). Tube pipes were recovered from strata ranging from 3500 to 1500 BCE (Switzer 1969:27). There were fragments of three tube pipes in the cave and one large, complete pipe, all of ground stone. Haury (1950:352) notes the intact pipe was caked with burned organic residue. This residue was found to fluoresce under UV light, consistent with burned tobacco, but was never subjected to more sophisticated analysis.

A contemporary stone tube with tobacco seeds was recovered from the aptly named Stone Pipe site near Tucson. Similar sites include human figurines, ear plugs, nose plugs, stone pallets, and stone atlatl finger loops (Ferg 1997). One site included a pithouse with nonutilitarian objects arrayed on the floor in a manner evocative of local rock art, interpreted as a shaman's structure (Gregory 1997). Tubular pipes were part of a ritual assemblage in much the same fashion as contemporary sites in the Eastern Woodlands.

Switzer speculates Southwest pipes were derived from California, where pipe smoking dated as early as 6000 years BP. Later, Hohokam deposits also contained evidence of tobacco in the form of cane cigarettes and cloud blower pipes (Nicolay 2012). Mogollon deposits from Bat Cave in Arizona include pipes as well as cane cigarettes. Pipes from Ventana and Bat Caves show tobacco smoking for achieving ASCs in cave-based rituals in Southern Arizona over 4,000 years.

Chapter 2 discussed ritual cave use with the creation of art and ingestion of intoxicants including tobacco. Blakeslee (2013:360) notes the inclusion of any object in a cave need not represent that object's use but may represent offering that object to spirits who inhabit the cave or whose realm can be accessed there. As discussed, tobacco was commonly sacrificed, and archaeological evidence indicates pipes were commonly sacrificed as well. When investigating caves containing intoxicant evidence, we must consider the entire context to determine whether the drugs were being consumed or whether they were left for the consumption of spirits.

There are also "artificial caves" such as at Casas Grandes in northern Mexico, dating to the thirteenth to fifteenth century CE. This site contains a well beneath a structure known as the "House of the Walk-In Well." VanPool (2009:185) describes the well's contents and function:

> The well's compound had two "shamanic caches" (jars with mineral concretions, quartz, and small fetishes), seven of the nine pipes found at Paquimé, large quantities of copper bells and shell tinklers (noisemakers), and a large jar (ca. 50 cm high) with depictions of two shamans transformed with their headdresses beside them. To enter into the well, one would literally have to step over a human skull embedded in the floor. The contexts of the pipes, the shamanic caches, and the olla decorated with shamans in the House of the Walk-in Well all have the expected characteristics of shamanic sacra and likely reflect a shamanic ritual space associated with tobacco use.

Much as smoking in Archaic and Adena/Hopewell cultures would become significant in the ritual lives of later societies, pipes and tobacco took a prominent role in later Southwestern cultures. Pueblo Bonito, an extensive Puebloan site, was occupied between 828 and 1126 CE. One room at Pueblo Bonito contained pipes, conch shell trumpets, as well as:

> "Copper, . . . turquoise ornaments, bird fetishes, grinding slabs, fossils, pigments, 14 parrot skulls, whole vessels with parrot bones, painted and unpainted wood, and dozens of fragments of ground stone . . . of inalienable objects too powerful and valuable to be stored in a living room [Mills and Ferguson 2008:346].

Farther south, Hohokam sites include pipe caches with figurines, crystals, shell ornaments, and animal bones (Bayman 2001:269) as early as 1500 BCE.

While the ritual significance of Southwest pipes is clear, this does not preclude secular use. Pipes are common in pithouse assemblages from 200 to 1000 CE (Diehl 1998:623). While we should not assume a lack of ritual importance in domestic contexts, we do see a parallel pattern to the segregated storage of pipes and other powerful objects.

There are tubes similar to Archaic/Early Woodland (ca. 4000–2000 BP) pipes in the East from undated burials in Montana. Nearby rock art may be historic or protohistoric (Frison and Van Norman 1993). Since the pipes have no residue, they may have been sucking tubes. Von Gernet (1992:178) argues sucking tubes and pipes are "symbolically and functionally equivalent." Additional tubes from Saskatchewan burial mounds date between 900 and 1500 CE (Wilson and Pendree 1984). These are often incised with geometric and/or "thunderbird" iconography. A Pueblo I (750–900 CE) cemetery has similar patterns in pipe internment as Adena/Hopewell pipes. Pipes in Colorado Pueblo I burials are differentially distributed, with some cemeteries including pipes, while cemeteries from other parts of the basin do not (Potter and Perry 2011:538). These differences are interpreted as having ethnic significance, indicating pipes were symbolic objects with implications for social identity.

Great Basin tube pipes have been recovered from sites associated with the Western Idaho Archaic Burial Complex. These sites are early for pipe smoking, ranging between approximately 4000 and 3000 BCE. The Olds Ferry Dunes site at the Idaho/Oregon border yielded five pipes in association with human remains, burned soil, red ocher, and elaborate flaked stone artifacts (Pavesic 2000). None of the pipes showed evidence of burning, as was the case with the Montana specimens, though one was shattered. Similar sites in the region have been dated to as early as 4000 BCE, older than any Eastern examples. These burials exhibit features similar to those from Glacial Kame sites, including cemeteries on hills, red ocher, and ritual objects, including pipes.

Several tobacco species grow in the vicinity, primarily *N. attenuata*, although *N. quadrivalvis* is also frequent (Goodspeed 1954:453). Pavesic identifies Olds Ferry as the site of funerals and healing rituals, associating pipes as cloud blowers. Bearberry was used in the Great Basin and Columbia Plateau, so tobacco may not have been the only plant smoked. Pavesic concludes the older pipes from Olds Ferry were associated with shamanistic practices. He also incorporates the role of smoke in Great Basin cultures, where it is associated with fog and clouds, and also the soul.

Furst (1976:30) relates observations by Tschopik (1941) of Navajo pipe making, where pipes were made in pairs to ensure balance, in male or female types, with different uses for each gender. Special clays are used and moistened by the pipe maker's own saliva. Grasses chewed by deer are used to mix the clay. Special songs are sung over completed pipes, and the pipes are named. Pipe makers take sweat baths after the process, and four days must pass prior to a pipe being used. Pipe colors have symbolic meanings of gender and sacred directionality. All of this shows the pipe's significance as a symbol well beyond its technical function.

NATIVE PIPES AND EUROPEAN CONTACT

As smoking became popular among Europeans during the sixteenth and seventeenth centuries, European pipes were traded in increasing numbers to North America. These had effects on Native smoking. There were changes in pipe use in the Northeast during the contact period, with areas around the Great Lakes using Native pipes and others adopting Euroamerican pipes (Trubowitz 1992). Other areas, such as Onondaga territory, show a hiatus in Native pipes followed by resurgence in the 1600s as a nativist response (Bradley 1987:122). This maintenance of Native tobacco technology, even while other technologies were abandoned, is a testament to the role of smoking pipes in Native culture. Pipes were intimately bound to Native religion, and religion tends to be the most conservative aspects of culture.

There may have been a decrease in the use of durable materials during the contact period with wooden pipes replacing clay or stone, as observed for the Seneca (Bradley 1987:61). Use of perishable materials for smoking is a possibility for all of prehistory, though they would of course be unlikely to preserve. It is possible that due to use of perishable materials during the contact period, evidence of smoking pipes may reflect preservation bias rather than a real change in smoking practices.

FINAL THOUGHTS ON TOBACCO AND SMOKING

Evidence presented in this chapter is a synopsis of available data on tobacco and pipes in North America. Even within the space allowed, several facts have been demonstrated. Tobacco is and always has been the most significant Native intoxicant. There is an unbroken chain of observations from modern ethnographies through contact-period accounts and from the archaeology of later prehistoric farming societies, earlier Archaic foraging populations, and even the early hunters of the Pleistocene. While additional intoxicants discussed in this volume have seen local significance, in every case they were used in addition to, not instead of, tobacco, as far back as we have evidence of tobacco use.

Smoking pipes became the dominant material symbol of tobacco for at least 4,500 years, though there is evidence at this point that tobacco itself predated the pipe, at least in the western regions of North America. From relatively crude early specimens, pipes became religious symbols with numerous sacred connotations. At the time of contact with Europeans, tobacco pipes had split into elaborate, curated sacred objects on one hand and ubiquitous items of personal reverence on the other. In both senses, Native Americans had become "people of the pipe."

Numerous species of tobacco, foreign and native, were consumed from Virginia to California, from the subarctic to Mesoamerica and South America. Either alone, or along with other intoxicants, tobacco was key to the ritual lives of Native North Americans. This is true even for areas where there never was any tradition of horticulture; those who did not or could not grow tobacco were beholden to their neighbors and other trading partners for the vital resource. Tobacco was a spiritual glue that held Native societies together. While all the intoxicants discussed in this volume have had great cultural significance, to understand Native North American cultures, you must also understand tobacco.

The final chapter considers what broad points about Native American culture are demonstrated by the evidence of the use of intoxicants discussed in preceding chapters.

CONCLUSION AND FUTURE DIRECTIONS

SUMMARY OF EVIDENCE

Based on the evidence presented in this volume, it is clear that Native North Americans were no different from any other human population in terms of innate desires for intoxication. The use of mind-altering substances, of a range of types and intensities, is a cultural fundamental in Native culture across North America. A wide variety of direct and indirect evidence supports this claim. There is abundant evidence from nineteenth- and twentieth-century anthropology that shows the central role of tobacco in all aspects of Native life. There are also numerous ethnographic examinations of the peyote religion(s) of the Southwest and Great Plains and their growth into the modern Native American Church. Less ethnographic data are available regarding what few other hallucinogenic plants or fungi there are in North America. These primarily relate to the use of datura in California and Mexico, which as a practice was on the wane by the time of the earliest true ethnographers.

Ethnohistoric data taken from the accounts of European observers during the sixteenth, seventeenth, and eighteenth centuries, with near unanimity, make often incredulous mention of Native American intoxicant consumption.

Again, the earliest of these European commentaries refer to Native tobacco use, which is also the most widespread intoxicant discussed in these earliest sources, encountered wherever European explorers traveled. Essentially every early Spanish, French, and English account of North America, whether written from firsthand experience or relating the observations of others, describes the importance of tobacco to Native religion and society. By the seventeenth century, descriptions of Native tobacco consumption were also comparisons to European tobacco use as the practice rapidly gained popularity and economic significance in the Old World. Native tobacco was seen as a curiosity and a vice while European tobacco was a vital and civilized commodity.

Likewise, sixteenth- and seventeenth-century Spanish and English sources provide the bulk of our objective knowledge about the use of ilex teas in southeastern North America, as well as datura across the continent, since these practices also were largely casualties of the contact process. Datura was primarily associated with puberty/initiation rituals that were undermined by Christianization, while ilex consumption was closely tied to indigenous sociopolitical structures that were also substantially disrupted through religious conversion, disease, and warfare. There are numerous references to unusual beverages in Northeastern sources, and the limited descriptions we have are broadly congruent with datura; but these accounts are generally lacking in any details that would allow a researcher to identify the substances in question.

Archaeological evidence for intoxicant use ranges from solid, physical, dated plant remains, to residue evidence from associated material culture, to material culture in general, and finally to indirect evidence in the form of various types of iconography. The botanical evidence for tobacco, primarily in the form of preserved, burned tobacco seeds, is the most widespread type of data, with the longest history. Tobacco seeds have been identified in very early contexts in the Southwest, perhaps as early as the first immigrants to North America over ten millennia ago. These migrants from Western Asia would have come from a prehistoric tradition of shamanic intoxication. They would have rapidly sought to replace the intoxicant plants they had left behind with new, local alternatives, taking advantage of native tobacco species soon after their entrance into the region. Tobacco thus came to replace intoxicants such as fly agaric mushrooms that played analogous roles in West Asia.

Preserved tobacco seeds from South America show the *Nicotiana* genus was being used as a smoke plant between 2000 and 1000 BCE; the data are still insufficient to give a solid origin for the selective breeding of either *N. rustica* or *N. tabacum* or for their introduction into North America. The number of preserved, securely dated and identified botanical specimens of tobacco is simply too small at this point to draw solid interpretations, and unfortunately may remain so due to limitations in recovery and preservation. Tobacco seeds are probably too small and fragile to preserve for the thousands of years necessary in most of North America (the possible exception being the arid Southwest). Even the molecular evidence found in organic residues may not survive long enough to be detected even with modern extraction and detection methods as fragile organic molecules decay over time.

Botanical evidence for other intoxicants besides tobacco are far more sporadic and recent in age. The oldest evidence in this category is for red "mescal" beans, which are quite durable and preserve for extended periods of time, especially in the arid Southwest where they were used. Questions remain as to how much these were used as intoxicants as opposed to decoration given the bean's known toxicity, as well as its relationship to the other hallucinogen in the region, peyote. Botanical evidence for other intoxicating substances, such as ilex or datura seeds, is comparatively rare and rarely older than late prehistoric contexts such as those associated with the Mississippian polities of the last few centuries prior to European contact. This does not in and of itself argue for a recent origin for those substances, and their use is likely far older than the physical evidence indicates; but there are significant challenges in recovering perishable data relating to relatively low-frequency practices. While intoxicant use was geographically extensive in North America, with the possible exception of tobacco, it does not seem to have been nearly as frequent as the use of food plants. Despite the greater cultural significance, intoxicants likely will always have a less intense archaeological footprint due to their relative rarity.

Some of the strongest direct evidence for intoxicant use so far recovered has not been botanical, but chemical. The extraction and analysis of organic residues is a highly promising but still underutilized method in general, and it is still mostly used to identify ancient food substances. There are few researchers actively pursuing research on chemical residues associated with intoxicants. Most of this research has focused on tobacco, for which there is a specific associated material culture in the form of smoking pipes.

There have also been useful pilot studies of chocolate and maize beer in the Southwest, looking at probable specialized pottery vessels used in consumption rituals based on those beverages. In the Eastern Woodlands of North America, there have been limited studies of pottery and smoking pipes associated with the consumption of ilex and datura. This author is still engaged in tobacco residue analysis, and hopefully we will see residue analysis of other intoxicants continue in greater frequency than has been the case so far. The relative lack of specialized research facilities conducting residue analysis continues to be a significant impediment in this regard. Hopefully there will come a time when organic residue analysis is as accessible and reliable as radiocarbon dating, and residue assays will be a standard item for any substantial archaeological project.

The most potentially informative type of evidence with regard to Native American intoxicants remains not the substances themselves but the material culture associated with their use. These data primarily consist of smoking pipes, which have an unbroken history going back at least 4,500 years. While cautions have been raised on many occasions that smoking pipes in and of themselves do not demonstrate tobacco use, the geographically widespread distribution and long history of botanical and organic residue evidence of tobacco indicates that most smoking pipes were used for tobacco. There is a thousand-year gap between the oldest residue evidence and the oldest smoking pipes that needs to be filled, but we can say with some confidence that tobacco likely was used during that period, especially in light of the recent Pleistocene tobacco discovery.

There is substantial ethnographic and ethnohistoric evidence of the use of various blends of other plants besides or in addition to tobacco across North America, as well as limited botanical and organic residue evidence. These mixtures generally include various components of what was known among the Algonquian speakers of the East as kinnikinnick. Also, botanical evidence shows one pipe from the Southeast was used for datura. But, this evidence notwithstanding, we can say with confidence now that the history of tobacco in North America is closely aligned with the history of smoking pipes at least for the past three thousand years, though the millennia preceding that period are still largely shrouded in uncertainty.

We should extend the material culture study of pipes to other types of intoxicant-related artifacts. The most obvious examples would be shell drinking cups or spoons for ilex and specialized ceramics associated potentially with ilex, datura, or alcohol. Caffeine, theobromine, scopolamine, atropine, and alcohol products are all known and detectable biomarkers that clearly identify particular intoxicant substances. Other possible examples would include stone pallets, grinding stones, or small stone cups, which could have been used in tobacco snuff production and consumption. While the range of uses of pottery vessels are not as clear as is the case for smoking pipes, in conjunction with residue analysis research we should be able to trace the development of intoxicant technology over time to a degree not yet attempted.

Evidence from Native American iconography can best be described as equivocal on the issue of intoxicant use. There are several rock art and ceramic art traditions that exhibit characteristics which have been associated with ASCs. A range of abstract and depictive artistic motifs are broadly congruent with reported hallucinatory imagery experienced from a range of stimuli, including intoxicants available in North America. A plausible argument can be made that some significant portion of this art was associated with shamanic or shamanistic practices and that these practices likely involved the consumption of various intoxicating substances. In a few rare instances, such as depictions of datura plants in the southwest, or rock art panels located immediately nearby growing wild tobacco, it is possible to directly associate the artwork with a particular intoxicant, and in these cases, the art should be taken as plausible evidence of the use of that substance in that region at that time.

However, using prehistoric art as evidence for intoxicant consumption must grapple with several significant challenges. For reasons of both cultural tendencies and natural preservation, the majority of extant Native rock art is located in the arid Southwest and northern Mexico. Eastern Native cultures were both historically less likely to engage in rock art, and what rock art was created was less likely to survive the temperate climate. That said, Western regions are home to some of the most potent psychoactive intoxicants in North America, the geographic distribution of which broadly corresponds to the distribution of major rock art traditions. So, despite the ambiguities in rock art depictions and the possible preservation bias, the distribution of rock art may be a real indicator of association with hallucinogen consumption.

Even for those artworks that are most evocative of neuropsychological interpretations of hallucination, a researcher must acknowledge that hallucinogenic intoxicants are only one way of inducing the perception of such imagery, albeit the simplest and most direct way available. The physical rigors and trauma involved in many Native rituals, the sensory deprivation of a cave environment, or continuous rhythmic noise and motion, all could induce ASCs. Finally, even a proponent of the neuropsychological approach to the study of past iconography must admit that not all such artwork was hallucinatory in nature, and that it is challenging to define objective criteria to discern between hallucinatory and non-hallucinatory images. How do you distinguish between a depiction of a figure experiencing bodily distortion due to hallucination and one of a mythical monster or spirit? So, while the iconographic evidence is fascinating and does provide useful insights on Native religious beliefs and rituals, its role should be to supplement the ethnographic, ethnohistoric, and archaeological records, not to replace or supersede them.

While it is abundantly clear that Native North Americans share in the psychic unity of humankind with regard to the ubiquity of intoxication, there is a fascinating regional twist to the story. According to the best evidence in the ethnographic and ethnohistoric record, a range of indigenous psychoactive plants and fungi have had local significance but have not seen widespread use on a continental scale. Red beans and peyote, for example, have been prominent in the desert Southwest/northern Mexico, though peyote extended into the Great Plains during the historic era and still is used within the rituals of the Native American Church. Ilex teas were commonplace throughout the Southeast and as far north as the mid-Atlantic region. Datura species were used across the temperate ranges of North America, but data are especially rich for areas of the Southeast, Southwest, and California. In all these cases, the use of the intoxicant in question was largely limited to the natural range of the plant from which it was derived. Trade in these substances to regions outside of the source areas seems to have been minimal based on current evidence.

However, a foreign cultigen—*Nicotiana rustica* tobacco—achieved a continental dominance sometime in the past three thousand years, if not earlier, and native species of tobacco have been used in the Southwest for at least as long, if not as long as human occupation of the continent. The Native American data on intoxicants seem to indicate that while powerful hallucinogens and stimulants can achieve widespread use, there are limits to their spread, and their ultimate distribution is largely determined by cultural affinities. In the absence of particular social institutions, such intoxicants are less likely to take hold outside of their natural range. Tobacco, however, clearly has qualities that allow it to transcend these limitations, the nature of which are explored below.

However, one of the most popular intoxicants in the rest of the world, alcohol, which widely transcends cultural divisions across the globe, has almost no presence at all in North America. Southwestern use of fermented maize, cacti, or other wild starchy plants have much in common with Mesoamerican traditions but disappear from the available record once you move away from northern Mexico and adjacent regions of the Southwest. While we cannot rule out the occasional use of fermented beverages from wild fruits in North American prehistory, or even the fermentation of Native starchy plants or maize, any such behavior does not seem to have left any significant footprint in the ethnographic, ethnohistoric, or archaeological record. Occasional propositions to the contrary have so far lacked evidentiary support beyond unsubstantiated anecdotes.

There has only been direct, chemical evidence of alcohol from a small number of late prehistoric sites in Arizona, though to be fair, such research has not been attempted in other regions. A research program to evaluate whether the apparent lack of a tradition of alcohol use is real might shed some light on the question, but this would be challenging. Even if no chemical evidence was found, it would not mean no past tradition existed, only that it was of a comparatively small scale.

Assuming that the lack of alcohol in North America is real, this absence can be attributed to two factors. First, the relatively late development of maize-based farming across most of North America, north of Mexico, means there was no surplus of starchy plants for fermentation. Second, the early spread of tobacco throughout the continent meant that the "cultural niche" of a mild, socially engaging intoxicant was already occupied before the origins of any farming, so there was no social need for alcohol's development or drive for its widespread acceptance. This situation continued until contact with Europeans.

Scholarly attention has only relatively recently been directed to the question of Native American intoxicant use in a scientifically rigorous way. While there was a burst of research primarily by cultural anthropologists during the 1960s and 1970s, with such researchers as Peter Furst, Gordon Wasson, or Weston La Barre expounding on human intoxicant use, the quality and objectivity of some of this work was uneven. Much of this seminal work was limited to the study of hallucinogens, while this volume has shown that this is only one class of intoxicants, and one that is less commonly used than milder stimulants, narcotics, or alcohol. One suspects the cultural preoccupation of the time with psychedelic drugs had some role in constraining academic focus, with counterculture figures such as Timothy Leary active in academic settings. While the research of the key figures mentioned above, and many others, was solid scholarship, the historical context led to the acceptance of substandard research, or even in the case of Castaneda, outright fraud. Castaneda's fraud, even after its exposure, was not decried by many anthropologists, and some notable figures went on to support Castaneda's work afterwards despite its known inaccuracy, presumably because it fit with the academic zeitgeist of the era. Even some seminal researchers of traditional hallucinogens and/or shamanism seemed to lose their objective distance from their subjects, "going native" and personally adopting the lifeways they were studying. While meaning no disrespect to anyone's life choices, this did not reflect favorably on the objectivity of the resulting research.

There was a general hiatus of research during the "just say no" era of the 1980s and 1990s, in part due to widespread cultural rejection of psychedelic culture, and in part due to the unobjective excesses of some contemporary researchers. With a few notable exceptions, the study of any drug culture became something serious academics did not work on. Scholarly attention is only gradually now turning back to the topic in a systematic and objective fashion.

The comparative absence of research specifically focused on intoxicants is particularly noticeable in the case of archaeology. While there has been substantial archaeological investigation of material culture associated with tobacco and smoking (i.e., smoking pipes), as we have seen, this is just one of many possible intoxicants used prehistorically. Tobacco research aside, there has been little in the way of research directed specifically at recovering data relating to intoxication; when recovered, such data have generally been incidental to unrelated research designs addressing questions typically related to diet and food production. Prehistoric evidence of intoxication has been a matter of convenience rather than a topic of preference. This has been gradually changing in recent years, and today there are several teams of researchers, often working in collaboration, exploring the question of the prehistoric use of intoxicants. Much data are left to uncover, the methodological challenges are real, and many questions still need to be answered. Future prospects are bright, however.

Residue analysis research is a rapidly expanding field with a great deal of potential. This methodology has provided direct evidence of the use of several prominent intoxicants even in contexts where conventional botanical evidence had not preserved. For example, several promising pilot studies on the detection of nicotine and other compounds in smoking pipe residue have been expanded by additional researchers, bringing more sophisticated methodology and more advanced technology to the question. So far, this research has supported the hypothesis that tobacco use was widespread in late prehistory, immediately prior to Native contact with Europeans, and has a significantly longer history before that time than had been previously supposed. Tobacco-related compounds have been positively identified in smoking pipes from the Northeast, Pacific Coast, and Southeast, from contexts over 2,000 years old. A promising avenue of research would be to conduct similar research on pipes from the Southwest, Texas, and northern Mexico, along the most likely path by which tobacco use was introduced into North America. This would allow us to clarify the chronology of the spread of this most widespread of American intoxicants. In addition, we should try to seek additional specimens from the regions already documented that date prior to the second millennium BP, both from new excavations and existing museum collections.

Molecular evidence of the association of smoking pipes with tobacco is sounder today than it previously was, even allowing for the prehistoric use of other plants in addition to or in place of tobacco as documented for multiple cultures historically. More and more artifacts are being investigated every year. The accuracy, precision, and availability of instruments are improving. Biomarker compounds and ratio patterns for less specific compounds for numerous plants, edible, medicinal, and intoxicant, are being isolated and published. This is likely to be especially promising for intoxicants that were used in relatively high volume in liquid form, particularly chocolate beverages in the Southwest and ilex beverages in the Southeast. Both substances are likely to have been made in large quantities, and so one would expect to see a relatively high sample size of vessels or sherds with residues. Also, some of these vessels may be stylistically or materially distinct; for example, the use of shell vessels and utensils associated with ilex production and consumption provide an interesting case study. Does shell absorb sufficient organic residue? Residue analysis of archaeological and experimental samples would address this question.

Residue analysis is least likely to be of much use for substances such as peyote, red bean, or hallucinogenic mushrooms that require little to no processing prior to consumption nor any specialized material culture in order to consume. Peyote, based on ethnographic observations, was most often eaten whole, but infusions were made occasionally; so residue evidence cannot be ruled out, which may be especially significant given the poor preservation characteristics of cacti.

Datura beverages remain a possibility, but the potency and toxicity of that substance likely kept the volume of its use low and specialized, leaving a small sample size of relevant ceramics for analysts to investigate. The vessels in question may be formally distinct, in this case evoking the form of the datura plant, giving researchers an initial clue to form a sample for analysis. But there is a strong possibility that datura was also processed frequently in fairly generic pottery vessels, indistinguishable from utilitarian forms, or even smoked in pipes as demonstrated for a late prehistoric pipe.

Additional research on intoxicant substances other than tobacco should continue, as should residue research on tobacco. These goals would be aided by a dedicated facility that could conduct residue analyses. While there have been efforts to establish such a facility, the availability of instrumentation and trained analysts remains a limiting factor.

Residue analysis may be the most promising method for research on intoxicants, but we should not overlook the importance of more conventional botanical research as well. Evidence for datura use in the Southeast, while derived from a smoking pipe, was in the form of pollen rather than nicotine residue. Perhaps a portion of pipe residues slated for residue analysis should be set aside for palynology, pollen having potentially more favorable preservation properties than organic residues, which degrade over time even in favorable climates. And, greater emphasis should be placed on recovering botanical evidence, particularly seeds. How much seed evidence of datura, for example, has been discarded from burial contexts because nobody thought to conduct flotation analysis on soil samples from non-domestic and non-food-related contexts? Or beyond botanical evidence entirely, is there overlooked evidence of red ant ordeals in prehistory, or faunal evidence of *Bufo* frog consumption that has been overlooked as intrusive or purely food-related? The materialist foundation of archaeology exists for a reason given the nature of the data, but this does not mean that there are no material data that relate to nonmaterial, mental elements of past human lives. We just have to make the effort to look for it.

GENERAL TRENDS IN NORTH AMERICAN INTOXICANTS

This volume has largely focused on data relating to the use of specific North American intoxicants. Any anthropological investigation should also seek broad generalizations that can be applied cross-culturally. By comparing patterns of use of all the intoxicants herein reviewed, some meaningful general patterns do emerge. These trends can be applied generally outside of North American contexts and likely represent common patterns in human behavior relating to intoxicant-induced ASCs. Two general trends stand out from the North American data: (1) the probable widespread and early use of intoxicants in human history and (2) the primarily nonutilitarian, ritual context of traditional intoxicant use.

As discussed in the introduction to this volume, evidence of intoxicant use in the Old World is historically early and likely was an evolved and adaptive trait of our earliest human ancestors. The occurrence of analogous behavior in nonhuman mammals indicates intoxication is an early and conserved trait among animals with complex nervous systems, primarily mammals. With these points in mind, I noted a common hypothesis among scholars of New World intoxicants that the first colonists of the Americas during the late Pleistocene epoch were already using drug-induced ASCs in their ritual practices. If this hypothesis is to be born out, we would expect to find evidence of intoxicants in the oldest archaeological contexts in North America. The evidence collected in this volume partially bears this out. The only intoxicant we can say with any confidence has Pleistocene roots is tobacco, and that is based on one discovery from Utah. The pan-continental distribution of tobacco use at contact is itself inferential evidence of antiquity, but only that. The only other intoxicant with a long prehistory is red bean, with reported examples going back as early as the dawn of the Holocene, over 8,000 years ago.

The true historical age of all the other intoxicants covered in the volume is as yet undetermined, with their oldest archaeological evidence at 2000 BCE or later, among the relatively sedentary, farming societies of late prehistory. We can again infer that the widespread geographic distributions of substances like ilex, used throughout its growth range, and datura, used from California to Virginia, indicate cultural practices of considerable age. But this assessment is as of now circumstantial. Hard evidence in the form of botanical or molecular evidence from reliably dated contexts has proven exceedingly rare if not altogether absent for most of the substances discussed in this volume. If, as is plausible given the historic evidence, the use of intoxicants is older than the physical data so far support, there are plausible causes for the lack of data.

The primary cause of this lack of ancient evidence is poor preservation, which can drop the archaeological visibility of already low-abundance substances below what we can detect with current methods and technology. This is a common pattern in paleontology, for example, where the origin, gradual expansion, and inevitable decline of a species are not documented in the fossil record, since that is when the abundance of the organism in question is at its lowest, below the threshold of preservation. This gives the false impression of a sudden origin and extinction, because it is only when the abundance of something is at its highest level that it preserves often enough to be recovered by researchers.

Similarly, intoxicant plants are high-value, but low-volume resources compared to food resources, and the amount of any given substance in circulation at one point in time is likely to be comparatively low. Most, if not all, of the little physical evidence there is would then likely be lost to decay over time, especially for substances such as cacti or fungi which are not physically durable even in ideal preservation environments. One may hold out some hope that the dry caves of the Southwest may yet yield evidence of intoxicants significantly earlier than what has so far been discovered. Analysis of pottery or stone artifacts may in the future lead to molecular evidence of intoxicant compounds in ancient contexts. Molecular evidence may also exist on previously excavated artifacts from museum collections, though such data do present their own array of challenges due to decay and/or contamination. Alternatively, developing methods of investigating human remains for similar molecular, pollen, or even botanical evidence could in the future provide physical evidence of ancient intoxicants. But, until such a time as these possibilities come to fruition, the pre-farming, "archaic" history of several varieties of North American intoxicants, and of hallucinogens in particular, is likely to remain speculative.

Equally as important as the history of intoxicants is the social context in which they were used. In the introduction, several hypotheses were presented as to the potential adaptive value intoxication might provide to humans and other mammals. While a biological adaptation is plausible, this volume adopts the perspective that it is the social value of intoxicants that has been largely responsible for their widespread use by human societies. Keeping that in mind, we can discuss the social value of intoxication and the social prescriptions and proscriptions associated with their use.

We have extensively documented how intoxicant use by Native Americans was consistently associated with ritual practices engaged in when interacting with spirits. The data also show patterning in the details of who was able to engage in these practices based on the nature of specific intoxicants. Specifically, the data indicate that the degree of social restriction of a given intoxicant seems to relate to the degree to which the substance in question altered consciousness. Paradoxically, while ASCs are a human universal, the more intense that altered state is (i.e., the more it deviates from normal cognition), the more likely it is to be subject to social regulation of some sort. Mild stimulants, like caffeine, are often nearly ubiquitous in society, restricted only by age and then often loosely. Even in our own society, which strongly limits or regulates intoxicants, caffeine is widely available to all members of society. Even children drink caffeinated soft drinks, and the only restrictions on more highly caffeinated coffee beverages or energy drinks are social conventions.

Under the influence of milder stimulants such as caffeine, a subject's personality is not substantially altered, and the effect may not even be noticeable to observers. Kola nut, beetle nut, coca leaf, or qat are used by sizeable cross sections of the cultures that use them, with some unofficial limitations based on age or sex. Qat, for example, is primarily chewed by adult men. Coffee, tea, and cacao are not only widespread but have become the foundations of multi-billion-dollar transnational industries. Alcohol and modern tobacco are likewise widespread but with a primary restriction to adults in most settings. This restriction, unlike the unofficial restrictions for mild stimulants, is generally legally defined with sanctions for violation, though of course there is substantial illicit underage use of both around the world. Some cultures make distinctions within these categories, for example, policing the use of high-proof alcoholic spirits more strictly than low-proof beer or wine.

Both alcohol and tobacco have more significant effects on the personality and cognition of the user than do milder stimulants, so it fits with the observed pattern that they are more severely restricted in their use. Alcohol's personality-altering effect is a major factor in its use, but it is also highly dose dependent. While a drink or two might do little more than loosen a subject's inhibitions, severe alcohol intoxication can render the user effectively a different person, one devoid of social inhibitions and impulse control. Tobacco likewise has significant personality-altering effects only in very large doses; the commercial tobacco products of today mostly induce relaxation, and that mostly by providing just enough nicotine to stave off withdrawal symptoms. The potential severe intoxication and even hallucinations produced by tobacco described in Chapter 5 occurred with noncommercial species of tobacco not widely marketed today, with much higher concentrations of nicotine, and often with consumption in much greater amounts. However, the health effects of both alcohol and tobacco use, especially chronic use, far outweigh those of mild stimulants, and this likely also plays a role in their age restriction. In both cases, today it tends to be the person who withholds from caffeine or alcohol who is the anomaly, and while smoking is declining precipitously in the United States, it is still a very common practice in the developing world.

By comparison, powerful hallucinogens or narcotics are commonly restricted to particular categories of user in specific, controlled circumstances. Fly agaric mushrooms in the shamanic cultures of Siberia are used by shamans or administered in controlled circumstances by shamans. *Banisteriopsis/ayahuasca* in South America is also typically administered by an individual who is well versed in the substance's use. Likewise, intoxicants with significant unpleasant or even life-threatening side effects, such as powerful narcotics, are typically restricted to special use as well. In modern societies, these two categories of powerful hallucinogens or drugs with significant side effects are typically proscribed legally, in part because the element of expert supervision has broken down and powerful and/or dangerous substances are now taken by individuals for recreational reasons. Even where modern science has hypothesized potentially therapeutic uses for hallucinogens, such as "microdosing" of LSD to treat PTSD or use of ketamine to treat severe, treatment-resistant depression, it has been difficult to conduct research due to the stringent legal restrictions placed on these substances. This is also likely again an effect of the hallucinatory excesses of the 1960s having a negative effect on the conduct of intoxicant research today.

While speculative, it is plausible that intoxicants that significantly alter a subject's personality, making oneself "other" in comparison with other members of society, or whose dangerous effects threaten the social collective, are more likely to be restricted or entirely proscribed. From a functionalist perspective, social norms within traditional cultures, and the laws of developed countries, exist in large part to protect the group from the actions of the individual and to protect the individual from exploitation by the group. Intoxicants which substantially alter an individual's personality and social persona, or which are seen as a threat to individual and public health, are not likely to become generalized in use and are more likely to be restricted or banned. From a more modern social theory perspective, those same norms and laws also function to perpetuate social hierarchies and inequalities. Powerful hallucinogens, with their ability to allow an individual insight into previously unconscious social relations, threaten those social hierarchies and are thus restricted or banned by the structure of authority.

Some substances exist in a gray zone between the two extremes of widespread use and restriction/proscription. Cannabis is an excellent example in this regard. It was once viewed as a dangerous narcotic in developed countries, in large part due to racist associations with immigrant populations and later with counterculture movements, but the relatively benign nature of its technically hallucinogenic effects has allowed it over time to enter an age-restricted but generalized category in much of the world. Within the past decade we have seen a radical shift in legal attitudes toward cannabis, from active prosecution of even low-level users leading to substantial jail terms, and a major investment in the national "war on drugs," to widespread decriminalization or outright legalization. Cannabis is on track to occupy an intoxicant niche parallel to tobacco and alcohol across most of the world, as a socially sanctioned and governmentally taxed legal intoxicant. Tobacco, on the other hand, has been seeing a reverse trend, from a widespread pattern of use in the early-to-mid-twentieth century to increasing legal restrictions on the locations it can be used and the ages of those who can use it.

A closely related factor is the degree of commensality associated with a given intoxicant's consumption. One can divide intoxicants into commensal and noncommensal types, those taken in group settings that encourage sociability as opposed to those either taken individually or that impede sociability. Commensal intoxicants are likely subject to strong social or legal restrictions less often than noncommensal intoxicants. In our own culture, caffeine, tobacco, or alcohol are highly commensal in their consumption and are less restricted legally, while strong hallucinogens such as LSD or opioids like heroin are noncommensal and are subject to strict, legal prohibition.

The examples of intoxicants from North America broadly follow these trends as well. Native tobacco, as opposed to commercial tobacco, is widespread and generalized in use, and while its use seems to have spread quite rapidly in prehistory, it does seem to have been more restricted in its early adoption within the societies that used it. Many early accounts indicate a gender segregation in its use, with all adult males partaking but female or childhood use being quite rare. The earliest smoking pipes (which still predate most evidence for tobacco itself) were high-energy investment tools, involving often exotic, rare materials and considerable craftmanship to manufacture; were rare in number; and were limited to special, nonutilitarian contexts such as caches or burials. These data indicate that tobacco was benign enough to be widely generalized in its use, if socially defined to certain categories, but that this generalization took time to develop from a highly specialized, socially restricted, and context-specific setting. The high degree of commensality associated with the social context of tobacco likely played a role in the rapid adoption and spread of tobacco use in prehistory.

Alcohol, cacao, and ilex are fairly generalized in use when available, though as with the earlier stages of tobacco, there appear to be rank and gender restrictions. The data regarding cacao and alcohol for North America are fairly limited, so the best we can say at this point is that there is the potential for social limitations by age (adults only) and possibly by gender, though there are observations of inebriated women. It is difficult to say whether these were remarked upon because they were anomalies or whether they were common occurrences. It is likely, though not proven, that these are substances reserved for high-ranking males. This certainly seems to be the case for ilex. All the historic sources make this a clear distinction, and the prehistoric associations of ilex-associated shell cups are generally with male burials. Again, the commensal nature of alcohol, cacao, and ilex consumption presumably played a role in each intoxicant's popularity.

Hallucinogens such as red bean, peyote, or datura were either taken only by specialists (shamans) or administered by specialists and were generally used for specific ritual events, most often healing or rites of passage. Red bean and datura have a double restrictive factor, both being not only hallucinogenic but also highly toxic. Expertise or expert supervision is thus required to prevent accidental poisoning. Peyote, while hallucinogenic, is more benign in its effects, with no examples of credible death due to toxicity, and we do see it historically being fairly widely used by adults, but generally under expert supervision in controlled circumstances. Peyote, at least in the historic context of the Native American Church, is the most commensal of these hallucinogens, taken often in group rituals involving substantial social interaction, and so is also the least restricted of the North American hallucinogens. At the other extreme, the significant dissociation and delirium associated with datura precludes any commensality, since users are often unaware of their surroundings, contributing further to the significant restrictions regarding the substance's use.

Another factor, closely related to the issue of commensality, and also relevant to the degree of social restriction in intoxicant use, is the nature of the cultural context in which that use took place. This essentially relates to the degree of Native religiosity involved in a drug's use. The guiding hypothesis outlined in the Introduction to this volume was that intoxicant use would be closely related to shamanism or shaman-like practices in traditional cultures. That seems to relate to the nature rather than the intensity of a given intoxicant. The cultural context of hallucinogens, including red bean, peyote, and datura, all closely model shamanic or shamanistic behavior, where a specialist ingests or administers the substance and translates the resultant ASC as a spiritual experience. The most generalized of these three in terms of use is peyote in the Native American Church, where numerous individuals periodically take the intoxicant together. Yet even while modern peyote use is not the explicit privilege of a shaman, peyote rituals are guided by senior practitioners, and the goal for all participants is a spiritual experience. While not narrowly shamanic, even the least specialized hallucinogenic rituals of this sort are still broadly shamanistic, following the distinction laid out in the Introduction.

Less intense intoxicants, such as caffeine or tobacco, are more likely to be socially restricted rather than functionally restricted. That is to say, their use may be monopolized by social norms relating to specific members of a society, such as males or members of high rank, but they are not used shamanistically to as great a degree as hallucinogens. This trend is what one might expect, since caffeine in black drink or cacao, or nicotine in tobacco, do not cause hallucinatory or dissociative ASCs of the sort sought by shamans or those engaging in shamanistic activities. As discussed in Chapter 5, while you do see Native American shamans using tobacco in the historic record, true hallucinatory tobacco shamanism, where one smokes massive amounts of tobacco to the point of stupefaction and hallucination, is more a South American practice than North American. While there is evidence that nicotine, and even caffeine, can have hallucinatory effects, these generally occur after very high, even life-threatening doses.

While there is a sacred component to the use of black drink in Native social rituals, the substance did not function to put individuals in direct contact with spirits via a hallucinatory ASC. In this regard, ilex, cacao, and even alcohol, were more likely to be used as indicators of status or elevated social status in general, which correlates with the ethnographic, ethnohistoric, and archaeological records. Nearly all the ethnohistoric sources for black drink depict it as the exclusive right of high-rank males; the archaeological record of ilex-associated vessels is likewise associated with high-rank burials. While the data available for cacao and alcohol are limited in North America north of Mesoamerica, what evidence we currently have indicates a similar pattern of high-rank association but not a shamanic function. Stimulants, then, seem to represent an exception to the hypothesis that Native American intoxicants were primarily tools of supernatural ritual practices; instead they were more likely to serve as symbols of status and facilitators of social interaction.

Tobacco is a different case, set in between the extremes of hallucinogens such as datura and stimulants such as ilex. The ethnographic and ethnohistoric sources are clear that Natives regarded tobacco and tobacco smoke as a means for communing with spirits. While mild tobacco intoxication is not anywhere near the dissociative delirium of datura or the hallucinations of peyote, it does include physical symptoms that Natives have interpreted as facilitating communication with the supernatural. Tobacco, for which we have the most direct physical evidence, has a twofold developmental pattern. Early tobacco use, based on archaeological evidence, does appear to be a restricted, likely shamanic practice. This element persists into the historic period. However, over time we also see greater and greater access to smoking and increasing secularization of tobacco. This indicates that over time, tobacco moved from a pattern similar to that of datura and peyote, restricted, shamanistic use for supernatural rituals, to a pattern more similar to ilex, relatively generalized use for demonstrating social status and facilitating social interactions within and between cultures.

THE FUTURE OF INTOXICANT STUDIES

While there are clearly methodological challenges to the study of intoxication due to poor preservation of a statistically rare but culturally significant practice, the greatest limitation to this research is a lack of scholarly attention. We need more researchers to recognize the insights systematic study of intoxicants and the social practices associated with them can provide on human cultures past and present. As with the study of human belief and ritual, the closely related study of intoxication should not be peripheral to the study of culture. Many elements of modern anthropology, archaeology in particular, are moving theoretically toward a "new materialism" focused on human ecology. While this approach is highly relevant in this age of environmental change, there is the danger that important aspects of the human story might be overlooked. Any anthropological study that does not take belief, ideology, and religion into account will be lacking vital elements. The study of intoxication is integral, or should be, to that ideological research.

The research presented in this volume shows that any study of Native American culture that does not include the role of intoxication is at best incomplete and at worst misleading. The study of intoxication is best achieved through a combination of approaches, including data drawn from ethnographic, ethnohistoric, archaeological, and archaeometric approaches. The resultant data then must be interpreted through a comprehensive theoretical framework regarding the sociocultural role of intoxicant use in any given setting. In this regard, we have seen how Native American intoxicants often played key roles in Native religion and spirituality and always played a role in Native social interactions. While this volume has barely scratched the surface of this topic, one hopes that additional research will be conducted, in North America, across the New World, and beyond the Americas to study the universal human practice of intoxication.

REFERENCES CITED

ABEL, E.

1980 *Marihuana: The First Twelve Thousand Years.* Plenum Press, New York.

ABERLE, D. F.

1991 *The Peyote Religion among the Navajo.* University of Oklahoma Press, Norman.

ABERLE, D. R., AND O. C. STEWART

1957 *Navaho and Ute Peyotism: A Chronological and Distributional Study.* Series in Anthropology No. 6. University of Colorado Studies, Boulder.

ABRAHAM, H.D., A. M. ALDRIDGE, AND P. GOGIA

1989 The Psychopharmacology of Hallucinogens. *Neuropsychopharmacology* 14(4):285–298.

ACOSTA, JOSÉ DE

1880 *The Natural and Moral History of the Indies.* Hakluyt Society, London.

ADAIR, J.

1930 [1775] In: Williams, Samuel Cole (ed.), *Adair's History of the American Indians.* The Watauga Press, Johnson City, Tennessee. Originally published 1775, Edward and Charles Dilly, London.

ADAIR, M.

2000 Tobacco on the Plains: Historical Use, Ethnographic Accounts, and Archaeological Evidence. In *Tobacco Use by Native North Americans: Sacred Smoke and Silent Killer,* edited by J. C. Winter, pp. 171–201. University of Oklahoma Press, Norman.

ADAMS, K., K. JOHNSON, AND T. MURPHY

2015 Prehistoric Puebloan Yucca Quids with Wild Tobacco Contents: Molecular and Morphological Evidence from Antelope Cave, Northwestern Arizona. *Journal of Field Archaeology* 40 (3):310–324.

ADAMS, K. R., AND M. S. TOLL

2000 Tobacco Use, Ecology, and Manipulation in the Prehistoric and Historic Southwestern United States. In *Tobacco Use by Native North Americans:*

Sacred Smoke and Silent Killer, edited by J. C. Winter, pp. 143–170. University of Oklahoma Press, Norman.

ADOVASIO, J., AND G. FRY

1976 Prehistoric Psychotropic Drug Use in Northeastern Mexico and Trans-Pecos Texas. *Economic Botany* 30(1):94–96.

ALDENDERFER, M.

1993 Ritual, Hierarchy, and Change in Foraging Societies. Journal of Anthropological Archaeology 12(1):1–40.

ANDERSON, D. G.

1998 Swift Creek in a Regional Perspective. In *A World Engraved: Archaeology of the Swift Creek Culture*, edited by J. M. Williams, pp. 274–300. University of Alabama Press, Tuscaloosa.

ANDERSON, E.

1995 Peyote and its Derivatives as Medicine. In *Sacred Plants, Consciousness, and Healing: Cross-cultural and Interdisciplinary Perspectives*, edited by M. Winkelman and W. Andritsky. Verlag für Wissenschaft und Bildung, Berlin.

1996 *Peyote: The Divine Cactus*. University of Arizona Press, Tucson.

ANYON, R., AND S. A. LEBLANC

1984 *The Galaz Ruin*. University of New Mexico Press, Albuquerque.

APPLEGATE, R.

1975 The Datura Cult among the Chumash. *Journal of California Anthropology* 2:6–17.

ARISS, R.

1939 Material Culture Notes: Distribution of Smoking Pipes in the Pueblo Area. *New Mexico Anthropologist* 3(3/4):53–57.

ASCH, D. L.

1991 *Tobacco Seeds in the Archaeobotanical Collections of the Center for American Archaeology*. Archaeobotanical Lab Report No. 82. Center for American Archaeology, Kampsville, Illinois.

1994 Aboriginal Specialty-Plant Cultivation in Eastern North America: Illinois Prehistory and a Post-Contact Perspective. In *Agricultural Origins and Development in the Midcontinent*, edited by W. Green, pp. 149–203. University of Iowa Press, Iowa City.

ASCH, D. L., AND N. B. ASCH

1985 Prehistoric Plant Cultivation in West–Central Illinois. In *Prehistoric Food Production in North America*, edited by R. I. Ford, pp. 149–203. University of Michigan, Ann Arbor.

BAKER, J. R.

1994 *The Old Woman and her Gifts: Pharmacological Bases of the Chumash Use of Datura*. Curare 17(2):253–276.

BAKER, M. A.

1981 *The Ethnobotany of the Yurok, Tolowa and Karok Indians of Northwest California*. MA thesis, Department of Biology, Humboldt State University, Arcata, California.

BALABANOVA, S., F. PARSCHE, AND W. PIRSIG

1992 First Identification of Drugs in Egyptian Mummies. *Naturwissenschaften* 79:358.

BALABANOVA, S., F. PARSCHE, G. BUHLER, AND W. PIRSIG

1993 Was Nicotine Known in Ancient Egypt? *Homo* 44(1):92–94.

BALABANOVA, S., B. WEI, AND M. KRAMER

1995 First Detection of Nicotine in Ancient Population of Southern China. *Homo* 46(1):68–75.

BALABANOVA, S., F. W. ROSING, G. BUHLER, W. SCHOETZ, G. SCHERER, AND J. ROSENTHAL

1997 Nicotine and Cotinine in Prehistoric and Recent Bones from Africa and Europe and the Origin of these Alkaloids. *Homo* 48(1):72–77.

BALL, E. K.

1962 *Early Uses of California Plants*. University of California Press, Berkeley.

BANDELIER, A. F.

1890 *Final Report of Investigations among the Indians of the Southwestern United States, Carried on Mainly in the Years from 1880 to 1885, Part I*. Papers of the Archaeological Institute of America, American Series III. University Press, Cambridge, Massachusetts.

BARBER, B.

1941 Acculturation and Messianic Movements. *American Sociological Review* 6(5):663–669.

BARBOUR, P. L. (ED.)

1969 *The Jamestown Voyages under the First Charter 1606–1609*, Vols. I & 2. Hakluyt Society, London.

BARROWS, D. P.

1967 *The Ethno-Botany of the Coahuilla Indians of Southern California*. Malki Museum Press, Banning, California.

BARTRAM, W.

1928 *The Travels of William Bartram*. Macy-Masius, New York.

BATESON, G.

1972 *Steps to an Ecology of the Mind*. Ballantine Books, New York.

BAYMAN, J. M.

2001 The Hohokam of Southwest North America. *Journal of World Prehistory* 15(3):257–311.

BEAGLEHOLE, E., AND P. BEAGLEHOLE

1935 Hopi of the Second Mesa. *Memoirs of the American Anthropological Association* 44:5–65.

BEAN, L. J., AND K. S. SAUBEL

1972 *Temalpakh (From the Earth): Cahuilla Indian Knowledge and Usage of Plants.* Malki Museum Press, Banning, California.

BECK, W., D. J. DONAHUE, A. J. T. JULL, G. BURR, W. S. BROECKER, G. BONANI, I. HAJDAS, AND E. MALOTKI

1998 Ambiguities in Direct Dating of Rock Surfaces using Radiocarbon Measurements. *Science* 280:2132–2139.

BELL, C.

1997 *Ritual: Perspectives and Dimensions.* Oxford University Press, Oxford.

BELL, W. H., AND E. F. CASTETTER

1937 Ethnobiological Studies in the American Southwest V: *The Utilization of Mesquite and Screwbean by the Aborigines in the American Southwest.* The University of New Mexico Biological Series, Vol. 5, No. 2. University of New Mexico Press, Albuquerque.

BENAVENTE MOTOLINIA, T.

1914 Historia de los Indios de la Nueva España. Heredores de J. Gili, Barcelona.

BENN, D. W.

1981 The Paleoethnobotany of the M.A.D. Sites (13CF101 and 13CF102) and Relationships with other Prairie Peninsula Sites. In *Archaeology of the M.A.D. Sites at Denison, Iowa,* edited by D. W. Benn, pp. 1–45. Iowa State Historical Society, Iowa City.

BENSE, J. A.

1994 *Archaeology of the Southeastern United States: Paleoindian to World War I.* Left Coast Press, Walnut Creek, California.

BENZONI, G.

1565 *Historia del Mondo Nuovo.* Venice.

BEVERLEY, R.

1855 The History of Virginia, in Four Parts. J. W. Randolph, Richmond, Virginia.

BEVERLEY, R.

1947 *The History and Present State of Virginia.* The Institute of Early American History and Culture, Williamsburg, Virginia.

BIGGAR, H. P.

1929 *The Works of Samuel de Champlain, Vol. 3.* The Champlain Society, Toronto.

BILLINGS, J. D.

1993 Coffee and Hardtack, or, the Unwritten Story of Army Life. University of Nebraska Press, Lincoln.

BISSET, N. G., J. G. BRUHN, AND M. H. ZENK

1996 The Presence of Opium in a 3,500 Year Old Cypriote Base-Ring Juglet. *Ägypten und Levante* 6:203–204.

BJORN, L.O.

1993 Responding to 'First Identification of Drugs in Egyptian Mummies'. *Naturwissenschaften* 80:244.

BLACKBURN, T.

1977 Biopsychological Aspects of Chumash Rock Art. *The Journal of California Anthropology* 4(1):88–94.

BLAKESLEE, D. J.

1981 The Origin and Spread of the Calumet Ceremony. *American Antiquity* 46(4):759–768.

2013 Caves and Related Sites in the Great Plains of North America. In *Sacred Darkness: A Global Perspective on the Ritual Use of Caves*, edited by H. Moyes, pp. 353–364. University of Colorado Press, Boulder.

BLANCHETTE, R., B. D. COMPTON, N. TURNER, AND R. L. GILBERTSON

1992 Nineteenth Century Shaman Grave Guardians are Carved *Fomitopsis officinalis* Sporophores. *Mycologia* 84(1):119–124.

BLANTON, D.

2015 *Mississippian Smoking Pipes in the Southern Appalachian Region*. University of Tennessee Press, Knoxville.

2016 Evolution of a Ritual: Pipes and Smoking in Etowah's Realm. In *Perspectives on the Archaeology of Pipes, Tobacco and other Smoke Plants in the Ancient Americas*, edited by E. A. Bollwerk and S. Tushingham, pp. 93–108. Springer Press, New York.

BLETZER K. V.

1976 Castaneda's Shaman Don Juan: 'Sorcerer' or Literary Vehicle? *Journal of Psychoactive Drugs* 8(4):327–329.

BLITZ, J. H.

2009 New Perspectives in Mississippian Archaeology. *Journal of Archaeological Research* 18:1–39.

BLOCH, M. AND BLOCH, M.E.

1986 From Blessing to Violence: History and Ideology in the Circumcision Ritual of the Merina. Cambridge University Press, Cambridge, United Kingdom.

BOCEK, B. R.

1984 Ethnobotany of Costanoan Indians, California, Based on Collections by John P. Harrington. *Economic Botany* 38(2):240–255.

BOHRER, V.

2004 *Flotation Analysis from High Rolls Cave (LA 114103), Otero County, New Mexico.* Southwest Ethnobotanical Enterprises Report 39. Portales, New Mexico.

BOLLWERK, E. A.

2012 *Seeing What Smoking Pipes Signaled: An Examination of Late Woodland and Early Contact Period (A.D. 900–1665) Native Social Dynamics in the Middle Atlantic.* PhD Dissertation, Department of Anthropology, University of Virginia. University Microfilms, Ann Arbor, Michigan.

BOREK, T, C. MOWRY, AND G. DEAN

2008 Analysis of Modern and Ancient Artifacts for the Presence of Corn Beer: Dynamic Headspace Testing of Pottery Sherds from Mexico and New Mexico. *Materials Research Society Symposium Proceedings* 1047:185–194.

BOSTWICK, T. W.

2002 *Landscape of the Spirits: Hohokam Rock Art at South Mountain Park.* University of Arizona Press, Tucson.

BOURGUIGNON, E.

1973 *Religion, ASCs, and Social Change.* Ohio University Press, Columbus.

1989 Trance and Shamanism: What's in a Name? *Journal of Psychoactive Drugs* 21(1):9–15.

BOYD, C. E.

1998 Pictographic Evidence of Peyotism in the Lower Pecos, Texas Archaic. In *The Archaeology of Rock Art,* edited by C. Chippendale and P. Taçon, pp. 229–246. Cambridge University Press, Cambridge, United Kingdom.

2003 *Rock Art of the Lower Pecos.* Texas A&M University Press, College Station.

BOYD, C. E., AND J. P. DERING

1996 Medicinal and Hallucinogenic Plants Identified in the Sediments and Pictographs of the Lower Pecos, Texas Archaic. *Antiquity* 70(268): 256–275.

BRADLEY, J. W.

1987 *Evolution of the Onondaga Iroquois: Accommodating Change, 1500–1655.* Syracuse University Press, Syracuse, New York.

BRAIDWOOD, R. J., J. D. SAUER, H. HELBAEK, P. C. MANGELSDORF, H. C. CUTLER, C. S. COON, R. LINTON, J. STEWARD, AND A. LEO OPPENHEIM

1953 Symposium: Did Man Once Live by Beer Alone? *American Anthropologist* 55(4):515–526.

BRANDT, C. B.

2000 Ethnobotanical Notes from Zuni Pueblo. In *Tobacco Use by Native Americans: Sacred Smoke and Silent Killer,* edited by J. C. Winter, pp. 81–83. University of Oklahoma Press, Norman.

BRANT, C. S.

1950 Peyotism among the Kiowa-Apache and Neighboring Tribes. *Southwestern Journal of Anthropology* 6(2):212–222.

BRASSER, T. J.

1980 Self-Directed Pipe Effigies. *Man in the Northeast* 19:95–104.

BRODY, J. J.

1977 *Mimbres Painted Pottery*. University of New Mexico Press, Albuquerque.

BROOKS, J. E.

1937 *Tobacco, Its History, Illustrated by the Books, Manuscripts and Engravings in the Library of George Arents, Jr., Vol. I, 1507–1615*. Rosenbach, New York.

BROSE, D. S.

1985 The Woodland Period. In *Ancient Art of the American Woodland Indians*, edited by D. Brose, J. Brown, and D. W. Penney, pp. 43–92. Harry N. Abrams, New York.

BROWN, I.

1989 The Calumet Ceremony in the Southeast and its Archaeological Manifestations. *American Antiquity* 54(2):311–331.

BROWN, J. A.

1985 The Mississippian Period. In *Ancient Art of the American Woodland Indians*, edited by D. Brose, J. Brown, and D. W. Penney, pp. 93–176. Harry N. Abrams, New York.

1997 The Archaeology of Religion in the Eastern Woodlands. *The Annual Review of Anthropology* 26:465–85.

BROWN, J. A., AND D. J. ROGERS

1999 AMS Dates on Artifacts of the Southeastern Ceremonial Complex from Spiro. *Southeastern Archaeology* 18(2):134–141.

BROWN, J. E.

1953 *The Sacred Pipe: Black Elk's Account of the Seven Rites of the Oglala Sioux*. University of Oklahoma Press, Norman.

BRUGGE, D. M.

1982 Western Navajo Ethnobotanical Notes. In *Navajo Religion and Culture*, edited by D. M. Brugge and Ch. J. Frisbie, pp. 89–97. University of New Mexico Press, Albuquerque.

BRUHN, J. G., J. F. LINDGREN, B. HOLMSTEDT, AND J. M. ADOVASIO

1978 Peyote Alkaloids: Identification in a Prehistoric Specimen of Lophophora from Coahuila, Mexico. *Science* 99(4336):1437–1438.

BUCKO, R. A.

1998 *The Lakota Ritual of the Sweat Lodge: History and Contemporary Practice*. University of Nebraska Press, Lincoln.

BUCKSKIN, F. AND A. BENSON

2005 The Contemporary Use of Psychoactive Mushrooms in Northern California. *Journal of California and Great Basin Anthropology* 25(1):87–92.

BUNZEL, R. L.

1929 *Zuñi Katcinas*. Forty-Seventh Annual Report, Bureau of American Ethnology (1929–1930). Smithsonian Institution, US Government Printing Office, Washington DC.

BURKS, J.

2001 Strait Site Radiocarbon Dates Revealed. *Ohio Archaeological Council Newsletter* 13(1):7.

BURLAGE, H. M.

1968 *Index of Plants of Texas with Reputed Poisonous or Medicinal Properties.* Burlage, Austin, Texas.

CABEZA DE VACA, A. N.

1983 [1542] *Cabeza de Vaca's Adventures in the Unknown Interior of America.* Translated and edited by Cyclone Covey. Reprinted. University of New Mexico Press, Albuquerque. Originally published 1961, Crowell-Collier, Springfield, Ohio.

CALABRESE, J. D., II

1994 Reflexivity and Transformation Symbolism in the Navajo Peyote Meeting. *Ethos* 22(4):494–527.

CAMPBELL, T. N.

1958 Origin of the Mescal Bean Cult. *American Anthropologist* 60(1):156–160.

CARMODY, S. B.

2015 Secrets in the Smoke: Prehistoric Tobacco Use in Tennessee. *Tennessee Council for Professional Archaeology*, posted September 23, 2015. https://tennesseearchaeologycouncil.wordpress.com/2015/09/23/30-days-of-tennessee-archaeology-2015-day-23/.

CARMODY, S. B., M. CAFFREY, B. S. LADY, AND S. P. HORN

2017 Palynological and Chemical Analyses of Prehistoric Pipe Residues as Evidence of Tobacco Use in Tennessee. *Tennessee Archaeology* 9(1):5–15.

CARMODY, S., J. DAVIS, S. TADI, J. S. SHARP, R. K. HUNT, AND J. RUSS

2018 Evidence of Tobacco from a Late Archaic Smoking Tube Recovered from the Flint River Site in Southeastern North America. *Journal of Archaeological Science: Reports* 21: 904–910.

CARMODY, S. B., R. HUNT, J. R. DAVIS, N. PRODANOVICH, AND J. RUSS

2017 Inhaling Prehistory: Exploring the Smoking Culture of the Eastern Woodlands. Paper Presented at the 2017 Annual Meeting of the Society for American Archaeology, Vancouver.

CARMODY, S. B., R. HUNT, J. RUSS, J. R. DAVIS, N. PRODANOVICH, B. MCKENZIE, AND C. VAN DE VEN

2016 Scraping the Bowl: New Data on Prehistoric Tobacco Use in the Southeast. *Tennessee Council for Professional Archaeology*, posted on September 30, 2016. https://tennesseearchaeologycouncil.wordpress.com/2016/09/30/scraping-the-bowl-new-data-on-prehistoric-tobacco-use-in-the-southeast/.

CAROD-ARTAL F. J., AND C. B. VÁZQUEZ-CABRERA

2006 Mescaline and the San Pedro Cactus Ritual: Archaeological and Ethnographic Evidence in Northern Peru. *Revista de Neurologia* 42(8):489–498.

CAROD-ARTAL F. J.

2015 Alucinógenos en las Culturas Precolombinas Mesoamericanas. *Neurología* 30:42–49.

CARPENTER, E. S.

1950 Five Sites of the Intermediate Period. *American Antiquity* 15(4):298–314.

CARR, L. G.

1947 Native Drinks in the Southeast and their Values, with Special Emphasis on Persimmon Beer. *Proceedings of the Delaware County Institute of Science* 10:29–43.

CARTIER, J.

1545 *Bref récit et succincte narration de la navigation faite en MDXXXV et MDXXXVI par le capitaine Jacques Cartier aux iles de Canada Hochelaga, Saguenay et autres.* Librairie Tross, Paris.

CASTETTER, E. F.

1943 Early Tobacco Utilization and Cultivation in the American Southwest. *American Anthropologist* 45(2): 320–325.

CASTETTER, E. F., AND W. H. BELL

1937 The Aboriginal Utilization of the Tall Cacti in the American Southwest. *University of New Mexico Bulletin, Biological Series* 5(1). University of New Mexico Press, Albuquerque.

1942 *Pima and Papago Indian Agriculture.* University of New Mexico Press, Albuquerque.

1951 *Yuman Indian Agriculture.* University of New Mexico Press, Albuquerque.

CASTETTER, E. F., W. H. BELL, AND A. R. GROVE

1938 Ethnobiological Studies in the American Southwest VI: The Early Utilization and the Distribution of Agave in the American Southwest. *University of New Mexico Bulletin, Biological Series* 5(4). University of New Mexico Press, Albuquerque.

CASTETTER, E. F., AND M. E. OPLER

1936 The Ethnobiology of the Chiricahua and Mescalero Apache: The Use of Plants for Foods, Beverages and Narcotics. *University of New Mexico Bulletin, Biological Series* 4(5). University of New Mexico Press, Albuquerque.

CASTETTER, E. F., AND R. M. UNDERHILL

1935 Ethnobiological Studies in the American Southwest II. The Ethnobiology of the Papago Indians. *University of New Mexico Bulletin* 4(3). University of New Mexico Press, Albuquerque.

CHAMBERLAIN, A. F.

1902 Algonkian Words in American English: A Study in the Contact of the White Man and the Indian. *The Journal of American Folklore* 15(59): 240–267.

CHAMBERLAIN, V. D.

1992 Chief and His Council: Unity and Authority from the Stars. In *Earth and Sky: Vision of the Cosmos in Native American Folklore,* edited by Ray A. Williamson and Claire R. Farrer. University of New Mexico Press, Albuquerque.

CHARLEVOIX, P.

1923 *Journal of a Voyage to North America, Vol. 2,* edited by Louise Phelps Kellogg. The Caxton Club, Chicago.

CHIPPINDALE, C., B. SMITH, AND P. TAÇON

2000 Visions of Dynamic Power: Archaic Rock Paintings, ASCs and "Clever Men" in Western Arhnem Land (NT) Australia. *Cambridge Archaeological Journal* 10(1):63–101.

CHIPPINDALE, C., AND P. S. C. TAÇON

1998 An Archaeology of Rock-Art through Informed Methods and Formal Methods. In *The Archaeology of Rock Art,* edited by C. Chippindale and P. S. C. Taçon, pp. 1–10. Cambridge University Press, Cambridge, United Kingdom.

CHOVANEC, Z.

2013 Products of Social Distinction: Organic Residue Analysis of Specialized Products in Bronze Age Cyprus. PhD dissertation, University at Albany, State University of New York.

CLAASSEN, C.

1998 *Shells.* Cambridge University Press, Cambridge, United Kingdom.

CLARK, A.

2013 Mississippian Objects on Permanent Display at St. Louis Art Museum. *Illinois Antiquity* 48(3):7–9.

CLARK, C. P.

1990 A Dog Burial from Isle Royale, Lake Superior: An Example of Household Ritual Sacrifice in the Terminal Woodland Period. *Midcontinental Journal of Archaeology* 15(2):265–278.

CLARKE, R.C., AND M. D. MERLIN

2013 *Cannabis Evolution and Ethnobotany.* University of California Press, Berkeley.

CLAVIGERO, ABBÉ D. F. S.

1787 *Istoria Antica del Mexico.* Translated into English by Charles Cullen, in Two Volumes. G. G. J. and J. Robinson, London. Originally published 1780–1781, Gregorio Biasini, Cesena, Italy.

CLOTTES, J., AND D. LEWIS-WILLIAMS

1996 *The Shamans of Prehistory: Trance and Magic in the Painted Caves.* Harry N. Abrams, New York.

CLOUGH, ALAN R.

2001 Does Kava Cause Hallucinations in Aboriginal Populations in Eastern Arnhem Land (Australia)? *South Pacific Journal of Psychology* 13:34–37.

COBB, C. R.

1991 Social Reproduction and the Longue Durée in the Prehistory of the Midcontinental United States. In *Processual and Postprocessual Archaeologies: Multiple Ways of Knowing the Past*, edited by R. W. Preucel, pp. 168–182. Occasional Paper No. 10, Center for Archaeological Investigations. Southern Illinois University, Carbondale.

2003 Mississippian Chiefdoms: How Complex? *Annual Review of Anthropology* 32:63–84.

COBO, P. B.

1890–1893 *Historia del Nuevo Mundo*. E. Rasco, Seville, Spain.

COE, S. D., AND M. D. COE

2007 *The True History of Chocolate*. Thames and Hudson, London.

COE, M. D., AND R. A. DIEHL

1980 *In the Land of the Olmec*. University of Texas Press, Austin.

COLLINS, J. M.

1990 *The Archaeology of the Cahokia Mounds ICT-II: Site Structure*. Illinois Cultural Resources Study No. 10. Illinois Historic Preservation Society, Springfield.

CONCANNON, M.

1993 Early Woodland Depopulation: A Review of the Evidence. *Bulletin of the Massachusetts Archaeological Society* 54(2):71–79.

CONWAY, T., AND J. CONWAY

1990 *Spirits on Stone: The Agawa Pictographs*. Heritage Discovery Books, Echo Bay, Ontario.

COOK, R.

1993 *The Voyages of Jacques Cartier*. University of Toronto Press, Toronto.

CORE, E. L.

1967 Ethnobotany of the Southern Appalachian Aborigines. *Economic Botany* 21(3):199–214.

COUES, E.

1900 *On the Trail of a Spanish Pioneer; the Diary and Itinerary of Francisco Garcés (Missionary Priest) in his travels through Sonora, Arizona, and California, 1775–1776, Vol. 2*. F. P. Harper, New York.

COUSINS, D., AND M. A. HUFFMAN

2002 Medicinal Properties in the Diet of Gorillas: An Ethno-Pharmacological Evaluation. *African Study Monographs* 23(2):65–89.

COX, I. J.

1905 *The Journeys of Réné Robert Cavelier, Sieur de la Salle*. A.S. Barnes, New York.

CROTHERS, G. M.

2012 Early Woodland Use of Caves in Eastern North America. *American Antiquity* 77(3):524–541.

CROTHERS, G. M., C. H. FAULKNER, J. F. SIMEK, P. J. WATSON, AND P. WILLEY

2002 Woodland Cave Archaeology in Eastern North America. In *The Woodland Southeast*, edited by D. G. Anderson and R. C. Mainfort Jr., pp. 502–524. University of Alabama Press, Tuscaloosa.

CROWE, S. F., J. BAROT, S. CALDOW, J. D'ASPROMONTE, J. DELL'ORSO, A. DI CLEMENTE, K. HANSON, M. KELLETT, S. MAKHLOTA, B. MCIVOR, L. MCKENZIE, R. NORMAN, A. THIRU, M. TWYEROULD, AND S. SAPEGA

2011 The Effect of Caffeine and Stress on Auditory Hallucinations in a Non-Clinical Sample. *Personality and Individual Differences* 50(5):626–630.

CROWN, P., AND W. J. HURST

2009 Evidence of Cacao Use in the Prehispanic American Southwest. *Proceedings of the National Academy of Science* 106:2110–2113.

CROWN, P. L., T. E. EMERSON, J. GU, W. J. HURST, T. R. PAUKETAT, AND T. WARD

2012 Ritual Black Drink Consumption at Cahokia. *Proceedings of the National Academy of Science* 109(35):13944–13949.

CROWN, P. L., J. GU, W. J. HURST, T. J. WARD, A. D. BRAVENEC, S. ALI, L. KEBERT, M. BERCH, E. REDMAN, P. D. LYONS, J. MEREWETHER, D. A. PHILLIPS, L. S. REED, AND K. WOODSON

2015 Ritual Drinks in the Pre-Hispanic US Southwest and Mexican Northwest. *Proceedings of the National Academy of Science* 112(37):11436–11442.

CUMMINGS, L. S.

2000 Prehistoric Tobacco Pollen in Southwestern Colorado: Distribution and Possible Contamination. In *Tobacco Use by Native Americans: Sacred Smoke and Silent Killer*, edited by J. C. Winter, pp. 205–222. University of Oklahoma Press, Norman.

CURTIN, J., AND J. N. B. HEWITT

1918 *Seneca Fiction, Legends and Myths*. Thirty-Second Annual Report, Bureau of American Ethnology (1910–1911). Smithsonian Institution, US Government Printing Office, Washington, DC.

CURTIN, L. S. M.

1984 *By the Prophet of the Earth: Ethnobotany of the Pima*. University of Arizona Press, Tucson.

CUSTER, J.

1987 New Perspectives on the Delmarva Adena Complex. *Midcontinental Journal of Archaeology* 12(1):33–53.

CUTLER, H. C., AND L. KAPLAN

1956 Some Plant Remains from Montezuma Castle and Nearby Caves. *Plateau* 28:98–100.

CYPHERS, A., B. ZÚÑIGA, AND A. DI CASTRO

2005 Another Look at *Bufo marinus* and the San Lorenzo Olmec. *Current Anthropology* 46(5):S129–S133.

DAIKER, F. H.

1914 *Liquor and Peyote: A Menace to the Indians.* Thirty-Second Report of the Annual Lake Mohonk Conference on the Indians and other Dependent Peoples. Philadelphia.

DANCEY, W. S., AND J. BURKS

2006 Middle Woodland Period Settlement as Seen from the Overly and Strait Sites in Central Ohio. Paper Presented at the Archaeological Society of Ohio Conference, Hopewell: Origins, Artistry and Culture. Columbus, Ohio.

DAVID, B.

2002 *Landscapes, Rock Art, and the Dreaming: An Archaeology of Preunderstanding.* Leicester University Press, Leicester.

DAVIS, J. T.

1961 Trade Routes and Economic Exchange among the Indians of California. *University of California Archaeological Survey Reports* 54:1–71.

DAVIS, W., AND A. WEIL

1992 Identity of a New World Psychoactive Toad. *Ancient Mesoamerica* 3(1):51–59.

DEAN, B.

2009 *Urarina Society, Cosmology, and History in Peruvian Amazonia.* University Press of Florida, Gainesville.

DE BAILLOU, C.

1965 A Test Excavation of the Hollywood Mound (9 RI 1), Georgia. *Southern Indian Studies* XVII:3–11.

DE BORHEGYI, S. F.

1961 Miniature Mushroom Stones from Guatemala. *American Antiquity* 26:498–504.

1963 Pre-Columbian Pottery Mushrooms from Mesoamerica. *American Antiquity* 28:328–338.

DE CARDENAS, J.

1591 *Primera parte de los problemas y secretos marauillosos de las Indias.* Pedro Ocharte, Mexico.

DE CASTELLANOS, J.

1886–1887 *Historia del Nuevo Reino de Granada.* A. Pérez Dubrul, Madrid.

DE MILLE, R. (ED.)

1980 The Don Juan Papers: Further Castaneda Controversies. Santa Barbara Press, Santa Barbara.

DENT, R. J., JR.

1995 *Chesapeake Prehistory: Old Traditions, New Directions*. The American University, Washington D.C.

DE ORTEGA, J.

1754 *Apostólicos afanes de la Compañia de Jesús en su Provincia de México*. P. Nadal, Barcelona.

DE RIOS, M. D.

1984 *Hallucinogens, Cross-cultural Perspectives*. University of New Mexico Press. Albuquerque.

DE RIOS, M. D. AND M. WINKELMAN

1989 Shamanism and Altered States of Consciousness: An Introduction. Journal of Psychoactive Drugs 21(1):1–7.

DE SMET, P. A. G. M.

1985 Ritual Enemas and Snuffs in the Americas. *Latin American Studies* 33.

DEVEREUX, P.

1997 *The Long Trip: A Prehistory of Psychedelia*. Penguin Putnam, New York.

DIAMOND, J.

2001 Anatomy of a Ritual. *Natural History* 110(6):16.

DIAZ, J.

1996 *How Drugs Influence Behavior*. Prentice Hall, Upper Saddle River, New Jersey.

DÍAZ-ROMO, P., AND S. S. ALVAREZ

2000 The Huichol Indians, Tobacco, and Pesticides. In *Tobacco Use by Native North Americans: Sacred Smoke and Silent Killer*, edited by J. C. Winter, pp. 342–352. University of Oklahoma Press, Norman.

DIEHL, M.

1998 The Interpretation of Archaeological Floor Assemblages: A Case Study from the American Southwest. *American Antiquity* 63(4):617–634.

DIETLER, M.

2011 Fasting and Feasting. In *The Oxford Handbook of the Archaeology of Ritual and Religion*, edited by T. Insoll, pp. 179–194. Oxford University Press, Oxford.

DI PESO, C.

1957 A Tubular Stone Pipe (?) from Sonora. *American Antiquity* 22(3):288–290.

DIXON, R. B.

1933 Tobacco Chewing on the Northwest Coast. *American Anthropologist* 35(1):146–150.

DIXON, R. B., AND J. B. STETSON JR.

1922 Analysis of pre-Columbian Pipe Dottels. *American Anthropologist* 24(2):245–246.

DOBYNS, H. F.

1988 Piman Indian Historic Agave Cultivation. *Desert Plants* 9(2):49–53.

DOCKSTADER, F. J.

1961 *Indian Art in America: The Arts and Crafts of the North American Indian.* New York Graphic Society, Greenwich.

DOWSON, T. A.

2007 Debating Shamanism in Southern African Rock Art: Time to Move On. . . . *South African Archaeological Bulletin* 62(185): 49–61.

DRAGOO, D.

1963 *Mounds for the Dead.* Annals of the Carnegie Museum, Pittsburg.

DRIVER H.

1937 Cultural Elements Distribution VI: Southern Sierra Nevada. *University of California Anthropological Records* 1(2):53–154.

DRIVER, H.

2011 *Indians of North America.* University of Chicago Press, Chicago.

DRIVER, H., AND MASSEY, W.

1957 Comparative Studies of North American Indians. *Transactions of the American Philosophical Society* 47(2):165–456.

DUBOIS, C. G.

1908 *The Religion of the Luiseño and Diegueño Indians of Southern California.* University of California Publications in American Archaeology and Ethnology, Vol. 8:69–186.

DU CREUX, F.

1969 *The History of Canada or New France.* Two Volumes. Greenwood Press, Westport, Connecticut.

DUDLEY, R.

2014 *The Drunken Monkey: Why We Drink and Abuse Alcohol.* University of California Press, Berkeley.

DUKE, D., S. K. RICE, D. C. YOUNG, AND R. BYERLY

2018 *The Playas Archaeological Inventory: 6,914 Acres on the Utah Test and Training Range Including Portions of the West Distal Delta of the Old River Bed and Test Excavations at the Wishbone Site (42TO6384), Tooele County, Utah.* Far Western Anthropological Research Group, Henderson, Nevada. Submitted to the Center for Integrated Research on the Environment, University of Montana, Missoula, and Hill Air Force Base.

DUNHAM, G. H.

1994 *Common Ground, Contesting Visions: The Emergence of Burial Mound Ritual in Late Prehistoric Central Virginia.* PhD dissertation, Department of Anthropology, University of Virginia. University Microfilms, Ann Arbor, Michigan.

DYE, D.

2007 Ritual, Medicine, and the War Trophy Iconographic Theme in the Mississippian Southeast. In *Ancient Objects and Sacred Realms: Interpretations of Mississippian Iconography*, edited by F. K. Reilly III and James F. Garber, pp. 289–320. University of Texas Press, Austin.

DYE, D.

In press Chiefly Warfare, Culture Heroes, and Religious Cults in the Lower Mississippi Valley. In *Visions of Other Worlds: Ideological and Ritual Functions of Mississippian Symbols*, edited by K. E. Smith. University of Florida Press, Tuscaloosa.

EARLE, R.

2014 Indians and Drunkenness in Spanish America. *Past and Present* 222 Supplement 9:81–99.

EERKENS, J., S. TUSHINGHAM, K. LENTZ, J. BLAKE, D. ARDURA, M. PALAZOGLU, AND O. FIEHN

2012 GC/MS Analysis of Residues Reveals Nicotine in Two Late Prehistoric Pipes from CA-ALA-554. *Society for California Archaeology Proceedings* 26:212–219.

EERKENS, J. W., S. TUSHINGHAM, K. BROWNSTEIN, R. GARIBAY, K. PEREZ, E. MURGA, P. KAIJANKOSKI, J. S. ROSENTHAL, AND D. R. GANG

2018 Dental Calculus as a Source of Ancient Alkaloids: Detection of Nicotine by LC-MS in Calculus Samples from the Americas. *Journal of Archaeological Science Reports* 18(April 2018):509–515.

ELFERINK, J. G. R.

1988 Some Little Known Hallucinogenic Plants of the Aztecs. *Journal of Psychoactive Drugs* 20(4):427–435.

EL-SEEDI, H., P. DE SMET, O. BECK, G. POSSNERT, AND J. BRUHN

2005 Prehistoric Peyote Use: Alkaloid Analysis and Radiocarbon Dating of Archaeological Specimens of Lophophora from Texas. *Journal of Ethnopharmacology* 101(1–3): 238–42.

ELIADE, M.

2004 *Shamanism: Archaic Techniques of Ecstasy*. Princeton University Press, Princeton, New Jersey.

ELLIS, H.

1898 Mescal: A New Artificial Paradise. *Contemporary Review* 73:131–134.

ELLIS, L.

2000 *Archaeological Method and Theory: An Encyclopedia*. Garland, New York.

ELMORE, F. H.

1944 *Ethnobotany of the Navajo*. School of American Research Monograph Series, Vol. 1, No. 7. University of New Mexico Press, Albuquerque.

EL SOHLY, M. A.

2007 *Marijuana and the Cannabinoids*. Springer, New York.

EMBODEN, W.

1979a Narcotic Plants. Macmillan, New York.

1979b *Nymphaea ampla* and other Narcotics in Maya Ritual and Shamanism. *Mexicon* 1(4):50–52.

EMERSON, T. E.

1982 *Mississippian Stone Images in Illinois*. Illinois Archaeological Survey, Circular No. 6, Urbana.

1989 Water, Serpents and the Underworld: An Exploration into Cahokia Symbolism. In *The Southeastern Ceremonial Complex: Artifacts and Analysis*, edited by P. Galloway, pp. 45–92. University of Nebraska Press, Lincoln.

2003 Materializing Cahokia Shamans. *Southeastern Archaeology* 22(2):135–154.

EMERSON, T. E., AND S. L. BOLES

2010 American Bottom Flint Clay Objects. *Illinois Archaeology* 22(2):473–490.

EMERSON, T. E., R. E. HUGHES, K. FARNSWORTH, S. WISSEMAN, AND M. HYNES

2005 Tremper Mound, Hopewell Catlinite, and PIMA Technology. *Midcontinental Journal of Archaeology* 30:189–216.

EMERSON, T. E., K. FARNSWORTH, S. WISSEMAN, AND R. HUGHES

2013 The Allure of the Exotic: Reexamining the Use of Local and Distant Pipestone Quarries in Ohio Hopewell Pipe Caches. *American Antiquity* 78(1):48–67.

EMERSON, T. E., AND T. PAUKETAT

2015 Identifying Black Drink Ceremonialism and Cahokia: Chemical Residue Analysis. *Illinois Antiquity* 50(3):6–7.

ERSPAMER, V., T. VITALI, M. ROSEGHINI, AND J. M. CEI

1967 5-Methoxy- and 5-Hydroxyindoles in the Skin of *Bufo alvarius*. *Biochemical Pharmacology* 16(7):1149–1164.

EVANS-PRITCHARD, E. E.

1969 *The Nuer*. Oxford University Press, Orxford.

FABING H. D.

1956 On Going Berserk: A Neurochemical Inquiry. *Scientific Monthly* 83(5):232–237.

FABING, H. D., AND J. R. HAWKINS

1956 Intravenous Bufotenine Injection in the Human Being. *Science* 123(3203):886–887.

FARRER, R. A., AND C. R. WILLIAMSON

1992 *Earth and Sky: Visions of the Cosmos in Native American Folklore*. University of New Mexico Press, Albuquerque.

FAULKNER, C. H.

1971 Adena and Copena: A Case of Mistaken Identity. In *Adena: The Seeking of an Identity*, edited by B. K. Swartz Jr., pp. 100–114. Ball State University, Muncie, Indiana.

1988 A Study of Seven Southeastern Glyph Caves. *North American Archaeologist* 9(3):223–246.

FENTON, W. N.

1941 Masked Medicine Societies of the Iroquois. *Smithsonian Institution Annual Report for 1940*, pp. 397–429. US Government Printing Office, Washington DC.

1953 *The Iroquois Eagle Dance: An Offshoot of the Calumet Dance*. Bureau of American Ethnology Bulletin 156. Washington, DC.

FERG, A.

1997 Cinega Phase Exotic Artifacts: Finding Their Place in History. *Archaeology in Tucson Newsletter* 11(3):8–9.

FERNANDEZ, J. W., AND R. L. FERNANDEZ

2001 "Returning to the Path": The Use of Iboga[ine] in an Equatorial African Ritual Context and the Binding of Time, Space and Social Relationships. *The Alkaloids*, Vol. 56. Academic Press, Cambridge, Massachusetts.

FEWKES, J. W.

1896 A Contribution to Ethnobotany. *American Anthropologist* 9:14–21.

1912 *Casa Grande, Arizona*. Twenty-Eighth Annual Report, Bureau of American Ethnology (1906–1907) 28:142–143. Smithsonian Institution, US Government Printing Office, Washington, DC.

1914 *Archaeology of the Lower Mimbres Valley, New Mexico*. Smithsonian Institution, Washington, DC.

FIKES, J. C.

1993 *Carlos Castaneda, Academic Opportunism and the Psychedelic Sixties*. Millennia Press, Santa Monica, California.

FISHER-CARROLL, R., AND R. C. MAINFORT JR.

2000 Late Prehistoric Mortuary Behavior at Upper Nodena. *Southeastern Archaeology* 19(2):105–119.

FITZPATRICK, S.

2018 *Ancient Psychoactive Substances*. University Press of Florida, Gainesville.

FORD, J. A., AND G. I. QUIMBY

1945 *The Tchefuncte Culture: An Early Occupation of the Lower Mississippi Valley*. Millwood, New York.

FORD, R. I.

1981 Gardening and Farming before A.D. 1000: Pattern of Prehistoric Cultivation North of Mexico. *Journal of Ethnobiology* 1(1):6–27.

1985 Patterns of Prehistoric Food Production in North America. In *Prehistoric Food Production in North America*, edited by R. I. Ford, pp. 341–364. Anthropological Papers, Vol. 75. Museum of Anthropology, University of Michigan, Ann Arbor.

FRISON, G. C., AND Z. VAN NORMAN

1993 Carved Steatite and Sandstone Tubes: Pipes for Smoking or Shaman's Paraphernalia. *Plains Anthropologist* 38(143):163–176.

FROESE, T.

2015 The Ritualized Mind Alteration Hypothesis of the Origins and Evolution of the Symbolic Human Mind. *Rock Art Research* 32(1):90–97.

FULLER, J. L.

1985 The Genetics of Alcohol Consumption in Animals. *Biodemography and Social Biology* 32(3–4):210–221.

FURST, P.

1965 West Mexican Tomb Art as Evidence for Shamanism in Pre-Hispanic Mesoamerica. *Anthropológica* 15:29–80.

1971 *Ariocarpus retusus*, the "False Peyote" of Huichol Tradition. *Economic Botany* 25:182–187.

1972a Introduction. In *Flesh of the Gods*, edited by P. Furst, pp. i–xiv. Praeger, New York.

1972b To Find Our Life: Peyote Among the Huichol Indians of Mexico. In *Flesh of the Gods*, edited by P. Furst, 136–184. Praeger, New York.

1974 *Archaeological Evidence for Snuffing in Prehistoric Mexico*. Harvard University Botanical Museum Leaflets, Vol. 24, No. 1. Cambridge, Massachusetts.

1976a *Hallucinogens and Culture*. Chandler and Sharp, Novato, California.

1976b Shamanistic Survivals in Mesoamerican Religion. *Actas del XLI Congreso Internacional de Americanistas* 3:149–157.

1989 The Water of Life: Symbolism and Natural History on the Northwest Coast. *Dialectical Anthropology* 14(2):95–115.

1995 Kiéri and the Solanaceae: Nature and Culture in Huichol Mythology. *Acta Americana* 3(2):43–57.

FURST, P., AND J. FURST

1982 *North American Indian Art*. Rizzoli, New York.

1983 The Sacred Pipe as Artifact and Prayer. *Terra* 22(2):11–17.

GAMBLE, L., P. WALKER, AND G. RUSSELL

2001 An Integrative Approach to Mortuary Analysis: Social and Symbolic Dimensions of Chumash Burial Practices. *American Antiquity* 66(2)185–212.

GANDHI, K. N., M. A. VINCENT, AND J. L. REVEAL

2011 *Dermatophyllum*, the correct name for *Calia* (Fabaceae). *Phytoneuron* 57:1–4.

GARDNER, L. G.

1907 *Narratives of Early Virginia, 1606–1625*. Charles Scribner's Sons, New York.

GARFINKEL, A. P., D. R. AUSTIN, D. EARLE, AND H. WILLIAMS

2009 Myth, Ritual and Rock Art: Coso Decorated Animal-Humans and the Animal Master. *Rock Art Research* 26(2):179–197.

GARFINKEL, A. P., AND S. J. WALLER

2012 Sounds and Symbolism from the Netherworld: Acoustic Archaeology at the Animal Master's Portal. *Pacific Coast Archaeological Society Quarterly* 46(4):37–60.

GARRITY, J. F.

2000 Jesus, Peyote, and the Holy People: Alcohol Abuse and the Ethos of Power in Navajo Healing. *Medical Anthropology Quarterly* 14(4): 521–542.

GATSCHET, A. S.

1884 *A Migration Legend of the Creek Indians: With a Linguistic, Historic, and Ethnographic Introduction*, Vols. 1–2. D. G. Brinton, Philadelphia.

1891 *The Karankawa Indians, the Coast People of Texas*. Papers of the Peabody Museum of Archaeology and Ethnology, Vol. 1, No. 2. Harvard University, Cambridge, Massachusetts.

1899 "Real," "True," or "Genuine," in Indian Languages. *American Anthropologist*, New Series 1(1):155–161.

GAYTON, A. H.

1928 *The Narcotic Plant Datura in Aboriginal American Culture*. PhD dissertation, Department of Anthropology, University of California, Berkeley.

GEETA, R., AND W. GHARAIBEH

2007 Historical Evidence for a Pre-Columbian Presence of Datura in the Old World and Implications for a First Millennium Transfer from the New World. *Journal of Biosciences* 32(1):1227–1244.

GEHLBACH, D. R.

1982 Ohio Pipe Chronology Chart. *Ohio Archaeologist* 32(4):8–9.

GERBER, P.

1982 Theoretical Explanations of the Peyote Religion. *Abstracts, 44th International Congress of Americanists in Manchester*.

GIANNINI, A. J., H. BURGE, J. M. SHAHEEN, AND W. A. PRICE

1986 Khat: Another Drug of Abuse? *Journal of Psychoactive Drugs* 18(2):155–158.

GIANNINI, A. J., AND A. E. SLABY

1989 Drugs of Abuse. *Medical Economics Books*:207–239.

GIBSON, J. L.

2001 *The Ancient Mounds of Poverty Point: Place of Rings*. University Press of Florida, Tuscaloosa.

GIFFORD, E. W.

1939 The Coast Yuki. *Anthropos* 34(1):292–375.

GILMORE, M. R.

1913 A Study in the Ethnobotany of the Omaha Indians. *Collections of the Nebraska State Historical Society* 17:314–357.

GISH, J. W.

2000 Morphologic Distinctiveness of *Nicotiana* Pollen and the Potential for Identifying Prehistoric Southwestern Tobacco through Pollen Analysis. In *Tobacco*

Use by Native North Americans: Sacred Smoke and Silent Killer, edited by J. C. Winter, pp. 223–261. University of Oklahoma Press, Norman.

GLADWIN, H. S., E. W. HAURY, E. B. SAYLES, AND N. GLADWIN

1938 *Excavations in Snaketown.* Medallion Papers No. XXV, Gila Pueblo, Globe, Arizona.

GLENNON R. A.

1994 Classical Drugs: An Introductory Overview. In *Hallucinogens: An Update,* edited by G. C. Lin and R. A. Glennon. National Institute on Drug Abuse, Rockville, Maryland.

GODELIER, M.

1986 The Mental and the Material: Thought, Economy and Society. Verso, London.

GODLASKI, T. M.

2013 Holy Smoke: Tobacco Use among Native American Tribes in North America. *Substance Use and Misuse* 48:1–8.

GODWIN, H.

1967 The Ancient Cultivation of Hemp. *Antiquity* 41:42–49.

GOGGIN, J. M.

1938 A Note on Cheyenne Peyote. *New Mexico Anthropologist* 3(2):26–30.

GONZALEZ DAVILA, J. M.

2012 An Alternative Interpretation of Some Iconographies Present in the Lower Pecos River Style Rock Art: An Ethnographic Study. *Journal of Big Bend Studies* 24:253–272.

GOODMAN, J.

1993 *Tobacco in History: The Cultures of Dependence.* Routledge, London.

1995 Excitantia: or, How Enlightenment Europe Took to Soft Drugs. In *Consuming Habits: Drugs in History and Anthropology,* edited by J. Goodman, P. E. Lovejoy, and A. Sherratt, pp. 121–141. Routledge, London.

GOODRICH, J., AND C. LAWSON

1980 *Kashaya Pomo Plants.* American Indian Studies Center, University of California, Los Angeles.

GOODSPEED, T. H.

1954 The Genus Nicotiana: Origins, Relationships and Evolution of its Species in the Light of their Distribution, Morphology and Cytogenetics. *Chronica Botanica* 16(1/6).

GRANT, W. L.

1907 *Voyages of Samuel De Champlain, 1604–1618.* Charles Scribner's Sons, New York.

GREER, M., AND J. GREER

2003 A Test for Shamanic Trance in Central Montana Rock Art. *Plains Anthropologist* 48(186):105–120.

GREGORY, D.

1997 A Ritual Array of Artifacts from a Cienega Phase Pit Structure. *Archaeology in Tucson Newsletter* 11(3):4–5.

GRIFFIN, J. B.

1983 George Irving Quimby: The Formative Years. *Anthropological Papers of the University of Michigan* 72:7–17.

GRIFFITH, R.

1897 The Hymns of the Rigveda. E. J. Lazarus and Co., Benares.

GRINNELL, G. B.

1905 Some Cheyenne Plant Medicines. *American Anthropologist*, New Series 7(1):37–43.

GROARK, K. P.

1996 Ritual and Therapeutic Use of "Hallucinogenic" Harvester Ants (*Pogonomyrmex*) in Native South-Central California. *Journal of Ethnobiology* 16(1):1–29.

2001 Taxonomic Identity of "Hallucinogenic" Harvester Ant (*Pogonomyrex californicus*) Confirmed. *Journal of Ethnobiology* 21(2):133–144.

GUERRA-DOCE, E.

2015 Psychoactive Substances in Prehistoric Times: Examining the Archaeological Evidence. *Time and Mind: The Journal of Archaeology, Consciousness and Culture* 8(1):91–112.

GUZMÁN, G., J. OTT, J. BOYDSTON, AND S. POLLOCK

1976 Psychotropic Mycoflora of Washington, Oregon, California, and British Columbia. *Mycologia* 69(6):1267–1271.

HABERMAN, T. W.

1984 Evidence of Aboriginal Tobaccos in Eastern North America. *American Antiquity* 49(2):268–287.

HALE, E. M.

1891 *Ilex Cassine: The Aboriginal North American Tea. Its History, Distribution, and Use among the Native North American Indians*. US Department of Agriculture, Division of Botany, Bulletin No. 14. US Government Printing Office, Washington, DC.

HALL, R.

1977 An Anthropocentric Perspective for Eastern United States Prehistory. *American Antiquity* 42(4): 499–518.

1987 Calumet Ceremonialism, Mourning Ritual, and Mechanisms of Inter-tribal trade. In *Mirror and Metaphor: Material and Social Constructions of Reality*, edited by D. W. Ingersoll and G. Bronitski. University Press of America, Lanham, Maryland.

1989 The Cultural Background of Mississippian Symbolism. *The Southeastern Ceremonial Complex: Artifacts and Analysis*, edited by P. Galloway, pp. 239–278. University of Nebraska Press, Lincoln.

1997 *An Archaeology of the Soul: North American Indian Belief and Ritual.* University of Illinois Press, Champagne.

HALLER, C., AND N. BENOWITZ

2000 Adverse Cardiovascular and Central Nervous System Events Associated with Dietary Supplements Containing Ephedra Alkaloids. *New England Journal of Medicine* 343(25):1833–1838.

HALLY, D.

1986 The Identification of Vessel Function: A Case Study from Northwest Georgia. *American Antiquity* 51(2):267–295.

HAMBLIN, N.

1981 The Magic Toads of Cozumel. *Mexicon* 3(1):10–14.

HAMELL, G. R.

1987 Strawberries, Floating Islands, and Rabbit Captains: Mythical Realities and European Contact in the Northeast during the Sixteenth and Seventeenth Centuries. *Journal of Canadian Studies* 21(4):72–94.

HAMILTON, R.

1970 *Marquette's Explorations: The Narratives Reexamined.* University of Wisconsin Press, Madison.

HAMMETT, J. E.

2000 Out of California: Cultural Geography of Western North American Tobacco. In *Tobacco Use by Native North Americans: Sacred Smoke and Silent Killer*, edited by J. C. Winter, pp. 128–140. University of Oklahoma Press, Norman.

HAMMOND, N., AND C. MIKSICEK

1981 Ecology and Economy of a Formative Maya Site at Cuello, Belize. *Journal of Field Archaeology* 8(3):259–269.

HAMPSON, J.

2016 Embodiment, Transformation and Ideology in the Rock Art of Trans-Pecos Texas. *Cambridge Archaeological Journal* 26(2):217–241.

HANN, J. H.

1986 The Use and Processing of Plants by Indians of Spanish Florida. *Southeastern Archaeology* 5(2):91–102.

HARDY, R. W. H.

1829 *Travels in the Interior of Mexico in 1825, 1826, 1827, & 1828.* Henry Colburn and Richard Bentley, London.

HARIOT, THOMAS.

1972 *A Briefe and True Report of the New Found Land of Virginia.* Dover Publications, New York.

HARNER, M.

1972 *The Jívaro: People of the Sacred Waterfalls.* University of California Press, Berkeley.

HARNER, M. J. (ED.)

1973 *Hallucinogens and Shamanism.* Oxford University Press, Oxford.

HART, G.

1980 Calumets and Their Pipes. *Prehistoric Art* 15(1):22–29.

HART, J. A.

1979 The Ethnobotany of the Flathead Indians of Western Montana. *Botanical Museum Leaflets* 27(10):261–307.

HASSAN, Z., M. MUZAIMI, V. NAVARATNAM, N. H. YUSOFF, F. W. SUHAIMI, R. VADIVELU, B. K. VICKNASINGAM, D. AMATOC, S. VON HÖRSTEND, N. I. W. ISMAIL, N. JAYABALAN, A. I. HAZIMA, S. M. MANSOR, AND C. P. MÜLLER

2013 From Kratom to Mitragynine and its Derivatives: Physiological and Behavioural Effects Related to Use, Abuse, and Addiction. *Neuroscience and Biobehavioral Reviews* 37(2):138–151.

HATCHER, M.

1927 Descriptions of the Tejas or Asinai Indians, 1691–1722. *Southwestern Historical Quarterly* 31(2):150–180.

HAURY, E. W.

1945 *The Excavation of Los Muertos and Neighboring Ruins in the Salt River Valley, Southern Arizona.* Papers of the Peabody Museum of American Archaeology and Ethnology, Vol. 24, No. 1. Harvard University, Cambridge, Massachusetts.

1950 *The Stratigraphy and Archaeology of Ventana Cave, Arizona.* University of Arizona Press, Tucson.

1976 *The Hohokam: Desert Farmers and Craftsmen. Excavations at Snaketown 1964–1965.* University of Arizona Press, Tucson.

HAVARD, V.

1896 Drink Plants of the North American Indians. *Bulletin of the Torrey Botanical Club* 23(2):33–46.

HAVILAND, W. A., AND M. A. POWER

1994 *The Original Vermonters: Native Inhabitants, Past and Present.* University Press of New England, Hanover, New Hampshire.

HAYES, A.

1940 Peyote Cult on the Goshiute Reservation at Deep Creek, Utah. *New Mexico Anthropologist* 4(2):34–36.

HAYS-GILPEN, K.

2006 North America: Pueblos. In *The Oxford Handbook of the Archaeology of Ritual and Religion*, edited by T. Insoll, pp. 600–606. Oxford University Press, Oxford.

HECKENBERGER, M. J., J. B. PETERSON, E. R. COWIE, A. E. SPEISS, AND L. A. BASA

1990 Early Woodland Mortuary Ceremonialism in the Far Northeast: A View from the Boucher Cemetery. *Archaeology of Eastern North America* 18:109–144.

HEDDEN, J.

2016 Central Plains Tradition Smoking Pipes in the Glenwood Locality of Iowa: Within a Landscape of the Rising and Falling Sky. In *Perspectives on the Archaeology of Pipes, Tobacco and other Smoke Plants in the Ancient Americas*, edited by Elizabeth Anne Bollwerk and Shannon Tushingham, pp. 135–156. Springer Press, New York.

HEDGES, K.

1982 Phosphenes in the Context of Native American Rock Art. *American Indian Rock Art* 7(8):1–10.

1994 Pipette Dreams and the Primordial Snake-Canoe: Analysis of a Hallucinatory Form Constant. In *Shamanism and Rock Art in North America*, edited by S. A. Turpin, pp. 103–124. Rock Art Foundation, San Antonio.

2007 *Images of the Spirit World: Vision Imagery and Spirit Beings in North American Rock Art*. Sunbelt Publications, El Cajon, California.

HEISTER, C.

1992 On Possible Sources of the Tobacco of Prehistoric Eastern North America. *Current Anthropology* 33(1):54–56.

HEIZER, R.

1940 The Botanical Identification of Northwest Coast Tobacco. *American Anthropologist* 42(4):704–706.

HELVENSTON, P. A., AND P. G. BAHN

2003 Testing the 'Three Stages of Trance' Model. *Cambridge Archaeological Journal* 13(2):213–224.

HERBERT, M., E. HERBERT, AND JAGIELLO-WÓJTOWICZ

2006 *Datura stramonium* L., Its Use over the Ages. *Acta Toxicologica* 14(1–2):4–9.

HERRICK, J. W.

1983 The Symbolic Roots of Three Potent Iroquois Medicinal Plants. In *The Anthropology of Medicine: From Culture to Method*, edited by L. Romanucci-Ross, D. E. Moerman, and L. R. Tancredi, pp. 134–155. Praeger, New York.

1995 *Iroquois Medical Botany*. Syracuse University Press, Syracuse, New York.

HICKOK, A., W. WHITE, K. RECALMA-CLUTESI, S. HAMM, AND H. KANIPE

2010 Mortuary Evidence of Coast Salish Shamanism? *Canadian Journal of Archaeology* 34(2):240–264.

HILGER, M. I.

1944 Chippewa Burial and Mourning Customs. *American Anthropologist*, New Series 46(4):564–568.

HILL, W. W.

1938 Navajo Use of Jimsonweed. *New Mexico Anthropologist* 3(2):19–21.

HIND, H. Y.

1860 *Narrative of the Canadian Red River Exploring Expedition of 1857 and of the Assiniboine and Saskatchewan Exploring Expeditions of 1858*. 2 Vol., Longman, Green, Longman, and Roberts, London.

HOCKINGS, K. J., M. ITO, AND G. YAMAKOSHI

2020 The Importance of Raffia Palm Wine to Coexisting Humans and Chimpanzees. In *Alcohol and Humans: A Long and Social Affair*, edited by K. J. Hockings, and R. Dunbar, pp. 45–59. Oxford University Press, Oxford.

HOFFER, A, AND H. OSMOND

1967 *The Hallucinogens*. Academic Press, Cambridge, Massachusetts.

HOFMANN, A.

1971 Teonanacatl and Ololiuqui: Two Ancient Magic Drugs of Mexico. *Bulletin on Narcotics*. United Nations: Division of Narcotic Drugs, Department of Economic and Social Affairs, New York.

HOFMANN, A., R. HEIM, A. BRACK, H. KOBEL, A. FREY, H. OTT, T. PETRZILKA, AND F. TROXLER

1959 Psilocybin und Psilocin. *Helvetica Chimica Acta* 42:1557–1572.

HOLLIMAN, S. E.

2000 Archaeology of the *'Aqi*: Gender and Sexuality in Prehistoric Chumash Society. *Archaeologies of Sexuality*, edited by R. A. Schmidt and B. L. Voss, pp. 179–196. Routledge, London.

HOLLMAN, J.

2002 Natural Models, Ethology and San Rock-Paintings: Pilo-Erection and Depictions of Bristles in Southeastern South Africa. *South African Journal of Science* 98(11–12):563–567.

HOLLOWAY, R. G.

1983 Diet and Medicinal Plant Usage of a Late Archaic Population from Culberson County, Texas. *Bulletin of the Texas Archaeological Society* 54:319–329.

HOLMES, W. H.

1883 *Art in Shell of the Ancient Americans*. Smithsonian Institution Bureau of Ethnology, Washington, DC.

HOWARD, J. H.

1957 The Mescal Bean Cult of the Central and Southern Plains: An Ancestor of the Peyote Cult? *American Anthropologist* 59(1):75–87.

1967 The Half Moon Way: The Peyote Ritual of Chief White Bear. *Museum News* 28(1–2):1–24.

HOWES, W. J.

1942 The Thin-Shelled Stone Tubes. *Bulletin of the Massachusetts Archaeological Society* III(2):11–17.

HRDLIČKA, A.

1908 *Physiological and Medical Observations among the Indians of Southwestern United States and Northern Mexico.* Smithsonian Institution Bureau of American Ethnology, Bulletin No. 34. US Government Printing Office, Washington, DC.

HU, S. Y.

1979 The Botany of Yaupon. In *The Black Drink: A Native American Tea,* edited by C. Hudson. University of Georgia Press, Athens.

HUCKELL, L. W., AND C. S. VANPOOL

2006 *Toloatzin* and Shamanic Journeys: Exploring the Ritual Role of Sacred Datura in the Prehistoric Southwest. In *Religion in the Prehispanic Southwest,* edited by C. S. VanPool, T. L. VanPool, and D. A. Phillips Jr., pp. 147–163. AltaMira Press, Walnut Creek, California.

HUDSON, C.

1976 *The Southern Indians.* University of Tennessee Press, Knoxville.

1979 Introduction. In *The Black Drink: A Native American Tea,* edited by C. Hudson, pp. 1–10. University of Georgia Press, Athens.

HUFFMAN, M.A., K. KOSHIMIZU, AND H. OHIGASHI

1996 Ethnobotany and Zoopharmacognosy of *Vernonia amygdalina*: A Medicinal Plant Used by Humans and Chimpanzees. In *Compositae: Biology and Utilisation* Vol. 2, edited by P. Caligari and D. J. N. Hind, pp. 351–360. The Royal Botanical Gardens, Kew, London.

HULTKRANTZ, Å.

1966 An Ecological Approach to Religion. *Ethos* 31:131–150.

1968 The Ecological and Phenomenological Aspects of Shamanism. In *Shamanism in Siberia,* edited by B. Dioszegi and M. Hoppal, pp. 27–58. Akademiai Kiado, Budapest.

1992 *Shamanic Healing and Ritual Drama: Health and Medicine in Native North American Religious Traditions.* Crossroad, New York.

1995 Some Viewpoints on the Peyote Religion in North America. *Acta Americana* 3(2):58–70.

1997 *The Attraction of Peyote: An Inquiry into the Basic Conditions for the Diffusion of the Peyote Religion in North America.* Almqvist and Wiksell International, Stockholm.

HUNTINGTON, W. R.

1973 Death and the Social Order: Bara Funeral Customs (Madagascar). *African Studies* 32(2):65–84.

HURST, J., R. A. MARTIN, S. M. TARKA JR., AND G. D. HALL

1989 Authentication of Cocoa in Maya Vessels Using High-Performance Liquid Chromatographic Techniques. *Journal of Chromatography* 466:279–289.

HURST, J., S. M. TARKA JR., T. G. POWIS, F. VALDEZ JR., AND T. HESTERM

2002 Cacao Usage by the Earliest Maya Civilization. *Nature* 418(6895):289.

HUSSEY, J. S.

1974 Some Useful Plants of Early New England. *Economic Botany* 28(3):311–337.

INSOLL, T. (ED.)

2011 *The Oxford Handbook of the Archaeology of Ritual and Religion*. Oxford University Press, Oxford.

IRWIN, J. D., W. C. J. BOYKO, J. M. HERBERT, AND C. BRALEY

1999 Woodland Burial Mounds in the North Carolina Sandhills and Southern Coastal Plain. *North Carolina Archaeology* 48:59–86.

JACKSON, H. E., AND S. L. SCOTT

2003 Patterns of Elite Faunal Utilization at Moundville, Alabama. *American Antiquity* 68(3):552–572.

JACOBS, D.

1995 The Use of Datura in Rites of Transition. In *Sacred Plants, Consciousness, and Healing: Cross-Cultural and Interdisciplinary Perspectives*, edited by M. Winkelman and W. Andritsky. Verlag für Wissenschaft und Bildung, Berlin.

JENNINGS, J. D., N. H. NICKERSON, E. K. REED, A. H. SCHROEDER, AND G. R. WENGER

1956 *A Reappraisal of the Fremont Culture, with a Summary of the Archaeology of the Northern Periphery*. Proceedings of the Denver Museum of Natural History, No. 1, Denver.

JERNIGAN, D. AND C. S. ROSS

2020 The Alcohol Marketing Landscape: Alcohol Industry Size, Structure, Strategies, and Public Health Responses. *Journal of Studies on Alcohol and Drugs*, Supplement 19:13–25.

JIANG, H., X. LI, Y. ZHAO, D. K. FERGUSON, F. HUEBER, S. BERA, Y. WANG, L. ZHAO, C. LIU, AND C. LI

2006 A New Insight into *Cannabis sativa* (Cannabaceae) Utilization from 2500-year-old Yanghai Tombs, Xinjiang, China. *Journal of Ethnopharmacology* 108:414–422.

JOHANNESSEN, S.

1984 Plant Remains. In *The Fish Lake Site (11-Mo-608)*, edited by A. C. Fortier, R. B. Lacampagne, and F. A. Finner, pp. 197–214. American Bottom Archaeology FAI-270 Site Reports 8. University of Illinois Press, Urbana.

JOHNSON, A.

1994 A Steed-Kisker Effigy Pipe. *Plains Anthropologist* 39(148):185–193.

JOHNSON, F. R.

1967 *The Tuscaroras: Mythology, Medicine, Culture.* Vol. I. Johnson, Chicago.

JOHNSTON, A.

1970 Blackfeet Indian Utilization of the Flora of the Northwestern Great Plains. *Economic Botany* 24:301–324.

JONAITIS, A.

1988 *From the Land of the Totem Poles: The Northwest Coast Indian Art Collection at the American Museum of Natural History.* American Museum of Natural History, New York.

JONES, B. C., D. T. PENTON, AND L. D. TESAR

1998 1973 and 1994 Excavations at the Block-Sterns Site, Leon County, Florida. In *A World Engraved: Archaeology of the Swift Creek Culture,* edited by J. M. Williams, pp. 222–246. University of Alabama Press, Tuscaloosa.

JONES, P.

1861 *History of the Ojebway Indians, with Especial Reference to their Conversion to Christianity.* A. W. Bennett, London.

JONES, P. N.

2006 Shamanism: An Inquiry into the History of the Scholarly Use of the Term in English-Speaking North America. *Anthropology of Consciousness* 17(2):4–32.

JONES, S., AND C. FERNYHOUGH

2009 Caffeine, Stress, and Proneness to Psychosis-Like Experiences: A Preliminary Investigation. *Personality and Individual Differences* 46(4):562–564.

JONES, V. H.

1935 Ceremonial Cigarettes. *Southwestern Monuments Monthly Report,* Supplement, October 1935:287–291.

JONES, V. H.

1944 Was Tobacco Smoked in the Pueblo Region in Pre-Spanish Times? *American Antiquity* 9(4):451–456.

JONIGER, O., AND M. DOBKIN DE RIOS

1973 Suggestive Hallucinogenic Properties of Tobacco. *Medical Anthropology Newsletter* 4(4):6–11.

JONIGER, O., AND M. DOBKIN DE RIOS

1976 Nicotiana an Hallucinogen? *Economic Botany* 30:149–151.

JORDAN, D.

1959 Adena and Blocked-end Tubes in the Northeast. *Bulletin of the Massachusetts Archaeological Society* 20(4):49–60.

JUAN-TRESSERRAS, J., AND M. J. VILLALBA

1999 Consumo de la adormidera (*Papaver somniferum* L.) en el Neolítico Peninsular: el enterramiento M28 del complejo minero de Can Tintorer. *Il Congrés del Neolític a la Península Ibèrica SAGVNTVM-PLAV*, Extra-2:397–404.

KAISER, P.

1984 The Lakota Sacred Pipe: Its Tribal Use and Religious Philosophy. *American Indian Culture and Research Journal* 8(3):1–26.

KAN, M., C. MEIGHAN, AND H. B. NICHOLSON

1989 *Sculpture of Ancient West Mexico: Nayarit, Jalisco, Colima*. Los Angeles County Museum of Art, Los Angeles.

KAPCHES, M.

1992 "Rude but Perfect": A Study of Miniature Smoking Pipes in Iroquoia. In *Proceedings of the 1988 Smoking Pipe Conference*, edited by C. F. Hays III, pp. 71–82. Rochester Museum and Science Center Records, Rochester, New York.

KAY, P.

2005 Ancient Voices . . . Murals and Pots Speak: Datura. Poster Presentation at the 70th Annual Meeting of the Society for American Archaeology, March 2005. Salt Lake City, Utah.

KEDDIE, G.

2016 Aboriginal Use and Context of Pipes, Tobacco and Smoking in Northwestern North America. In *Perspectives on the Archaeology of Pipes, Tobacco and other Smoke Plants in the Ancient Americas*, edited by Elizabeth Anne Bollwerk and Shannon Tushingham, pp. 157–181. Springer Press, New York.

KEENE, D. A.

2004 Reevaluating Late Prehistoric Coastal Subsistence and Settlement Strategies: New Data from Grove's Creek Site, Skidaway Island, Georgia. *American Antiquity* 69(4):671–688.

KEEWAYDINOQUAY

1979 The Legend of Miskwedo. *Journal of Psychedelic Drugs* 11(1–2):29–31.

KEHOE, A. B.

2000 *Shamanism and Religion: An Anthropological Exploration in Critical Thinking*. Waveland Press, Long Grove, Illinois.

KELLY, J. E., AND J. A. BROWN

2010 Just in Time: Dating Mound 34 at Cahokia. *Illinois Antiquity* 54(1):3–9.

KENNEDY, A.

1982 Ecce Bufo: The Toad in Nature and in Olmec Iconography. *Current Anthropology* 23(3):273–290.

KEUR, D. L.

1941 Big Bead Mesa. An Archaeological Study of Navaho Acculturation 1745–1812. *Memoirs of the Society for American Archaeology* No. 1:(ii–vi, 1–90).

KING, A.

2001 Long-Term Histories of Mississippian Centers: The Developmental Sequence of Etowah and its Comparison to Moundville and Cahokia. *Southeastern Archaeology* 20(1):1–17.

KING, A., T. POWIS, K. CHEONG, AND N. GAIKWAD

2017 Absorbed Residue Evidence of Datura Use in Mississippian Contexts. Paper presented at the 2017 Annual Meeting of the Society for American Archaeology, Vancouver.

KING, D. H. (ED.)

2007 *The Memoirs of Lieutenant Henry Timberlake: The Story of a Soldier, Adventurer, and Emissary to the Cherokees, 1756–1765*. Museum of the Cherokee Indian Press, Cherokee, North Carolina.

KING, J. C.

1977 *Smoking Pipes of the American Indian*. BMP, London.

KIRKLAND, F., AND W. W. NEWCOMB JR.

1967 *The Rock Art of Texas Indians*. University of Texas Press, Austin.

KITCHELL, J. A.

2010 Basketmaker and Archaic Rock Art of the Colorado Plateau: A Reinterpretation of Paleoimagery. *American Antiquity* 75(4):819–840.

KLEIN, C., E. GUZMAN, E. MANDELL, AND M. STANFIELD MAZZI

2002 The Role of Shamanism in Mesoamerican Art: A Reassessment. *Current Anthropology* 43(3):383–419.

KLÜVER, H.

1966 *Mescal and Mechanisms of Hallucinations*. University of Chicago Press, Chicago.

KNIGHT, V. J., JR.

1975 Some Observations Concerning Plant Materials and Aboriginal Smoking in Eastern North America. *Journal of Alabama Archaeology* 21:120–144.

1986 The Institutional Organization of Mississippian Religion. *American Antiquity* 51(4):675–687.

KNIGHT, V. J., JR., J. A. BROWN, AND G. E. LANKFORD

2001 On the Subject Matter of Southeastern Ceremonial Complex Art. *Southeastern Archaeology* 20(2):129–141.

KNOLL, M., J. KUGLER, O. HOFNER, AND S. D. LAWDER

1963 Effects of Chemical Stimulation of Electrically-Induced Phosphenes on Their Bandwidth, Shape, Number and Intensity. *Confinia Neurologica* 23(3):201–226.

KOSCHEL, K.

1996 Opium Alkaloids in a Cypriote Base Ring I Vessel (Bilbil) of the Middle Bronze Age from Europe. *Ägypten und Levante* 6:159–166.

KOZUCH, L.

2013a Ceramic Effigies of Lightning Whelk Shell Cups. *Illinois Antiquity* 48(3):14.

2013b Ceramic Shell Cup Effigies from Illinois and Their Implication. *Southeastern Archaeology* 32(1):29–45.

KRAFT, H. C.

1976 The Rosenkrans Site, an Adena-Related Mortuary Complex in the Upper Delaware Valley, New Jersey. *Archaeology of Eastern North America* 4:9–49.

KRIPPNER, S.

2000 The Epistemology and Technologies of Shamanic States of Consciousness. *Journal of Consciousness Studies* 7(11–12):93–118.

KROEBER, A. L.

1925 *Handbook of the Indians of California*. Bureau of American Ethnology, Bulletin 78.

KUHN, R. D.

1986 *Trade and Exchange among the Mohawk-Iroquois: A Trace Element Analysis of Ceramic Smoking Pipes*. PhD dissertation, Department of Anthropology, State University of New York, Albany. University Microfilms, Ann Arbor, Michigan.

LA BARRE, W.

1938 Native American Beers. *American Anthropologist*, New Series 40(2):224–234.

1947 Primitive Psychotherapy in Native American Cultures: Peyotism and Confession. *Journal of Abnormal and Social Psychology* 42(3):294–309.

1957 Mescalism and Peyotism. *American Anthropologist*, New Series 59(4)708–711.

1960 Twenty Years of Peyote Research. *Current Anthropology* 1(1):45–60.

1970 Review of Soma: Divine Mushroom of Immortality. *American Anthropologist* 72(2):368–372.

1972 Hallucinogens and the Shamanic Origin of Religion. In *Flesh of the Gods: The Ritual Use of Hallucinogens*, edited by P. T. Furst, pp. 261–278. Waveland Press, Long Grove, Illinois.

1975 *The Peyote Cult*. 4th ed. Archon Books, Hamden, Connecticut. Originally published 1938, Yale University Press, New Haven, Connecticut.

1979 Peyotl and Mescaline. *Journal of Psychoactive Drugs* 11(1–2):33–39.

LAME DEER, J. F., AND R. ERDOES

1972 *Lame Deer: Seeker of Visions*. Simon and Schuster, New York.

LANKFORD, G. E.

2012 Weeding out the Noded. *The Arkansas Archeologist* 50:50–68.

LARSON, L. H.

1971 Archaeological Implications of Social Stratification at the Etowah Site, Georgia. In *Approaches to the Social Dimensions of Mortuary Practices*, edited by James A. Brown, pp. 58–67. Society for American Archaeology, Memoirs 25. Washington, DC.

LATTA, F. F.

1977 *Handbook of Yokuts Indians*. Bear State Books, Santa Cruz, California.

LAWSON, J.

1903 *History of North Carolina*. Observer Printing House, Raleigh, North Carolina.

LEE, G., AND W. D. HEIDER

1991 Prehistoric Rock Art as an Indicator of Cultural Interaction and Tribal Boundaries in South-Central California. *Journal of California and Great Basin* Anthropology 13(1)15–28.

LEMAISTRE, D.

1996 The Deer That is Peyote and the Deer That is Maize: The Hunt in the Huichol "Trinity." In *People of the Peyote: Huichol Indian History, Religion and Survival*, edited by E. Schafer and P. T. Furst, 306–329. University of New Mexico Press, Albuquerque.

LE MOYNE, J.

1875 Narrative of Le Moyne, an Artist who Accompanied the French Expedition to Florida Under Laudenière, 1564. James R. Osgood and Go., Boston.

LEONARD, I. A.

1942 Peyote and the Mexican Inquisition, 1620. *American Anthropologist* 44(2):324–326.

LE PAGE DU PRATZ, A.

2006 *The History of Louisiana*. Reprint edition. BiblioBazaar, Charleston, South Carolina. Originally published 1774, T. Becket, London.

LEPOFSKY, D., M. L. MOSS, AND N. LYONS

2001 The Unrealized Potential of Paleoethnobotany in the Archaeology of Northwestern North America: Perspectives from Cape Addington, Alaska. *Arctic Anthropology* 38(1):48–59.

LEROI-GOURHAN, A.

1967 *The Art of Prehistoric Man in Western Europe*. Thames and Hudson, London.

LESCARBOT, M.

1914 *The History of New France*, Vol. 3, edited and translated by W. L. Grant. Champlain Society, Montreal.

LÉVI-STRAUSS, C.

1963 *Structural Anthropology*. Basic book, New York.

LEWIS, G.

1980 *Day of Shining Red. An Essay on Understanding Ritual*. Cambridge University Press, Cambridge, United Kingdom.

LEWIS, T. M., AND M. KNEBERG LEWIS

1961 *Eva, an Archaic Site*. University of Tennessee Press, Knoxville.

LEWIS-WILLIAMS, J. D.

2001 Brainstorming Images: Neuropsychology and Rock Art Research. In *Handbook of Rock Art Research*, edited by D. S. Whitley, pp. 332–350. AltaMira, Walnut Creek, California.

2002 *The Mind in the Cave*. Thames and Hudson, London.

LEWIS-WILLIAMS, J. D., AND T. A. DOWSON

1988 The Sign of All Times: Entoptic Phenomena and Upper Paleolithic Art. *Current Anthropology* 29:201–45.

LEWIS-WILLIAMS, J. D., AND T. A. DOWSON

1989 Theory and Data: A Brief Critique of A. Marshack's Research Methods and Position on Upper Paleolithic Shamanism [comment on Marshack (1989)]. *Rock Art Research* 6(1):38–53.

LINTON, R.

1924a Totemism and the A.E.F. *American Anthropologist* 26:296–300.

1924b *The Use of Tobacco among North American Indians*. Field Museum of Natural History Anthropological Leaflets, 15.

LIPPERT, J.

1886–1887 *Kulturgeschichte der Menscheit in Ihrem Organischem Aufbau*, Vol. 1. F. Enke, Stuttgart.

LITZINGER, W. J.

1981 Ceramic Evidence for Prehistoric Datura Use in North America. *Journal of Ethnopharmacology* 4(1):57–74.

LOEB, E. M.

1943 Primitive Intoxicants. *Quarterly Journal of Studies on Alcohol* 4(2):387–398.

LOENDORF, L.

1994 Finnegan Cave: A Rock Art Vision Quest Site in Montana. In *Shamanism and Rock Art in North America*, edited by S. A. Turpin, pp. 125–137. Rock Art Foundation, San Antonio, Texas.

LOENDORF, L., M. WILLIS, L. WHITE, P. REYNOSA, AND R. ABDULLAYEV

2015 The Dona Ana Site (LA66667): Formative Period Abstract Rock Art. *American Indian Rock Art* 41:99–109.

LOFTIN, J. D.

1991 Religion and Hopi Life. Indiana University Press, Bloomington.

LOMNITZ, LARISSA A.

1969 Patterns of Alcohol Consumption among the Mapuche. *Human Organization* 28(4):287–296.

LOPINOT, N. H.

1991 Archaeobotanical Remains. In *The Archaeology of the Cahokia Mounds ICT-II: Biological Remains*, edited by N. H. Lopinot, L. S. Kelly, G. Milner, and R.

Paine, pp. 1–268. Illinois Cultural Resources Study No. 13. Illinois Historic Preservation Agency, Springfield.

LORING, S.

1985 Boundary Maintenance, Mortuary Ceremonialism and Resource Control in the Early Woodland. *Archaeology of Eastern North America* 13:93–127.

LOVEJOY, P. E.

1980 Kola in the History of West Africa. *Cahiers d'Études Africaines* 20(77/78): 7–134.

LOWELL, E. S.

1990 Paletas and Tabletas: Comparison of Hohokam Stone Palettes with Snuff Trays of South America. *Kiva* 55(4):321–355.

LOWIE, R. H.

1919 *Tobacco Society of the Crow Indians.* Anthropological Papers of the American Museum of Natural History, Vol. XXI, Part II. American Museum of Natural History, New York.

LOWY, B.

1971 New Records of Mushroom Stones from Guatemala. *Mycologica* 63:983–993.

LUMHOLTZ, C.

1900 *Symbolism of the Huichol Indians.* Memoirs of the American Museum of Natural History 3:1–228. American Museum of Natural History, New York.

1902 Unknown Mexico. Macmillan and Co., Limited, London.

LYNN, C. D.

2005 Adaptive and Maladaptive Dissociation: An Epidemiological and Anthropological Comparison and Proposition for an Expanded Dissociation Model. *Anthropology of Consciousness* 16(2):16–49.

LYNN, C. D., J. PARIS, C. A. FRYE, AND L. M. SCHELL

2010 Salivary Alpha-Amylase and Cortisol among Pentecostals on a Worship and Nonworship Day. *American Journal of Human Biology* 22(6):819–822.

LYONS, T., AND R. L. CARHART-HARRIS

2018 Increased Nature Relatedness and Decreased Authoritarian Political Views after Psilocybin for Treatment-Resistant Depression. *Journal of Psychopharmacology* 32(7):811–819.

MACLEAN, H.,

2001 Sacred Colors and Shamanic Vision among the Huichol Indians of Mexico. *Journal of Anthropological Research* 57(3):305–323.

MACNUTT, A. F.

1912 *De Orbe Novo: The Eight Decades of Peter Martyr D'Anghera,* Vol. 2. G. P. Putnam's Sons, New York and London.

MALOTKI, E.

1999 The Use of Hallucinogenic Plants by Archaic Basketmaker Rock Art Creators of the Palavayu, Northeast Arizona: The Case for Datura. *American Indian Rock Art* 25:101–120.

MALOTKI, E., AND K. GARY

2001 *Hopi Stories of Witchcraft, Shamanism, and Magic.* Taylor and Francis, Oxford.

MALOTKI, E., AND M. LOMATUWAY'MA

1987 *Maasaw: Profile of a Hopi God.* University of Nebraska Press, Lincoln.

MANGHI, R. A., B. BROERS, R. KHAN, D. BENGUETTAT, Y. KHAZAAL, AND D. F. ZULLINO

2009 Khat Use: Lifestyle or Addiction? *Journal of Psychoactive Drugs* 41(1):1–10.

MARLEY, M., B. LEPPER, D. GANG, J. SIX, W. PICKARD, K. BROWNSTEIN, S. TUSHINGHAM, S. RAFFERTY, K. LEONE, AND L. PANSING

2018 Analyses of Organic Residue from a Conical Pipe from the Niles-Wolford Mound (33Pi3), Pickaway County, Ohio. *Journal of Archaeological Sciences Reports* 19, June 2018:658–668.

MARQUARDT, W., AND L. KOZUCH

2016 The Lightning Whelk: An Enduring Icon of Southeastern North American Spirituality. *Journal of Anthropological Archaeology* 42:1–26.

MARQUARDT, W., AND P. J. WATSON

2005 *Archaeology of the Middle Green River Region, Kentucky.* Monograph No. 5, Institute of Archaeology and Paleoenvironmental Studies. Florida Museum of Natural History, University of Florida, Gainesville.

MARSHACK, A.

1989 Methodology in the Analysis and Interpretation of Upper Palaeolithic Image: Theory Versus Contextual Analysis, with comment by J. D. Lewis-Williams and T. A. Dowson (1989). *Rock Art Research* 6(1):17–53.

MARTIN, P., L. ROYS, AND G. VON BONIN

1936 Archaeology of Southwestern Colorado: Lowry Ruin in Southwestern Colorado. *Publications of the Field Museum of Natural History, Anthropological Series* 23(1):1–216. Field Museum, Chicago.

MATHEWS, Z. P.

1980 Of Man and Beast: The Chronology of Effigy Pipes Among Ontario Iroquoians. *Ethnohistory* 27(4):295–307.

MCBRIDE, M.

2000 Bufotenine: Toward an Understanding of Possible Psychoactive Mechanisms. *Journal of Psychoactive Drugs* 32(3): 321–331.

MCCLEAN, S., R. C. ROBINSON, C. SHAW, AND W. F. SMYTH

2002 Characterization and Determination of Indole Alkaloids in Frog-Skin

Secretions by Electrospray Ionization Ion Trap Mass Spectrometry. *Rapid Communications in Mass Spectrometry* 16(5):346–354.

MCCLEARY, J. A., P. S. SYPHERD, AND D. L. WALKINGTON

1960 Antibiotic Activity of an Extract of Peyote (*Lophophora williamii* [Lemaire] Coulter). *Economic Botany* 14:247–249.

MCCREERY, P., AND E. MALOTKI

1994 *Tapamveni: The Rock Art Galleries of Petrified Forest and Beyond.* Petrified Forest Museum Association, Petrified Forest, Arizona.

MCELWAIN, T.

1992 Asking the Stars: Seneca Hunting Ceremonial. In *Earth and Sky: Visions of the Cosmos in Native American Folklore,* edited by R. A. Williamson and C. R. Farrer, pp. 260–277. University of New Mexico Press, Albuquerque.

MCGOVERN, P.

2009 *Uncorking the Past: The Quest for Wine, Beer, and Other Alcoholic Beverages.* University of California Press, Berkeley.

MCGUIRE, J. D.

1899 *Pipes and Smoking Customs of the American Aborigines, Based on Material in the U. S. National Museum.* Report of the U.S. National Museum for 1897, pp. 361–645. US Government Printing Office, Washington DC.

MCGUIRE, T. M.

1982 Ancient Mayan Mushroom Connections: A Transcendental Interaction Model. *Journal of Psychoactive Drugs* 14(3):221–238.

MCLEOD, W. C.

1930 The Chewing of Tobacco in Southeastern North America. *American Anthropologist* 32(3):574–575.

MENTZNER, R.

1998 Hallucinogenic Drugs and Plants in Psychotherapy and Shamanism. *Journal of Psychoactive Drugs* 30(4):333–341.

MERCK AND CO., INC.

1983 *Merck Index,* 10th ed., Edited by Martha Winholz, Merck, Rahway, New Jersey.

MERLIN, M. D.

2003 Archaeological Evidence for the Tradition of Psychoactive Plant Use in the Old World. *Economic Botany* 57(3):295–323.

2018 Ancient Use of *Ephedra* in Eurasia and the Western Hemisphere. In *Ancient Psychoactive Substances,* edited by S. M. Fitzpatrick, pp. 71–111. University Press of Florida, Tuscaloosa.

MERRIAM, A. P., AND W. L. D'AZEVEDO

1957 Washo Peyote Songs. *American Anthropologist* 59(4):615–641.

MERRILL, W. L.

1979 The Beloved Tree: *Ilex vomitoria* Among the Indians of the Southeast and Adjacent Regions. In *Black Drink: A Native American Tea,* edited by C. Hudson, pp. 40–82. University of Georgia Press, Athens.

MERRILLES, R. S.

1962 Opium Trade in the Bronze Age Levant. *Antiquity* 36:287–292.

MEUSER, G. F.

1952 Tube Pipes. *Ohio Archaeologist* 2(3):14–15.

MICHEAUX, H.

1963 *Light through Darkness.* The Orion Press, New York.

MILANICH, J. T.

1979 Origins and Prehistoric Distribution of Black Drink and the Ceremonial Shell Drinking Cup. In *The Black Drink: A Native American Tea,* edited by C. Hudson, pp. 83–119. University of Georgia Press, Athens.

MILANICH, J. T., AND S. MILBRATH (EDS.)

1989 *First Encounters: Spanish Explorations in the Caribbean and the United States, 1492–1570.* University of Florida Press, Gainesville.

MILLER, J.

2015 Interior Carbonization Patterns as Evidence of Ritual Drink Preparation in Powell Plain and Ramey Incised Vessels. *American Antiquity* 80(1):170–183.

MILLS, B., AND T. FERGUSON

2008 Animate Objects: Shell Trumpets and Ritual Networks in the Greater Southwest. *Journal of Archaeological Method and Theory* 15(4):338–361.

MILLSPAUGH, C. F.

1974 *American Medicinal Plants.* Dover, New York.

MINNIS, P. E.

2004 *People and Plants in Ancient Western North America.* University of Arizona Press, Tucson.

MOERMAN, D. E.

1998 *Native American Ethnobotany.* Timber Press, Portland, Oregon.

MONARDES, N.

1925 *Joyfull Newes Out of the Newe Founde Worlde.* Alfred A. Knopf, New York.

MOONEY, J.

1897 The Kiowa Peyote Rite. *Der Urquell* 1:329–333.

1932 *The Swimmer Manuscript: Cherokee Sacred Formulas and Medicinal Prescriptions.* US Government Printing Office, Washington, DC.

MORGAN, L. H.

1972 *League of the Iroquois.* Citadel Press, Secaucus, New Jersey.

MORTON, JULIA F.

1977 *Major Medicinal Plants: Botany, Culture and Uses*. Charles C. Thomas, Springfield, Illinois.

MOTLEY, T. J.

1994 The Ethnobotany of Sweet Flag, *Acorus calamus* (Araceae). *Economic Botany* 48:397–412.

MOUNTJOY, J. B.

1982 An Interpretation of the Pictographs at La Pena Pintada, Jalisco, Mexico. *American Antiquity* 47(1):110–126.

MURRAY, E.

1988 *Ghosts of the Old West: Desert Spirits, Haunted Cabins, Lost Trails, and Other Strange Encounters*. Contemporary Books, Chicago.

MYERHOFF, B. G.

1974 *Peyote Hunt: The Sacred Journey of the Huichol Indians*. Cornell University Press, Ithaca, New York.

NAVET É.

1988 Les Ojibway et l'Amanite tue-mouche (*Amanita muscaria*). Pour une ethnomycologie des Indiens d'Amérique du Nord. *Journal de la Société des américanistes* 74:163–180.

NEAL, J. M., P. T. SATO, W. N. HOWALD, AND J. L. MCLAUGHLIN

1972 Peyote Alkaloids: Identification in the Mexican Cactus *Pelecyphora aselliformis*. *Science* 176:1131–1133.

NESSE, R. M., AND K. C. BERRIDGE

1997 Psychoactive Drug Use in Evolutionary Perspective. *Science* 278:63–66.

NEWCOMB, W. W., JR.

1967 *The Rock Art of Texas Indians*. University of Texas Press, Austin.

NICOLAY, S.

2012 Footsteps in the Dark Zone: Ritual Cave Use in Southwest Prehistory. In *Sacred Darkness: A Global Perspective on the Ritual Use of Caves*, edited by H. Moyes, pp. 171–183. University of Colorado Press, Boulder.

NIELSEN-GRIMM, G. B., M. BROWN, D. MATHENY, R. MATHENY, C. BALZOTTI, AND R. E. TERRY

2017 Residue Analysis for Cacao in Southeastern Utah Ancestral Puebloan Ceramics, Montezuma Canyon, Utah. Paper presented at the 2017 Annual Meetings of the Society for American Archaeology, Vancouver.

NOBLE, W. C.

1992 Neutral Iroquois Smoking Pipes. In *Proceedings of the 1988 Smoking Pipe Conference*, edited by C. F. Hays III, pp. 41–50. Rochester Museum and Science Center Research Records, Rochester, New York.

NORTON, S.A.

1998 Betel: Consumption and Consequences. *Journal of the American Academy of Dermatology* 38(1):81–88.

O'BRIEN, P.

2003 A Human Effigy Pipe of the Smoky Hill Phase. *Plains Anthropologist* 48(184):35–38.

O'CONNOR, M. M.

1995 *Lost Cities of the Ancient Southeast.* University Press of Florida, Gainesville.

OLSEN, S., AND J. OLSEN

1970 A Preliminary Report on the Fish and Herpetofauna of Grasshopper Ruin. *Kiva* 36(2):40–43.

OSTER, G.

1970 Phosphenes. *Scientific American* 222(2):82–87.

OTT, J.

1977 A Brief History of Hallucinogenic Mushrooms. In *Teonanacatl: Hallucinogenic Mushrooms of North America,* edited by J. Ott and J. Bigwood, pp. 5–26. Madrona, Seattle.

OTT, J., P. WHEATON, AND W. SCOTT CHILTON

1975 Fate of Muscimol in the Mouse. *Physiological Chemistry and Physics* 7:381–384.

OTTO, M. P.

1992 A Prehistoric Menagérie: Ohio Hopewell Effigy Pipes. In *Proceedings of the 1988 Smoking Pipe Conference,* edited by C. F. Hays III, pp. 1–14. Rochester Museum and Science Center Research Records, Rochester, New York.

OVIEDO Y VALDÉS, G. F.

1535 *La Historia general de las Indias.* J. Cromberger, Seville, Spain.

PAPER, J.

1987 Cosmological Implications of Pan-Indian Sacred Pipe Ritual. *The Canadian Journal of Native Studies* VII(2):297–306.

PAPER, J.

1988 *Offering Smoke: The Sacred Pipe and Native American Religion.* University of Idaho Press, Moscow, Idaho.

1992 The Iroquoian and Pan-Indian Sacred Pipes: Comparative Ritual and Symbolism. In *Proceedings of the 1989 Smoking Pipe Conference,* edited by C. F. Hayes III, pp. 163–170. Rochester Museum and Science Center Research Records, Rochester, New York.

PARKER, K. E.

1992 Archaeobotany. In *The Sponemann Site 2: The Mississippian and Oneota Occupations,* edited by D. K. Jackson, A.C. Fortier, and J. A. Williams, pp.

305–324. American Bottom Archaeology FAI-270 Site Reports, XXIV. University of Illinois Press, Springfield.

PARROTT A.C.

1998 Nesbitt's Paradox Resolved? Stress and Arousal Modulation during Cigarette Smoking. *Addiction* 93(1): 27–39.

PARSONS, E. C.

1996 *Pueblo Indian Religion*. University of Chicago Press, Chicago.

PATTERSON, A.

1992 *A Field Guide to Rock Art Symbols of the Greater Southwest*. Johnson Books, Boulder, Colorado.

PAUKETAT, T.

2010 *Cahokia: Ancient America's Great City on the Mississippi*. Penguin Books, London.

PAUKETAT, T., L. KELLY, G. FRITZ, N. LOPINOT, S. ELIAS, AND E. HARGRAVE

2002 The Residues of Feasting and Public Ritual at Early Cahokia. *American Antiquity* 67(2):257–279.

PAVESIC, M. G.

2000 Prehistoric Pipes from the Olds Ferry Dunes Site (10-WN-557), Western Idaho. *Journal of California and Great Basin Anthropology* 22(2):321–331.

PEARSALL, D. M.

1992 The Origins of Plant Cultivation in South America. In *The Origins of Agriculture: An International Perspective*, edited by C. W. Cowan and P. J. Watson. Smithsonian Institution Press, Washington DC.

PEARSON, J. M.

2002 *Shamanism and the Ancient Mind*. AltaMira Press, Walnut Creek, California.

PEEBLES, C. S.

1971 Moundville and Surrounding Sites: Some Structural Considerations of Mortuary Practices II. In *Approaches to the Social Dimensions of Mortuary Practices*, edited by James A. Brown, pp. 68–91. Society for American Archaeology, Memoir 25.

PEGG, R. B., A. RYBARCZYK, AND R. AMAROWICZ

2008 Chromatographic Separation of Tannin Fractions from a Bearberry-Leaf (*Arctostaphylos uva-ursi* L. Sprengel) Extract by SE-HPLC—a Short Report. *Polish Journal of Food and Nutrition Sciences* 58(4):485–490.

PEGO, C. M., R. F. HILL, G. W. SOLOMON, R. M. CHISHOLM, AND S. E. IVEY

1995 Tobacco, Culture and Health among American Indians: A Historical Review. *American Indian Culture and Research Journal* 19(2):143–64.

PENDLETON, M. W., B. B. PENDLETON, AND T. STEPHENS, T.

2003 Acacia Pollen Associated with the Abandonment of a Prehistoric Mimbres Archeological Site. *Microscopy and Microanalysis* 9(S02):648–649.

PENNEY, D. W.

1985 The Late Archaic Period. In *Ancient Art of the American Woodland Indians,* edited by D. S. Brose, J. Brown, and D. W. Penney, pp. 15–42. Harry N. Abrams, New York.

PHILLIPS, P. A., AND J. A. BROWN

1975 *Pre-Columbian Shell Engravings from Spiro,* Vol. I. Peabody Museum Press, Harvard University, Cambridge, Massachusetts.

1978 *Pre-Columbian Shell Engravings from the Craig Mound at Spiro, Oklahoma.* Peabody Museum Press, Harvard University, Cambridge, Massachusetts.

PINXTEN, R. AND I. VAN DOOREN

1992 Navaho Earth and Sky and the Celestial Life-Force. In *Earth and Sky: Visions of the Cosmos in Native American Folklore,* edited by R. A. Williamson and C. R. Farrer, pp. 101–109. University of New Mexico Press, Albuquerque.

PLUCKHAHN, T. J., J. M. COMPTON, AND M. T. BONHAGE-FREUND

2006 Evidence of Small-Scale Feasting from the Woodland Period Site of Kolomoki, Georgia. *Journal of Field Archaeology* 31(3):263–284.

POKOTYLO, D. L., AND P. D. FROESE

1983 Archaeological Evidence for Prehistoric Root Gathering on the Southern Interior Plateau of British Columbia: A Case Study from Upper Hat Creek Valley. *Canadian Journal of Archaeology* 7(2):127–157.

PONTIERI, F. E., G. TANDA, F. ORZI, AND G. DI CHIARA

1996 Effects of Nicotine on the Nucleus Accumbens and Similarity to those of Addictive Drugs. *Nature* 382:255–257.

POPE, HARRISON G.

1969 *Tabernanthe iboga*: An African Narcotic Plant of Social Importance. *Economic Botany* 23(2):174–184.

POTTER, J., AND E. PERRY

2011 Mortuary Features and Identity Construction in an Early Village Community in the American Southwest. *American Antiquity* 76(3):529–546.

PRENTICE, G.

1986 An Analysis of the Symbolism Expressed by the Birger Figurine. *American Antiquity* 51(2): 239–266.

1987 Marine Shells as Wealth Items in Mississippian Exchange. *Midcontinental Journal of Archaeology* 12(2):193–223.

PRIESTLEY, H. I.

1937 *A Historical, Political and Natural Description of California by Pedro Fages, Soldier of Spain.* University of California Press, Berkeley.

PURCHAS, S.

1626 *Purchas His Pilgrimes.* Vol. V. William Stansby for Henrie Fetherstone, London.

QUINLAN, A. R.

2000 The Ventriloquist's Dummy: A Critical Review of Shamanism and Rock Art in Far Western North America. *Journal of California and Great Basin Anthropology* 22(1):92–108.

RADIN, P.

1920 *The Autobiography of a Winnebago Indian.* University of California Publications in American Archaeology and Ethnology 16(7). University of California Press, Berkeley.

1923 *The Winnebago Tribe.* Thirty-Seventh Annual Report, Bureau of American Ethnology (1915–1916). Smithsonian Institution, US Government Printing Office, Washington DC.

RAFFAUF, R. F.

1960 Persistence of Alkaloids in Plant Tissue. *Science* 131(306):1010–1048.

RAFFERTY, S. M.

2002 Chemical Analysis of Early Woodland Period Smoking Pipe Residue. *Journal of Archaeological Science* 29(8):897–907.

2004 They Pass Their Lives in Smoke, and at Death, Fall into the Fire: Smoking Pipes and Mortuary Ritual during the Early Woodland Period. In *Smoking and Culture: Recent Developments in the Archaeology of Tobacco Pipes in Eastern North America,* edited by S. M. Rafferty and R. Mann, pp. 1–42. University of Tennessee Press, Knoxville.

2006 Evidence of Early Tobacco in Northeastern North America? *Journal of Archaeological Science* 33(4):453–458.

2007 The Archaeology of Alkaloids. In *Theory and Practice of Archaeological Residue Analysis,* edited by H. Barnard and J. W. Eerkens. British Archaeological Reports International Series 1650:179–188. Archaeopress, Oxford.

2008 Smoking Pipes and Early Woodland Mortuary Ritual. In *Transitions: Archaic and Early Woodland Research in the Ohio Country,* edited by M. P. Otto and B. G. Redmond, pp. 271–283. Ohio University Press, Athens.

2009 Evidence of Rituals at the Pethick Site, Schoharie County, New York. *Bulletin of the New York State Archaeological Association* No. 124:47–55.

2016 Smoking Pipes of Eastern North America. In *Perspectives on the Archaeology of Pipes, Tobacco and other Smoke Plants in the Ancient Americas,* edited by Elizabeth Anne Bollwerk and Shannon Tushingham, pp. 13–26. Springer Press, New York.

2018 Prehistoric Intoxicants of North America. In Fitzpatrick S., *Ancient Psychoactive Substances*, pp. 112–127. University Press of Florida Press, Gainesville.

RAFFERTY, S. M., I. LEDNEV, K. VIRKLER, AND Z. CHOVANEC

2012 Current Research on Smoking Pipe Residues. *Journal of Archaeological Science* 39(7):1951–1959.

RAHMAN, E.

2015 Tobacco and Water: Everyday Blessings. In *The Master Plant: Tobacco in Lowland South America*, edited by A. Russel and E. Rahman, pp. 131–152. Bloomsbury Academic, London.

RAPPAPORT, R. A.

1968 *Pigs for the Ancestors*. Yale University Press, New Haven, Connecticut.

1992 *Ritual, Time, and Eternity*. Zygon 27(1)5–30.

RÄTSCH, C.

2005 *The Encyclopedia of Psychoactive Plants: Ethnopharmacology and its Applications*. Park Street Press, Rochester, Vermont.

REAGAN, A. B.

1929 Plants Used by the White Mountain Apache Indians of Arizona. *Wisconsin Archeologist* 8:143–161.

REBER, E. A.

2014 Gas Chromatography-Mass Spectrometry (GC-MS): Applications in Archaeology. In *Encyclopedia of Global Archaeology*, Vol. 5, edited by C. Smith, pp. 2953–2959. Springer Reference, New York.

REBER, E. A., AND M. T. KERR

2012 The Persistence of Caffeine in Experimentally Produced Black Drink Residues. *Journal of Archaeological Science* 39(7):2312–2319.

REED, N. A.

2009 Excavations on the Third Terrace and Front Ramp of Monks Mound, Cahokia: A Personal Narrative. *Illinois Archaeology* 21:1–89.

REICHEL-DOLMATOFF, G.

1978 *Beyond the Milky Way. Hallucinatory Imagery of the Tukano Indians*. UCLA Latin American Center Publications, University of California, Los Angeles.

REICHEL-DOLMATOFF, G.

1987 *Shamanism and Art of the Eastern Tukanoan Indians, Columbian Northwest Amazon*. E. J. Brill, Leiden, The Netherlands.

RIPINSKY-NAXON, M.

1993 *The Nature of Shamanism: Substance and Function of a Religious Metaphor*. State University of New York Press, Albany.

RITCHIE, W.

1980 *The Archaeology of New York State*. Harbor Hill Books, Harrison, New York.

RITCHIE, W. AND D. DRAGOO

1960 *The Eastern Dispersal of Adena*. New York State Museum and Science Service. Bulletin, 379. Albany.

ROBBINS, W. W., J. P. HARRINGTON, AND B. FREIRE-MARRECO

1916 *Ethnobotany of the Tewa Indians*. Bureau of American Ethnology, Bulletin 55. Smithsonian Institution, US Government Printing Office, Washington, DC.

ROBERT, J. C.

1949 *The Story of Tobacco in America*. A. A. Knopf, New York.

ROBERTS, B. K., M. G. ARONSOHN, B. L. MOSES, R. L. BURK, J. TOLL, AND F. R. WEEREN

2000 *Bufo marinus* intoxication in dogs: 94 cases (1997–1998). *Journal of the American Veterinary Medical Association* 216(12):1941–1944.

ROBERTS, M. F., AND M. WINK

1998 Introduction. In *Alkaloids: Biochemistry, Ecology and Medicinal Applications*. Plenum Press, New York.

ROBICSEK, F.

1978 *Smoking Gods: Tobacco in Maya Art, History, and Religion*. University of Oklahoma Press, Norman.

ROBINSON, S.

2016 *Apache Voices: Their Stories of Survival as Told to Eve Ball*. University of New Mexico Press, Albuquerque.

RODNING, C. B.

2014 Cherokee Towns and Calumet Ceremonialism in Eastern North America. *American Antiquity* 79(3):425–443.

RODNING, C. B., AND A. M. VANDERWARKER

2002 Revisiting Coweeta Creek: Reconstructing Ancient Cherokee Lifeways in Southwestern North Carolina. *Southeastern Archaeology* 21(1):1–9.

ROGERS, E. S.

1966 *The False Face Society of the Iroquois*. Royal Ontario Museum, Toronto.

ROGERS, S. L., AND L. EVERNHAM

1983 Shamanistic Healing Among the Diegueño Indians of Southern California. In *The Anthropology of Medicine: From Culture to Method*, edited by L. Romanucci-Ross, D. E. Moerman, and L. R. Tancredi, pp. 103–118. Praeger, New York.

ROMAIN, W. F.

2009 *Shamans of the Lost World: A Cognitive Approach to the Prehistoric Religion of the Ohio Hopewell*. AltaMira Press, Walnut Creek, California.

ROWE, M. W.

2001 Dating by AMS Radiocarbon Analysis. In *Handbook of Rock Art Research*, edited by D. S. Whitley, pp. 139–166. AltaMira Press, Walnut Creek, California.

ROWE, M. W., AND K. L. STEELMAN

2002 Radiocarbon Dating of Rock Paintings Using Plasma-Chemical Extraction. *American Laboratory* 34:15–19.

RUDGLEY, R.

1999 *The Encyclopedia of Psychoactive Substances*. St. Martin's Press, New York.

RUSSELL, F.

1908 *The Pima Indians*. Twenty-Sixth Annual Report, Bureau of American Ethnology (1904–1905) 26:3–389. Smithsonian Institution, US Government Printing Office, Washington, DC.

SACKS, O.

2012 *Hallucinations*. Alfred A. Knopf, New York.

SAFFORD, W. E.

1915 *Identification of Teonanacatl of the Aztecs with the Narcotic Cactus L. williamsii*. Botanical Society of Washington DC.

1917 *Narcotic Plants and Stimulants of the Ancient Americans*. Smithsonian Report for 1916, US Government Printing Office, Washington DC.

1922 *Daturas of the Old World and New: An Account of Their Narcotic Properties and Their Use in Oracular and Initiatory Ceremonies*. Smithsonian Report for 1920:537–567. US Government Printing Office, Washington, DC.

SAGARD, G.

1939 *The Long Journey to the Country of the Hurons*. The Champlain Society, Toronto.

SAGGERS, S., AND GRAY, D.

1998 Explanations of Indigenous Alcohol Use. In *Dealing with Alcohol: Indigenous Usage in Australia, New Zealand and Canada*, edited by S. Saggers and D. Gray, pp. 68–88. Cambridge University Press, Cambridge, United Kingdom.

SAHAGÚN, FRAY BERNARDINO DE

1953 *Florentine Codex: General History of the Things of New Spain*, Book 2. Translated by Arthur J. O. Anderson and Charles E. Dibble. School of American Research, Santa Fe, New Mexico, and the University of Utah Press, Salt Lake City.

SAHAGÚN, FRAY BERNARDINO DE

1963 *Florentine Codex: General History of the Things of New Spain*, Book 11. Translated by Arthur J. O. Anderson and Charles E. Dibble. School of American Research, Santa Fe, New Mexico, and the University of Utah Press, Salt Lake City.

SALKIN, P. H.

1986 The Lake Farms Phase: The Early Woodland Stage in South-Central Wisconsin as Seen from the Lake Farms Archaeological District. In *Early*

Woodland Archaeology, edited by K. B. Farnsworth and T. E. Emerson, pp. 92–120. Center for American Archaeology, Kampsville, Illinois.

SAMET, J.

2000 Health Effects of Tobacco Use by Native Americans. *Tobacco Use by Native North Americans: Sacred Smoke and Silent Killer*, edited by J. C. Winter, pp. 331–341. University of Oklahoma Press, Norman.

SAMORINI, G.

2002 *Animals and Psychedelics: The Natural World and the Instinct to Alter Consciousness*. Park Street Press, Rochester, Vermont.

SANIOTIS, A.

2010 Evolutionary and Anthropological Approaches Towards Understanding Human Need for Psychotropic and Mood-Altering Substances. *Journal of Psychoactive Drugs* 42(4):477–484.

SCARRY, C. M.

2003 Food Plant Remains from Excavations in Mounds A, B, C, D and L at Bottle Creek. In *Bottle Creek: A Pensacola Culture Site in South Alabama*, edited by I. W. Brown, pp. 102–113. University of Alabama Press, Tuscaloosa.

SCHAAFSMA, P.

1994 Trance and Transformation in the Canyons: Shamanism and Early Rock Art on the Colorado Plateau. In *Shamanism and Rock Art in North America*, edited by S. Turpin, pp. 45–72. Rock Art Foundation, San Antonio, Texas.

SCHAEFER, S. B.

1996 The Crossing of the Souls: Peyote, Perception and Meaning among the Huichol Indians. In *People of the Peyote*, edited by S. B. Shaefer and P. T. Furst, pp. 136–168. University of New Mexico Press, Albuquerque.

1997 Peyote and Pregnancy. *Yearbook for Ethnomedicine and the Study of Culture* 1996(5):67–68.

SCHAEFER, S. B., AND P. T. FURST

1996 Introduction. In *People of the Peyote: Huichol Indian History, Religion and Survival*, edited by S. B. Schaefer and P.T. Furst, pp. 1–25. University of New Mexico Press, Albuquerque.

SCHAFER, T.

1993 Responding to 'First Identification of Drugs in Egyptian Mummies'. *Naturwissenschaften* 80:243–244.

SCHENCK, S. M., AND E. W. GIFFORD

1952 Karok Ethnobotany. *Anthropological Records* 13(6):377–392.

SCHLEIFFER, H.

1973 *Sacred Narcotic Plants of the New World Indians: An Anthology of Texts from the 16th Century to Date*. Hafner Press, New York.

SCHLESINGER, R., AND A. P. STABLER

1986 *André Thevet's North America*. McGill-Queens University Press, Kingston, Ontario.

SCHOENWETTER, J.

2001 Paleoethnobotanical Expressions of Prehistoric Ritual: an Early Woodland Case. In *Fleeting identities: Perishable Material Culture in Archaeological Research*, edited by P. B. Drooker, pp. 273–282. Center for Archaeological Investigations, Carbondale, Illinois.

SCHULTES, R. E.

1938 The Appeal of Peyote (*Lophophora williamsii*) as a Medicine. *American Anthropologist* 40:698–715.

SCHULTES, R. E.

1963 Hallucinogenic Plants of the New World. *Harvard Review* 1:18–32.

1967 The Botanical Origin of South American Snuffs. *Public Health Service Publication* No. 1645, pp. 291–305. Washington, DC.

1972 An Overview of Hallucinogens in the Western Hemisphere. In *Flesh of the Gods: The Ritual Use of Hallucinogens*, edited by P. T. Furst, pp. 3–54. Praeger Press, New York.

1976 Indole Alkaloids in Plant Hallucinogens. *Journal of Psychedelic Drugs* 8(1):7–25.

1979 Solanaceous Hallucinogens in the New World. In *The Biology and Taxonomy of the Solanaceae*, edited by J. G. Hawkes, R. N. Lester, and A. D. Skelding, pp. 137–160. Academic Press, Cambridge, Massachusetts.

SCHULTES, R. E., AND N. R. FARNSWORTH

1980 Ethnomedical, Botanical and Phytochemical Aspects of Natural Hallucinogens. *Botanical Museum Leaflets, Harvard University* 28(2):123–214.

SCHULTES, R. E., AND A. HOFMANN

1980 *The Botany and Chemistry of Hallucinogens*. Charles C. Thomas, Springfield, Illinois.

1987 *Plants of the Gods: Origins of Hallucinogenic Use*. Vanderbilt University Press, Nashville.

SCHULTES, R. E., AND M. WINKELMAN

1995 The Principal American Hallucinogenic Plants and their Bioactive and Therapeutic Effects. In *Sacred Plants, Consciousness, and Healing: Cross-Cultural and Interdisciplinary Perspectives*, edited by M. Winkelman and W. Andritsky, pp. 205–240. Verlag für Wissenschaft und Bildung, Berlin

SEBASTIAN, L.

1985 *Archaeological Excavation Along the Turquoise Trail: the Mitigation Program*. Office of Contract Archaeology, University of New Mexico, Albuquerque.

SEEMAN, M. F.

1981 A Late Woodland Steatite Pipe from the Catlin Site, Vermillion Co., Indiana: The Implications for East-West Trade. *Archaeology of Eastern North America* 9:103–109.

SELMAR, D., S. GROCHOLEWSKI, AND D. S. SEIGLER

1990 Cyanogenic Lipids: Utilization During Seedling Development of *Ungnadia speciose. Plant Physiology* 93(2):633–636.

SETCHEL, W. A.

1923 Aboriginal Tobaccos. *American Anthropologist,* New Series 23(4):397–414.

SHAFER, H. J.

2003 *Mimbres Archaeology and the NAN Ranch Ruin.* University of New Mexico Press, Albuquerque.

SHAFFER, B., AND J. NEELY

1992 Intrusive Anuran Remains in Pit House Features: A Test of Methods. *Kiva* 57(4):343–351.

SHERMER, M.

2011 *The Believing Brain: From Ghosts and Gods to Politics and Conspiracies—How We Construct Beliefs and Reinforce Them as Truths.* Times Books, New York.

SHERWOOD, S. C., J. H. BLITZ, AND L. E. DOWNS

2013 An Integrated Geoarchaeology of a Late Woodland Sand Mound. *American Antiquity* 78(2):344–358.

SHIROKOGOROFF, S. M.

1935. *Psychomental Complex of the Tungus.* Kegan Paul, Trench, Trubner, London.

SHONLE, R.

1925 Peyote, the Giver of Visions. *American Anthropologist* 27(1):53–75.

SHRIVER, P. R.

1983 Mississippian and Fort Ancient Pipes. *Ohio Archaeologist* 33(2):18–19.

SIEGEL, R. K.

2005 *Intoxication: Life in Pursuit of Artificial Paradise.* Inner Traditions/Bear and Co., Rochester, Vermont.

SIEGEL, R. K., AND M. E. JARVIK

1975 Drug-Induced Hallucinations in Animals and Man. In *Hallucinations: Behavior, Experience and Theory,* edited by R. K. Siegel and L. J. West, pp. 81–161. John Wiley and Sons, New York.

SIEVERT, A. K.

2003 Spiro Painted Maces and Shell Cups: The Scientific Use of Artifacts without Context. In *Theory, Method and Practice in Modern Archaeology,* edited by R. J. Jeske and D. K. Charles, pp. 182–195. Praeger, Westport, Connecticut.

SKINNER, A.

1915 *Societies of the Iowa, Kansa, and Ponca Indians.* Anthropological Papers of the American Museum of Natural History Vol. XI, Part IX, American Museum of Natural History, New York.

SLOTKIN, J. S.

1955 Peyotism 1521–1891. *American Anthropologist* 57:202–230.

SLOTKIN, J. S., AND D. P. MCALLESTER

1952 Menomini Peyotism, a Study of Individual Variation in a Primary Group with a Homogeneous Culture. *Transactions of the American Philosophical* Society 42(4):565–700.

SMALLEY, J., AND M. BLAKE

2003 Sweet Beginnings: Stalk Sugar and the Domestication of Maize. *Current Anthropology* 44(5):675–703.

SMART, R. G., AND A. C. OGBORNE

1986 *Northern Spirits: Drinking in Canada Then and Now.* Addiction Research Foundation, Toronto.

SMITH, J.

1630 The True Travels, Adventures, and Observations of Captain John Smith into Europe, Asia, Africa, and America From Ann. Dom. 1593 to 1629. Awnsham and John Churchill, London.

SNEADER, W.

2005 *Drug Discovery: A History.* John Wiley and Sons, Hoboken, New Jersey.

SOBOLIK, K. D., AND D. J. GERIK

1992 Prehistoric Medicinal Plant Usage: A Case Study from Coprolites. *Journal of Ethnobiology* 12(2):203–211.

SOLECKI, R.

1975 Shanidar IV, a Neanderthal Flower Burial in Northern Iraq. *Science* 190:880–881.

SPENCE, M. W. AND W. A. FOX

1986 The Early Woodland Occupations of Southern Ontario. In *Early woodland Archaeology*, edited by K. B. Farnsworth and T. E. Emerson, pp. 4–46. Center for American Archaeology, Kampsville, Illinois.

SPRINGER, J. W.

1981 An Ethnohistoric Study of the Smoking Complex in Eastern North America. *Ethnohistory* 28(3):217–235.

STAHL, P. W.

1985 The Hallucinogenic Basis of Early Valdivia Phase Ceramic Bowl Iconography. *Journal of Psychoactive Drugs* 17(2):105–123.

1986 Hallucinatory Imagery and the Origin of Early South American Figurine Art. *World Archaeology* 18(1):134–150.

STECKLEY, J.

1985 An Ethnolinguistic Analysis of Tobacco Among the Huron. *Arch Notes* 85(2):13–17.

STEEN, C.

1943 Some Notes on the Use of Tobacco and Cane Pipes by the Pimas of the Gila Valley. *American Anthropologist* 45(4):641–642.

STEIN, R. L., AND P. L. STEIN

2011 *The Anthropology of Magic, Religion and Witchcraft.* Routledge, London.

STEINMETZ, P. B.

1984 The Sacred Pipe in American Indian Religions. *American Indian Culture and Research Journal* 8(3):27–80.

STEPHENS, B. W.

1957 Tube Pipes. *Central States Archaeological Journal* 4:30–33.

STEVENSON, M. C.

1915 *Ethnobotany of the Zuñi Indians.* Thirtieth Annual Report, Bureau of American Ethnology (1908–1909). Smithsonian Institution, US Government Printing Office, Washington DC.

STEWARD, J.

1929 Petroglyphs of California and Adjoining States. *University of California Publications in American Archaeology and Ethnology* 24(2):47–238.

STEWART, O. C.

1942 Washo–Northern Paiute Peyotism. *University of California Publications in American Archaeology and Ethnology* 40:63–142.

1956 Three Gods for Joe. *Tomorrow, Quarterly Review of Psychical Research* 4(3):71–76.

1980 Peyotism and Mescalism. *Plains Anthropologist* 25(90):297–309.

1982 The History of Peyotism in Nevada. *Nevada Historical Society Quarterly* 25(3):197–209.

1987 *Peyote Religion: A History.* University of Oklahoma Press, Norman.

STEWART, R. M.

1989 Trade and Exchange in Mid-Atlantic Prehistory. *Archaeology of Eastern North America* 17:47–78.

STONE, C. U.

1955 Peace Pipes of Prehistoric American Indians. *Central States Archaeological Journal* 1:93.

STRACHEY, W.

1967 *The Historie of Travaile into Virginia Britannia (1612).* Hakluyt Society, London.

STURTEVANT, W. C.

1954 *The Mikasuki Seminole: Medical Beliefs and Practices.* PhD Dissertation, Department of Anthropology, Yale University, New Haven, Connecticut.

1979 Black Drink and other Caffeine-Containing Beverages Among Non-Indians. In *The Black Drink: A Native American Tea*, edited by C. Hudson, pp. 250–265. University of Georgia Press, Athens.

SULLIVAN, R. J., E. H. HAGEN, AND P. HAMMERSTEIN

2008 Revealing the Paradox of Drug Reward in Human Evolution. *Proceedings of the Royal Society* B 275:1231–1241.

SUTTON, M. Q., D. W. ROBINSON, G. GRASSE-SPRAGUE, AND J. SPRAGUE

2011 Cupules as Containers: A Hypothesis. *Pacific Coast Archaeological Society Quarterly* 45(3–4):87–93.

SWANTON, J. R.

1922 Early History of the Creek Indians and Their Neighbors. Smithsonian Institution Bureau of American Ethnology, Bulletin No. 73. US Government Printing Office, Washington DC.

SWANTON, J. R.

1928 *Religious Beliefs and Medical Practices of the Creek Indians.* Forty-Fourth Annual Report, Bureau of American Ethnology (1926–1927) 44:473:672. Smithsonian Institution, US Government Printing Office, Washington, DC.

1946 *The Indians of the Southeastern United States.* Smithsonian Institution Bureau of American Ethnology, Bulletin No. 137. US Government Printing Office, Washington DC.

SWITZER, R. R.

1969 *Tobacco, Pipes and Cigarettes of the Prehistoric Southwest.* El Paso Archaeological Society, El Paso, Texas.

TARROW, S.

1970 Translation of the Cèllere Codex. In T*he Voyages of Giovanni da Verrazano*, edited by L. C. Wroth, pp. 133–144. Yale University Press, New Haven, Connecticut.

TAYLOR, W. W.

1972 The Hunter-Gatherer Nomads of Northern Mexico: A Comparison of the Archival and Archaeological Records. *World Archaeology* 4(2):167–178.

TERRY, M. K.

2005 *A Tale of Two Cacti: Studies in Astrophytum asterias and Lophophora williamsii.* PhD dissertation, Department of Biology, Texas A&M University, College Station.

TERRY, M., K. L. STEELMAN, T. GUILDERSON, P. DERING, AND M. W. ROWE

2006 Lower Pecos and Coahuila Peyote: New Radiocarbon Dates. *Journal of Archaeological Science* 33:1017–1021.

TEUFEL, C., N. SUBRAMANIAM, V. DOBLER, J. PEREZ, J. FINNEMANN, P. MEHTA, I. GOODYER, AND P. FLETCHER

2015 Shift toward Prior Knowledge Confers a Perceptual Advantage in Early Psychosis and Psychosis-Prone Healthy Individuals. *Proceedings of the National Academy of Sciences* 112(43):13401–13406.

THATCHER, J. B.

1912 *Christopher Columbus*. G.P. Putnam's Sons, New York.

THEVET, A.

1558 *Les Singularitez de la France Antarctique*. Plantin, Antwerp.

THOMAS, C.

1985 *Report on the Mound Explorations of the Bureau of Ethnology*. Smithsonian Institution Press, Washington DC.

THOMAS, L., AND J. RAY

2002 Exchange at the Dahlman Site (23LA259), a Late Prehistoric Neosho Phase Settlement in Southwest Missouri. *Plains Anthropologist* 47(182):207–229.

THOMAS, R. A.

1971 Adena Influences in the Middle Atlantic States. In *Adena: The Seeking of an Identity*, edited by B. K. Swartz, pp. 55–87. Ball State University, Muncie, Indiana.

THOMPSON, V. D., AND T. J. PLUCKHAHN

2018 Pipes, Cups, Platform Mounds and Mortuary Ritual in the Lake Okeechobee Basin of South Florida. In *Ancient Psychoactive Substances*, edited by Scott M. Fitzpatrick, pp. 128–148. University Press of Florida, Gainesville.

THWAITES, R. G.

1902 *Father Marquette*. D. Appleton, New York.

THWAITES, R. G. (ED.)

1959 *The Jesuit Relations and Allied Documents: Travels and Explorations of the Jesuit Missionaries in New France 1610–1791*. Volumes 3, 7, 10, 13, 59, 61, 70. Pageant Books, New York

TIMBROOK, J.

1987 Virtuous Herbs: Plants in Chumash Medicine. *Journal of Ethnobiology* 7(2):171–180.

1990 Ethnobotany of the Chumash Indians, California, Based on the Collections of John P. Harrington. *Economic Botany* 44(2):236–253.

TORRES, C. M., AND D. B. REPKE

2006 Anadenanthera: Visionary Plant of Ancient South America. Haworth Herbal Press, New York.

TOTH, A.

1979 *The Marksville Connection*. Kent State University Press, Kent, Ohio.

TOUW, M.

1981 The Religious and Medicinal Uses of Cannabis in China, India and Tibet. *Journal of Psychoactive Drugs*, 13(1):23–34.

TRAIN, P., J. R. HENRICHS, AND W. A. ARCHER

1941 *Medicinal Uses of Plants by Indian Tribes of Nevada*. US Department of Agriculture, Washington DC.

TROIKE, R. C.

1962 The Origins of Plains Mescalism. *American Anthropologist* 64(5):946–963.

TRUBIT, M. B.

2000 Mound Building and Prestige Goods Exchange: Changing Strategies in the Cahokia Chiefdom. *American Antiquity* 65(4):669–690.

TRUBOWITZ, N.

1992 Thanks, But We Prefer to Smoke Our Own: Pipes in the Great Lakes–Riverine Region During the Eighteenth Century. In *Proceedings of the 1988 Smoking Pipe Conference*, edited by C. F. Hays III, pp. 97–112. Rochester Museum and Science Center Records, Rochester, New York.

TSCHOPIK, H., JR.

1941 *Navajo Pottery Making, Part III: Pipes*. Papers of the Peabody Museum of American Archaeology and Ethnology, Vol. 17, No. 1. Harvard University, Cambridge, Massachusetts.

TURNER, J. W.

2012 Listening to the Ancestors: Kava and the Lapita Peoples. *Ethnology* (Winter 2012):31–53.

TURNER, N. C., AND M. A. M. BELL

1971 The Ethnobotany of the Coast Salish Indians of Vancouver Island. *Economic Botany* 25(1):63–104.

1973 The Ethnobotany of the Southern Kwakiutl Indians of British Columbia. *Economic Botany* 27(3):257–310.

TURNER, N. J., AND D. C. LOEWEN

1998 The Original "Free Trade": Exchange of Botanical Products and Associated Plant Knowledge in Northwestern North America. *Anthropologica* 40(1):49–70.

TURNER, V. W.

1968 *The Drums of Affliction: a Study of Religious Processes among the Ndembu of Zambia*. Clarendon Press, Oxford.

1969 *The Ritual Process: Structure and Anti-Structure*. Aldine, Chicago.

TURNBAUGH, W. A.

1979 Calumet Ceremonialism as a Nativistic Response. *American Antiquity* 44(4):685–691.

1980 Native North American Smoking Pipes. *Archaeology* 33(1):15–22.

TURPIN, S.

1990 Rock Art and Hunter-Gatherer Archaeology: A Case Study from SW Texas and Northern Mexico. *Journal of Field Archaeology* 17(3):263–281.

1994 On a Wing and a Prayer: Flight Metaphors in Pecos River Art. In *Shamanism and Rock Art in North America*, edited by S. A. Turpin, pp. 73–102. Rock Art Foundation, San Antonio, Texas.

TUSHINGHAM, S., D. ARDURA, J. EERKENS, M. PALAZOGLU, S. SHAHBAZ, AND O. FIEHN

2013 Hunter-Gatherer Tobacco Smoking: Earliest Evidence from the Pacific Northwest Coast of North America. *Journal of Archaeological Science* 40(2):1397–1407.

2010 Gas Chromatography-Mass Spectrometry Analysis of Alkaloid Residues in Ancient and Experimental Pipes. Paper presented at the 75th annual meeting of the Society for American Archaeology, St. Louis, Missouri.

TUSHINGHAM, S. AND J. W. EERKENS

2016 Hunter-gatherer Tobacco Smoking in Ancient North America: Current Chemical Evidence and a Framework for Future Studies. In *Perspectives on the Archaeology of Pipes, Tobacco and other Smoke Plants in the Ancient Americas*, edited by E. A. Bollwerk and S. Tushingham, pp. 211–230. Springer, Cham.

TUSHINGHAM, S., M. PALUMBO, C. H. MCNUTT, AND U. ANDERSON

2011 The Biomolecular Archaeology of the Black Drink: Alkaloid Residue Analysis of *Ilex vomitoria* on Experimental Vessels and Applications for Prehistoric Specimens. Paper presented at the 68th annual meeting of the Southeastern Archaeology Conference, Jacksonville, Florida.

UNDERHILL, R.

1936 *The Autobiography of a Papago Woman*. Memoirs, American Anthropological Association, No. 46, Lancaster, Pennsylvania.

UNDERWOOD, J.

2002 Pipes and Tobacco Use among Southern California Yuman Speaker. *Journal of California and Great Basin Anthropology* 24(1):1–12.

UNITED NATIONS FOOD AND AGRICULTURE ORGANIZATION

2004 *Higher World Tobacco Use Expected by 2010—Growth Rates Slowing Down.* Press Release, January 8, 2004. UNFAO, Rome.

UNITED NATIONS OFFICE ON DRUGS AND CRIME

2008 *2008 World Drug Report*. United Nations Publications, Sales No. E.08.XI.1. United Nations, New York.

2013 *World Drug Report 2012*. United Nations Publications, Sales No. E.12.XI.1. United Nations, New York.

VAN DEN BERGHE, P. L.

1978 El Cargo De Las Animas: Mortuary Rituals and the Cargo System in Highland Peru. *Anthropological Quarterly* 51(2):129–136.

VANDERWARKER, A., AND B. STANYARD

2009 Bearsfoot and Deer Legs: Archaeobotanical and Zooarchaeological Evidence of a Special-Purpose Encampment at the Sandy Site, Roanoke, Virginia. *Journal of Ethnobiology* 29(1):129–148.

VAN DEYSEN, K.

2004 *Sing Story Healing Drum: Shamans and Storytellers of Turkic Siberia.* McGill-Queen's University Press, Montreal and Kingston, and University of Washington Press, Seattle.

VANPOOL, C.

2009 The Signs of the Sacred: Identifying Shamans Using Archaeological Evidence. *Journal of Anthropological Archaeology* 28(2):177–190.

VANSTONE, J. W.

1996 Ethnographic Collections from the Assiniboine and Yanktonia Sioux in the Field Museum of Natural History. *Fieldiana, Anthropology New Series* 26:1–91

VARNUM, R.

2014 *Álvar Núñez Cabeza de Vaca: American Trailblazer.* University of Oklahoma Press, Norman.

VECSEY, C.

1988 *Imagine Ourselves Richly: Mythic Narratives of North American Indians.* Crossroad, New York.

VESTAL, P. A.

1945 *The Ethnobotany of the Ramah Navaho.* Papers of the Peabody Museum of American Archaeology and Ethnology, Vol. 40, No. 4. Harvard University, Cambridge, Massachusetts.

VITEBSKY, P.

2001 *Shamanism.* University of Oklahoma Press, Norman.

VON GERNET, A.

1992 Hallucinogens and the Origins of the Iroquoian Pipe/Tobacco/Smoking Complex. In *Proceedings of the 1989 Smoking Pipe Conference,* edited by C. F. Hayes III, pp. 171–186. Rochester Museum and Science Center Records, Rochester, New York.

1995 Nicotian Dreams: The Prehistory and Early History of Tobacco in Eastern North America. In *Consuming Habits: Drugs in History and Anthropology,* edited by J. Goodman, P. E. Lovejoy, and A. Sherratt, pp. 67–87. Routledge, London.

2000 North American Indigenous Nicotiana Use and Tobacco Shamanism: The Early Documentary Record, 1520–1660. In *Tobacco Use by Native North Americans: Sacred Smoke and Silent Killer,* edited by J. C. Winter, pp. 59–83. University of Oklahoma Press, Norman.

VON GERNET, A. AND P. TIMMINS

1987 Pipes and Parakeets: Constructing Meaning in an Early Iroquoian Context. In *Archaeology as Long-term History*, edited by M. Waelkens, pp. 31–42. Cambridge University Press, Cambridge, United Kingdom.

WADLEY, G.

2016 How Psychoactive Drugs Shape Human Culture: A Multi-Disciplinary Perspective. *Brain Research Bulletin* 126(1)138–151.

WAGNER, G. E.

1987 *Uses of plants by the Fort Ancient Indians.* Washington University, St. Louis, Missouri.

2000 Tobacco in Prehistoric Eastern North America. In *Tobacco Use by Native Americans: Sacred Smoke and Silent Killer*, edited by J. C. Winter, pp. 185–203. University of Oklahoma Press, Norman.

WAGNER, R. M.

1975 Some Pragmatic Aspects of Navaho Peyotism. *Plains Anthropologist* 20(69):197–205.

WALDSEEMÜLLER, M.

1507 *Cosmographiae Introductio.* Walter and Nikolaus Lud, St. Dié, France.

WALKER, J R.

1991 *Lakota Belief and Ritual.* University of Nebraska Press, Lincoln.

WALLIS, R. J.

2013 Animism and the Interpretation of Rock Art. *Time and Mind* 6(1):21–28.

WALTHALL, J. A.

1979 Hopewell and the Southern Heartland. In *Hopewell Archaeology*, edited by D. S. Brose and N. Greber, pp. 200–208. Kent State University Press, Kent, Ohio.

1980 *Prehistoric Indians of the Southeast: Archaeology of Alabama and the Middle South.* University of Alabama Press, Tuscaloosa.

WARF, B.

2014 High Points: An Historical Geography of Cannabis. *Geographical Review* 104(4):414–438.

WASHBURN, D. K., W. N. WASHBURN, AND P. A. SHIPKOVA

2011 The Prehistoric Drug Trade: Widespread Consumption of Cacao in Ancestral Pueblo and Hohokam Communities in the American Southwest. *Journal of Archaeological Science* 38:1634–1640.

2012 Cacao Consumption during the 8th Century at Alkali Ridge, Southeastern Utah. *Journal of Archaeological Science* 40:2007–2013.

WASHBURN, D. K., W. N. WASHBURN, P. A. SHIPKOVA, AND M. A. PELLEYMOUNTER

2014 Chemical Analysis of Cacao Residues in Archaeological Ceramics from North America: Considerations of Contamination, Sample Size and Systematic Controls. *Journal of Archaeological Science* 50:191:207.

WASSÉN, S. H.

1967 Anthropological Survey of the Use of South American Snuffs. *U.S. Public Health Service Publication* No. 1645, pp. 233–289. Washington, DC.

WASSON, R. G.

1968 *Soma-Divine Mushroom of Immortality*. Harcourt Brace Jovanovich, New York.

1971 The Soma of the Rig Veda: What Was It? *Journal of the American Oriental Society* 91(2):169–187.

1979 Traditional Use in North America of *Amanita muscaria* for Divinatory Purposes. *Journal of Psychedelic Drugs* 11(1–2):25–28.

WATERMAN, P. G.

1998 Chemical Taxonomy of Alkaloids. In *Alkaloids: Biochemistry, Ecology and Medicinal Applications*. Plenum Press, New York.

WAUCHOPE, R.

1948 The Ceramic Sequence in the Etowah Drainage, Northwest Georgia. *American Antiquity* 13(3): 201–209.

WEBB, C. H.

1959 *The Belcher Mound: A Stratified Caddoan Site in Caddo Parish, Louisiana*. Memoirs of the Society for American Archaeology No. 16:iii–xiii, 1–212.

WEBB, C.

1982 *The Poverty Point Culture*. Louisiana State University, Baton Rouge.

WEBB, W. S., AND R. S. BABY

1957 *The Adena People, No. 2*. Ohio State University Press, Columbus.

WEBB, W. S., AND C. E. SNOW

1974 *The Adena People*. University of Tennessee Press, Knoxville.

WEBER, S. A., AND P. D. SEAMAN

1985 *Havasupai Habitat: A. F. Whiting's Ethnography of a Traditional Indian Culture*. University of Arizona Press, Tucson.

WECKERLE, C. S., V. TIMBUL, AND P. BLUMENSHINE

2012 Medicinal, Stimulant and Ritual Plant Use: An Ethnobotany of Caffeine-Containing Plants. In *Plants, Health and Healing: On the Interface of Ethnobotany and Medical Anthropology*, edited by E. Hsu and S. Harris, pp. 262–301. Berghahn Books, Oxford.

WEETS, J., C. CARR, D. PENNEY, AND G. CARRIVEAU

2005 Smoking Pipe Compositions and Styles as Evidence of the Social Affiliations of Mortuary Ritual Participants at the Tremper Site, Ohio. In *Gathering*

Hopewell: Society, Ritual and Ritual Interaction, edited by C. Carr and D. Troy Case, pp. 533–553. Plenum, New York.

WEIL, A. T.

1977 The Use of Psychoactive Mushrooms in the Pacific Northwest: An Ethnopharmacological Report. *Botanical Museum Leaflets, Harvard University* 25(5):131–149.

WEIL, A. T., AND W. DAVIS

1994 *Bufo alvarius*: A Potent Hallucinogen of Animal Origin. *Journal of Ethnopharmacology* 41(1–2):1–8.

WELLMANN, K. F.

1978 North American Rock Art and Hallucinogenic Drugs. *Journal of the American Medical Association* 239(15):1524–1527.

1981 Rock Art, Shamans, Phosphenes and Hallucinogens in North America. *Bollettino del Centro Camuno di Studi Preistorica* 18:89–103.

WEST, G. A.

1970 *Tobacco, Pipes and Smoking Customs of the American Indians*. Greenwood Press, Westport, Connecticut. Originally published 1934, Bulletin of the Public Museum of the City of Milwaukee, Vol. 17.

WEST, R., W. ZATONSKI, M. CEDZYNSKA, D. LEWANDOWSKA, J. PAZIK, P. AVEYARD, AND J. STAPLETON

2011 Placebo-Controlled Trial of Cytisine for Smoking Cessation. *The New England Journal of Medicine* 365(13):1193–1200.

WHALLEY, L.

1984 Plant Remains from the Stirling Phase. In *The BBB Motor Site*, edited by T. E. Emerson and D. K. Jackson, pp. 321–335. University of Illinois Press, Champagne.

WHITE, L.

1942 Further Data on the Cultivation of Tobacco among the Pueblo Indians. *Science* 96:59–60.

WHITE, N. M.

2013 *Pierce Mounds Complex: An Ancient Capital in Northwest Florida*. Final Report to George J. Mahr, Apalachicola, Florida.

WHITE, N. M., AND R. A. WEINSTEIN

2008 The Mexican Connection and the Far West of the U.S. Southeast. *American Antiquity* 73(2):227–277.

WHITING, A. F.

1939 *Ethnobotany of the Hopi*. Museum of Northern Arizona Bulletin No. 15. Northern Arizona Society of Science and Art, Flagstaff.

1978 AF Whiting: Ethnographic Notes and Papers. Northern Arizona University.

WHITLEY, D. S.

1987 Socioreligious Context and Rock Art in East-Central California. *Journal of Anthropological Archaeology* 6:159–188.

1992 Shamanism and Rock Art in Far Western North America. *Cambridge Archaeological Journal* 2(1):89–113.

1994 Shamanism, Natural Modeling, and the Rock Art of Far Western North American Hunter Gatherers. In *Shamanism and Rock Art in North America*, edited by S. A. Turpin, pp. 1–44. Rock Art Foundation, San Antonio, Texas.

1996 *A Guide to Rock Art Sites: Southern California and Southern Nevada.* Mountain Press, Missoula, Montana.

1998a Meaning and Metaphor in the Coso Petroglyphs: Understanding Great Basin Rock Art. In *Coso Rock Art: A New Perspective*, edited by E. Younkin, pp. 109–176. Maturango Press, Ridgecrest, California.

1998b Shamanism and the Rock Art of Native California. *Anthropology of Consciousness* 9(1):22–37.

2006a Rock Art and Rites of Passage in Far Western North America. In *Talking with the Past: The Ethnography of Rock Art*, edited by J. D. Keyser, G. Poetschat, and M. W. Taylor, pp. 295–326. Oregon Archaeological Society, Portland.

2006b Ethnohistory and Rock Art in South-Central California. In *1994 IRAC Proceedings, Rock Art World Heritage*, edited by F. Bock and A. J. Bock, pp. 241–258. American Rock Art Research Association, San Jose, California.

2011 Rock Art, Religion and Ritual. In *The Oxford Handbook of the Archaeology of Ritual and Religion*, edited by T. Insoll, pp. 307–326. Oxford University Press, Oxford.

WIEDMAN, D.

1985 Staff, Fan, Rattle and Drum: Spiritual and Artistic Expressions of Oklahoma Peyotists. *American Indian Art Magazine* 10(3):38–45.

2012 Upholding Indigenous Freedoms of Religion and Medicine Peyotists at the 1906–1908 Oklahoma Constitutional Convention and First Legislature. *American Indian Quarterly* 36(2):215–246.

WIEGAND, T., AND C. SMOLLIN

2007 Ingestion of Mescal Beans (*Sophora secundiflora*) Causing Agitation in an Adolescent—A New Intoxicant. *Clinical Toxicology* 45(4):344.

WIERCINSKI, A.

1989 On the Origins of Shamanism. *Shamanism: Past and Present* 1:19–25.

WIHR, W. S.

1995 "You Toad-Sucking Fool": An Inquiry into the Possible Use of Bufotenine by Northern Northwest Coast Shamans. *Northwest Anthropological Research Notes* 29(1):51–59.

WILBERT, J.

1987 *Tobacco and Shamanism in South America.* Yale University Press, New Haven, Connecticut.

1994 The Cultural Significance of Tobacco Use in South America. In *Ancient Traditions: Shamanism in Central Asia and the Americas*, edited by G. Seaman and J. S. Day, pp. 44–76. University of Colorado and Denver Museum of Natural History, Denver.

1995 El Significado Cultural del Uso de Tabaco en Sudamérica. *Acta Americana* 3(2):71–100.

WILLCOX, A.

1973 The Rock Art of North America: Some Impressions and Comparisons. *The South African Archaeological Bulletin* 28(109/110):27–31.

WILLIAMSON, R. A.

1992 An Alabama Myth of the Stars. In *Earth and Sky: Visions of the Cosmos in Native American Folklore*, edited by R. A. Williamson and C. R. Farrer. University of New Mexico Press, Albuquerque.

WILSON, CAPT.

1866 Report on the Indian Tribes Inhabiting the Country in the Vicinity of the 49th Parallel of North Latitude. *Transactions of the Ethnological Society of London* 4:275–332.

WILSON, J., AND E. PENDREE

1984 Further Tubular Pipes from the Northern Plains Periphery. *Plains Anthropologist* 29(106):339–342.

WINKELMAN, M.

1989 A Cross-cultural Study of Shamanistic Healers. *Journal of Psychoactive Drugs* 21(1):17–24.

1992 *Shamans, Priests and Witches: Cross-Cultural Study of Magio-Religious Practitioners.* Anthropological Research Papers. No. 44. Arizona State University, Tempe.

1996 Psychointegrator Plants: Their Roles in Human Culture, Consciousness and Health. In *Sacred Plants, Consciousness, and Healing: Cross-Cultural and Interdisciplinary Perspectives*, edited by M. Winkelman and W. Andritsky, pp. 9–53. Verlag für Wissenschaft und Bildung, Berlin.

2002 *Shamanism and Cognitive Evolution.* Cambridge Archaeological Journal 12(1):71–101.

2010 *Shamanism: The Neural Ecology of Consciousness and Healing.* Praeger, New York.

WINSHIP, G. P.

1896 *The Coronado Expedition, 1540–1542.* Extract from the Fourteenth Annual Report of the Bureau of Ethnology, US Government Printing Office, Washington, DC.

WINTER, J. C.

2000a Introduction to the North American Tobacco Species. In *Tobacco Use by Native North Americans: Sacred Smoke and Silent Killer*, edited by J. C. Winter, pp. 3–8. University of Oklahoma Press, Norman.

2000b Traditional Uses of Tobacco. In *Tobacco Use by Native North Americans: Sacred Smoke and Silent Killer*, edited by J. C. Winter, pp. 9–58. University of Oklahoma Press, Norman.

2000c Botanical Description of the North American Tobacco Species. In *Tobacco Use by Native North Americans: Sacred Smoke and Silent Killer*, edited by J. C. Winter, pp. 87–127. University of Oklahoma Press, Norman.

2000d From Earth Mother to Snake Woman: The Role of Tobacco in the Evolution of Native American Religious Organization. In *Tobacco Use by Native North Americans: Sacred Smoke and Silent Killer*, edited by J. C. Winter, pp. 265–303. University of Oklahoma Press, Norman.

2000e Food of the Gods: Biochemistry, Addiction, and the Development of Native American Tobacco Use. In *Tobacco Use by Native North Americans: Sacred Smoke and Silent Killer*, edited by J. C. Winter, pp. 305–328. University of Oklahoma Press, Norman.

2004 Creating Tobacco: Native American Origins, Beliefs and Uses. Paper presented at Beloit College. Beloit, Wisconsin.

WINTER, J. C., G. W. SOLOMAN, R. F. HILL, C. M. PEGO, AND S. E. VICTORIA

2000 Native Americans and Tobacco: Deer Person's Gift or Columbus's Curse? In *Tobacco Use by Native North Americans: Sacred Smoke and Silent Killer*, edited by J. C. Winter, pp. 353–381. University of Oklahoma Press, Norman.

WINTERS, H. D.

1969 *The Riverton Culture*. Reports of Investigations No. 13. Illinois State Museum, Springfield.

WITHINGTON, P.

2014 Introduction: Cultures of Intoxication. *Past and Present* Vol. 222, Supplement 9:9–33. Oxford University Press, Oxford.

WONDERLEY, A.

2005 Effigy Pipes, Diplomacy, and Myth: Exploring Interaction between St. Lawrence Iroquoians and Eastern Iroquois in New York State. *American Antiquity* 70(2):211– 240.

WOODWARD, A., T. FROESE, AND T. IKEGAMI

2015 Neural Coordination Can Be Enhanced by Occasional Interruption of Normal Firing Patterns: A Self-Optimizing Spiking Neural Network Model. *Neural Networks* 62:39–46.

WYCKOFF, D. G.

1985 Images on Shell: Spiro Symbolism and Ceremonial Art. *Reviews in Anthropology* 12(4):329–337.

YARNELL, R. A.

1959 Prehistoric Pueblo Use of Datura. *El Palacio* 66:176–178.

1964 *Aboriginal Relationships between Culture and Plant Life in the Upper Great Lakes Region*. University of Michigan, Ann Arbor.

1965 Implications of Distinctive Flora on Pueblo Ruins. *American Anthropologist* 67(3):662–674.

ZARRILLO, S., AND B. KOOYMAN

2006 Evidence for Berry and Maize Processing on the Canadian Plains from Starch Grain Analysis. *American Antiquity* 71(3):473–499.

ZIGMOND, M. L.

1980 *Kawaiisu Mythology: An Oral Tradition of South-Central California*. Ballena Press, Menlo Park, California.

1981 *Kawaiisu Ethnobotany*. University of Utah Press, Salt Lake City.

ZIGMOND, M. L., C. BOOTH, AND P. MUNKO

1990 *Kawaiisu: A Grammar and Dictionary with Texts*. University of California Publications in Linguistics, Vol. 119. University of California Press, Berkeley and Los Angeles.

ZINGG, R. M.

1938 *The Huichols, Primitive Artists*. G. E. Stechert, New York.

ZOLNIKOV, T. R.

2013 Let's Talk about Culture! Experiencing a Disco Funeral in Western Kenya. *Journal of Public Health*, October 17, 2013, pp. 1–3. DOI:10.1093/pubmed/fdt102.

ZUARDI, A. W.

2006 History of Cannabis as a Medicine: A Review. *Revista Brasileira de Psiquiatria* 28(2):153–157.

INDEX

www.ingramcontent.com/pod-product-compliance
Lightning Source LLC
LaVergne TN
LVHW102008210926
848483LV00010B/164

* 9 7 8 1 6 2 1 9 0 6 3 0 8 *